Next Generation Kinase Inhibitors

Paul Shapiro
Editor

Next Generation Kinase Inhibitors

Moving Beyond the ATP Binding/Catalytic Sites

Springer

Editor
Paul Shapiro
Department of Pharmaceutical Sciences
University of Maryland School of Pharmacy
Baltimore, MD, USA

ISBN 978-3-030-48282-4 ISBN 978-3-030-48283-1 (eBook)
https://doi.org/10.1007/978-3-030-48283-1

This Springer imprint is published by the registered company Springer Nature Switzerland AG
The registered company address is: Gewerbestrasse 11, 6330 Cham, Switzerland

Preface

The last 50 years of biomedical research has provided significant insight into the mechanisms of disease. Discoveries in genetic mutations and cell and molecular biology have incentivized the development of new precision medicines that target specific features of the disease while limiting unwanted toxic effects on normal tissue. While significant progress has been made in the treatment of diseases such as cancer, long-term durable therapeutic responses are often lacking, or effective drugs have yet to be developed for a specific disease.

Protein kinases have emerged as important drug targets for treating disease. Genetic mutations and other mechanisms resulting in protein kinase dysregulation or constitutive activation drive the progression of proliferative disorders such as cancer, chronic and acute inflammation-related disorders, and neurodegenerative disorders such as Alzheimer disease. The initial development of protein kinase inhibitors used the adenosine triphosphate (ATP) binding site as a logical starting point. It was reasonable to hypothesize that disruption of ATP interactions would prevent the protein kinase from transferring phosphate from naturally occurring ATP onto substrate and disable signaling pathways that promoted disease. Precedent for this had already been established in the early 1950s with drugs such as mercaptopurine that mimic naturally occurring nucleotides, disrupt DNA synthesis, and inhibit cell proliferation in a variety of cancers and autoimmune diseases. However, drugs like mercaptopurine are nonspecific, and off-target side effects on normal proliferating cells limit their effectiveness.

Imatinib (brand name Gleevec) was the first small-molecular-weight inhibitor to enter the clinic in the early 1990s which prevented the binding of ATP to a mutated protein kinase essential for the proliferation of a specific type of leukemia. While imatinib turned out to inhibit several protein kinases, it provided significant benefits to many cancer patients and opened the door to the development of many more small-molecule inhibitors targeting a variety of protein kinases. Today there are several dozen protein kinase inhibitors approved for clinical uses, and many more are in various stages of preclinical testing. Most of the protein kinase inhibitors that have been approved for clinical use interfere with ATP binding and are used to treat various types of cancer. However, in most cases, these types of protein kinase inhibitors do not provide sustained benefits to patients. Major barriers to an effective patient response are undesirable off-target effects, and the invariable development of drug resistance is observed with long-term use. Overcoming these barriers is nontrivial and will require new treatment regimens, knowledge of patient-specific factors, and new drugs that act through different mechanisms of action at the intended tissue site.

This book project will focus on new approaches at blocking protein kinase functions associated with disease. While it may be inferred that the lack of effective or sustained clinical responses with the current inhibitors suggests that protein kinases are not good drug targets, the subsequent chapters will emphasize that protein kinases are valid drug targets. However, the experiences over the last 30 years have provided compelling evidence that the current approach at inhibiting protein kinases, primarily targeting the ATP binding site, has its limitations, and better ways to inhibit protein kinase functions that promote disease are needed. Drugs that block ATP binding are typically promiscuous protein kinase inhibitors. This may have advantages in treating multi-factorial diseases such as cancer where polypharmacologic drugs may be more effective. However, ATP-competitive inhibitors may promote the development of drug resistance by blocking both pro-disease and anti-disease signaling. Protein kinases typically have many substrates that regulate a diverse set of functions, some of which may be desirable to maintain. Off-target effects of ATP-competitive inhibitors on protein kinases in normal cardiac and liver tissue can offset potential benefits.

The book will provide an overview of the current approaches and alternative ideas for developing effective protein kinase inhibitors. Many of these alternative approaches consider the conserved nature of the ATP binding site and the complexity of protein kinases in terms of the number of substrates they regulate and their control of cellular functions. The first objective of this project is to provide a general overview of the biological processes regulated by protein kinases and current therapeutic approaches to inhibit protein kinase activities relevant to disease. The amount of literature on these topics is extensive. Using the search terms "protein kinase and inhibitors" and "protein kinase and inhibitors and review" in the PubMed.gov database yielded ~200,000 and ~20,000 publications, respectively. It would be a daunting task to cover all the relevant studies in a single book, and apologies are extended to researchers of relevant studies that were not cited. However, it is hoped that the information provided in these chapters will help guide the reader in gathering additional details on specific topics of interest.

The second objective is to provide specific examples of emerging areas of protein kinase inhibitor development. However, not all emerging areas of research will be discussed. For example, new approaches at eliminating dysregulated proteins through targeted degradation using novel proteolysis-targeting chimeras (PROTACs) will not be discussed. While this approach entered clinical trials in 2019 to target the degradation of androgen receptor in prostate cancer, it will be interesting to see if clinical applications for targeted degradation of protein kinases are soon to follow. Accumulating details about the structure of protein kinases and functions in regulating substrates and biological processes provide opportunities to identify new approaches that avoid complete ablation of protein kinase activity and are more precise in their mechanisms of inhibition. Experts in this area of research will provide examples of the potential to inhibit specific protein kinase functions by disrupting key protein–protein interactions associated with disease while preserving other desirable kinase functions. In keeping with the movement toward more precision medicine and optimal patient outcomes, the next generation of protein kinase inhibitors will likely include compounds that target a subset of functions as opposed to complete enzyme inhibition observed with the current drugs.

Baltimore, MD, USA Paul Shapiro

Contents

Contributors

George N. Bendzunas Department of Pharmaceutical and Biomedical Sciences, University of Georgia, College of Pharmacy, Augusta, GA, USA

Philip E. Bourne Department of Biomedical Engineering, University of Virginia, Charlottesville, VA, USA

Data Science Institute, University of Virginia, Charlottesville, VA, USA

Kevin N. Dalby Targeted Therapeutic Drug Discovery and Development Program, The University of Texas at Austin, Austin, TX, USA

Division of Chemical Biology and Medicinal Chemistry, College of Pharmacy, The University of Texas at Austin, Austin, TX, USA

Department of Oncology, Dell Medical School, The University of Texas at Austin, Austin, TX, USA

Amy Defnet Department of Pharmaceutical Sciences, University of Maryland-School of Pharmacy, Baltimore, MD, USA

Leah G. Helton Department of Pharmaceutical and Biomedical Sciences, University of Georgia, College of Pharmacy, Augusta, GA, USA

Justin M. Holub Department of Chemistry and Biochemistry, Ohio University, Athens, OH, USA

Molecular and Cellular Biology Program, Ohio University, Athens, OH, USA

Edison Biotechnology Institute, Ohio University, Athens, OH, USA

Eileen J. Kennedy Department of Pharmaceutical and Biomedical Sciences, University of Georgia, College of Pharmacy, Augusta, GA, USA

Ameya J. Limaye Department of Pharmaceutical and Biomedical Sciences, University of Georgia, College of Pharmacy, Augusta, GA, USA

Alexander D. MacKerell Jr Department of Pharmaceutical Sciences, School of Pharmacy, University of Maryland, Baltimore, MD, USA

Institute for Bioscience and Biotechnology Research (IBBR), Rockville, MD, USA

Center for Biomolecular Therapeutics (CBT), School of Medicine, University of Maryland, Baltimore, MD, USA

SilcsBio LLC, Baltimore, MD, USA

Ramon Martinez III Department of Pharmaceutical Sciences, University of Maryland-School of Pharmacy, Baltimore, MD, USA

Rachel M. Sammons Targeted Therapeutic Drug Discovery and Development Program, The University of Texas at Austin, Austin, TX, USA

Paul Shapiro Department of Pharmaceutical Sciences, University of Maryland-School of Pharmacy, Baltimore, MD, USA

David J. Weber Institute for Bioscience and Biotechnology Research (IBBR), Rockville, MD, USA

Center for Biomolecular Therapeutics (CBT), School of Medicine, University of Maryland, Baltimore, MD, USA

Wenbo Yu Department of Pharmaceutical Sciences, School of Pharmacy, University of Maryland, Baltimore, MD, USA

Institute for Bioscience and Biotechnology Research (IBBR), Rockville, MD, USA

Center for Biomolecular Therapeutics (CBT), School of Medicine, University of Maryland, Baltimore, MD, USA

Zheng Zhao Department of Biomedical Engineering, University of Virginia, Charlottesville, VA, USA

Introduction to Kinases, Cellular Signaling, and Kinase Inhibitors

Paul Shapiro, Ramon Martinez III, and Amy Defnet

Abstract Protein kinases are essential regulators of cellular functions and responses to extracellular signals. Through phosphorylation of substrates, protein kinases control cell proliferation and survival. Proliferative disorders, such as cancer, are often observed to have excess protein kinase activity due to genetic mutations. Thus, the development of specific drugs to inhibit protein kinases in cancer cells has been a major goal of academic and pharmaceutical industry research during the last three decades. This chapter will provide a brief historical overview of groundbreaking discoveries describing the importance of protein kinases and the identification of clinically relevant kinase inhibitors. An outline of protein kinase classes, signaling pathways, and structural features will introduce current kinase inhibitor approaches and provide the rationale for identifying alternative approaches to block excess protein kinase activities that promote disease.

Keywords Kinase · Inhibitors · Disease · Drug discovery

Historical Overview of Protein Kinases and Targeted Inhibition

Kinases, derived from the Greek word *kinein* meaning "to move," are ubiquitous enzymes that have become prominent therapeutic targets in the treatment of a variety of diseases. Kinase enzymatic activity is in every cell of every species and facilitates physiological responses to both intracellular and extracellular signals. Through the process of phosphorylation, kinases move or transfer cellular information that regulates a variety of other proteins essential for the survival of the organism. The presence and appreciation of phosphorylated proteins and their importance in biological processes began in the early 1900s. It was in Phoebus Levene's laboratory at

P. Shapiro (✉) · R. Martinez III · A. Defnet
Department of Pharmaceutical Sciences, University of Maryland School of Pharmacy, Baltimore, MD, USA
e-mail: pshapiro@rx.umaryland.edu; rmartinez@umaryland.edu; amy.defnet@umaryland.edu

P. Shapiro (ed.), *Next Generation Kinase Inhibitors*,
https://doi.org/10.1007/978-3-030-48283-1_1

the Rockefeller Institute for Medical Research where phosphorylated serine residues were identified on the proteins casein and phosvitin, which are abundant in milk and egg yolks, respectively [1]. Subsequently, in the 1940s, Gerty and Carl Cori's research at Washington University in St. Louis discovered active and inactive forms of the phosphorylase enzymes that transfer inorganic phosphate to acceptor molecules and are involved in the process of glycogen metabolism. Cori's research was awarded a Nobel Prize in Physiology or Medicine in 1947 and provided the foundation for understanding the process of reversible phosphorylation [2]. Following this award, the significance of the enzymatic activity of kinases and the process of phosphorylation received a significant boost from the pioneering work of George Burnett and Gene Kennedy at the University of Chicago. Their 1954 publication in the *Journal of Biological Chemistry* conclusively demonstrated that rat liver mitochondria extracts contained a protein enzymatic activity, which the authors referred to as a phosphokinase, that extracts a phosphate group from the energy molecule ATP and covalently links it to another protein [3]. These studies revealed a new area of biology that describes how cells use the mineral phosphorus, and its biological form phosphate, to convey information and regulate biological molecules via phosphorylation to accomplish specific cellular functions.

Subsequent discoveries by Edmond Fischer and Edwin Krebs in 1956, at the University of Washington, demonstrated that kinases regulate protein functions in response to extracellular signals and that kinase-mediated phosphorylation events are reversible [4]. The significance of the work by Dr. Fischer and Dr. Krebs, who had trained in the previously mentioned Cori laboratory, was recognized with the Nobel Prize in Physiology or Medicine in 1992. The balance between the activities of kinases that mediate phosphorylation and phosphatase enzymes that facilitate de-phosphorylation is essential for regulation and maintenance of most cellular functions. There are numerous genetic alterations, which will be highlighted in subsequent chapters, responsible for dysregulated kinase activity and the disruption of the balance between phosphorylation and dephosphorylation events. These dysregulated phosphorylation events alter the steady state, or homeostasis, of cellular functions and, ultimately, contribute to the pathology of a variety of diseases.

Over the last several decades, a vast amount of research has discovered and described specific kinases and their functions in regulating specific physiological functions. These findings have revolutionized our understanding of the role of kinases in disease processes and the development of kinase-specific drug therapies. In most cases, the therapeutic objective is to inhibit constitutively active kinase activity found in proliferative disorders, like cancer. Despite a detailed understanding of kinase structures and functions, as well as the availability of potent and selective kinase inhibitors, the ability to achieve sustained patient responses to most of the current kinase inhibitors is limited. This raises the questions of how much is really known about the regulation of kinases in complex biological systems and their role in regulating disease. Furthermore, the multifaceted nature of diseases like cancer may limit the use of potent and selective kinase inhibitors that only target one aspect of the disease but allow compensatory kinase signals that protect cancer cell proliferation and survival. In contrast to the development of very selective kinase inhibitors, there is growing interest in developing inhibitors that target multiple kinases simultaneously or polypharmacologic properties that are uniquely effective against several dysregulated kinases associated with specific diseases [5].

The first, and arguably most successful, program to develop specific small-molecule kinase inhibitors to treat a specific type of cancer was realized by Drs. Nicholas Lydon and Brian Druker in the 1990s with the drug imatinib for the treatment of chronic myelogenous leukemia (CML) [6]. It was well known that CML cells contained a genetic translocation resulting in the fusion of the breakpoint cluster region (BCR) gene on chromosome 22 with the Abelson tyrosine kinase (ABL) gene from chromosome 9. The resulting BCR-Abl fusion protein is constitutively active, and this mutant tyrosine kinase drives the proliferation of white blood cells in nearly every CML patient. Dr. Druker hypothesized that BCR-Abl is a viable drug target and that inhibition of BCR-Abl would improve the therapeutic outcomes of CML patients. Dr. Lydon, working on drug discovery programs at Ciba-Geigy (now part of Novartis), provided the compound STI571, also referred to as imatinib mesylate (brand name Gleevec® or Glivec®), which is an ATP competitive inhibitor of BCR-Abl and other tyrosine kinases. As Drs. Lydon and Druker pointed out, there was skepticism from other scientists and the pharmaceutical industry that specific kinases inhibitors could be developed and that targeted inhibition of a single kinase would be effective against cancer cells with multiple genetic defects [7]. However, the results of the first clinical trials in 1998 and 1999 testing imatinib in CML patients had remarkable outcomes with almost every patient showing improvement. Moreover, the patients had very few side effects and a 5-year follow-up showed patient survival approaching 90% compared to 50% for patients on traditional chemotherapies [7]. While the success of imatinib in treating CML patients could be partially attributed to its off-target effects on other tyrosine kinases, these groundbreaking trials provided the justification for the Food and Drug Administration (FDA)'s approval in 2001 for clinical use. Imatinib remains one of the top-grossing cancer drugs with over $1.5 billion in sales in 2018. Importantly, the introduction of tyrosine kinase inhibitors such as imatinib has significantly improved the survival of CML patients as compared to before these drugs were available [8]. With the therapeutic success of imatinib, scientists and the pharmaceutical industry were provided the framework to pursue the development of other kinase-selective inhibitors for treating disease.

Despite the clinical success of imatinib in treating CML, sustained treatment responses using inhibitors of kinases for other cancer types or diseases have been difficult to achieve. The current approaches used to inhibit protein kinases involved in disease consist of small-molecular-weight compounds (e.g., small molecules) or monoclonal antibodies. As of June 2019, there were approximately 50 small-molecule inhibitors of protein kinases approved by the FDA for clinical use. The number of FDA-approved small-molecule kinase inhibitors from 1999 to 2018 shows an increasing trend over the last decade (Fig. 1). An excellent comprehensive description of the pharmacological properties of FDA approved small-molecule kinase inhibitors is available [9]. In addition, there are more than 30 FDA-approved monoclonal antibodies developed to block the activity of mostly receptor and non-

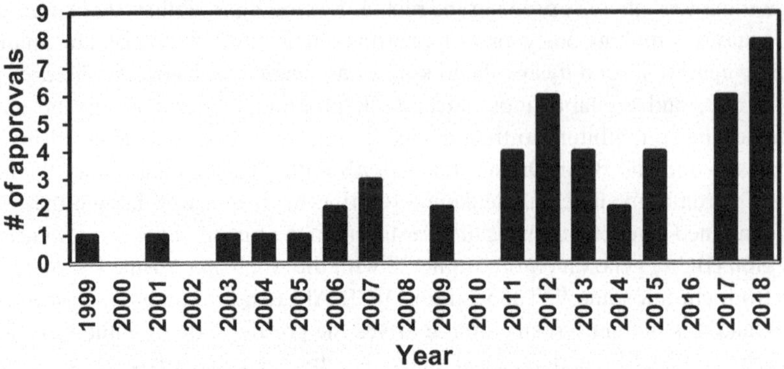

Fig. 1 FDA-approved small-molecule kinase inhibitors (1999–2018)

receptor tyrosine kinases involved in disease. Several reviews outline the development of monoclonal antibodies along with their therapeutic potential and limitations [10, 11]. However, the development of kinase-targeted monoclonal antibodies will not be the focus of subsequent chapters.

A major goal of this book project is to convey that the current approaches to block kinases, with either small molecules or monoclonal antibodies, have mostly failed to produce effective or sustained clinical responses despite the significant evidence supporting kinases as key drivers of disease. As such, new approaches to block important kinase activities involved in disease need to be explored. It is reasonable to suggest that the lack of effective kinase inhibitors can be explained by an inadequate understanding of the biological and genetic determinants that drive the disease. As such, inhibition of a key kinase predicted to drive the pathology of a specific disease is not enough and additional biological targets need to be considered. While this is likely true for many conditions, it can also be argued that the kinase being targeted is appropriate; it is just that the approach used to target a specific kinase is ineffective at producing durable clinical responses. To set the stage for the discovery of new approaches to inhibit kinases, the first chapters will provide an overview of the kinase structure, kinase-signaling networks, and the current approaches to develop small-molecule inhibitors of kinases involved in disease. Therapeutic uses and limitations of the current kinase inhibitors, including the emergence of drug resistance will be highlighted.

Small-molecule kinase inhibitors are classified into six categories commonly referred to as type I–VI kinase inhibitors that are grouped largely based on the structural interactions between the inhibitor and target kinase [12]. Chapter 2 provides a concise summary of the basic features of the type I and II kinase inhibitors, which are currently the most common approach to target kinases, and act by preventing interactions with ATP when the enzyme is in an active or inactive state, respectively. Chapter 3 will summarize recent developments in the type III–VI kinase inhibitors. Type III kinase inhibitors target allosteric sites in the kinase domain but do not affect ATP binding whereas type IV kinase inhibitors target allosteric sites outside the kinase domain and are generally designed to interfere with the interactions between kinases and other regulatory proteins or substrates. Type V kinase inhibitors are referred to as bivalent compounds that target both the ATP-binding site and unique allosteric sites outside the kinase domain. Finally, type VI kinase inhibitors form covalent interactions with cysteine and other amino acids in the ATP-binding site or other regions of the kinase. A recent review of approaches to target the extracellular signal-regulated kinases-1 and 2 (ERK1/2) provides an excellent visual description of the mechanism of action for type I–VI kinase inhibitors [13].

The second major goal of this book will be to highlight new approaches to target protein kinases, including the development of novel type IV small-molecule kinase inhibitors and kinase-targeted peptides that selectively inhibit specific kinase functions. Function-selective kinase inhibitors account for the diversity of protein substrates that are regulated by kinases involved in proliferative diseases, such as cancer, or inflammatory disorders. There are documented examples of how kinase-mediated regulation of substrates can drive a cellular response, but regulation of other substrates is involved in modulating that response through negative feedback mechanisms. Thus, kinases contribute to maintaining homeostasis in normal and diseased cellular responses through both positive and negative feedback regulation. Inhibition of kinase activity with the current type I and II inhibitors block all positive and negative enzyme activity whereas disruption of key kinase-substrate interactions has the potential to block undesirable kinase functions (e.g., protumorigenic) while maintaining desirable kinase functions (e.g., antitumorigenic negative feedback). Lack of durable responses of many kinase inhibitors used in the clinic may be attributed to inhibition of both positive and negative kinase functions. It will be interesting to see whether novel proteolysis targeting chimera (PROTAC) approaches that can be designed to selectively degrade kinases and other proteins involved in disease [14] will also have similar issues with efficacy.

The design of function-selective kinase inhibitors is based on a large body of information describing the structural features that determine specific protein-protein interactions (PPIs) and the biological consequences of those interactions. Chapter 4 will provide examples of PPIs focusing on specific kinase interactions with substrate proteins. These studies have helped in the design of new approaches to target key PPIs involved in disease. In addition, Chap. 4 will overview the emergence of acquired drug resistance to current kinase inhibitors used in the clinic, which presents a major barrier to sustained and durable patient responses. It is hypothesized that function-selective kinase inhibitors will prevent or mitigate the emergence of drug resistance observed with current kinase inhibitors that block all enzyme activity.

The final chapters will describe specific examples of theoretical and experimental approaches to develop kinase inhibitors that act outside of the ATP/catalytic site and inhibit specific kinase functions. Chapter 5 describes how computational models can facilitate the rationale design and analysis of new compounds that target specific PPIs and, in particular, those that involve kinase interactions with specific protein substrates. Chapter 6 provides a comprehensive description of known substrate-docking sites on the extracellular signal-regulated kinases (ERK1/2) and opportunities to develop type IV inhibitors that target these sites for treating cancer. Chapter 7 will describe the synthesis of novel peptide sequences that lock into secondary structures that recognize specific kinase sites involved in substrate recognition. Finally, Chap. 8 expands on the use of peptides that selectively modify kinase functions and outlines the challenges that need to be overcome before these agents can be used in the clinic. In conclusion, the evidence presented in these chapters will provide support for the discovery and development of novel kinase inhibitors that selectively block some, but not all, enzymatic functions. The development of new approaches aimed at partial inhibition of kinase functions involved in disease is predicted to lead to more effective and sustained therapeutic responses.

Overview of Protein Kinase Signaling Pathways

Protein kinases are essential regulators of cellular functions and responses to external signals. Protein kinases accomplish their regulatory role mostly, but not always, by catalyzing the transfer of phosphate from ATP onto substrates. Of the more than 500 distinct genes that encode for human protein kinases [15], it is estimated that ~80% fall into the category of serine or threonine kinases while the remaining 20% consist of tyrosine or histidine kinases [16]. However, it is estimated that roughly 90% of all phosphorylation events in human cells occur on serine residues while approximately 10% occurs on threonine residues, and less than 1% of phosphorylation events occur on tyrosine residues [16]. Given that most of the kinase inhibitors used in the clinic today block the actions of tyrosine kinases, these numbers suggest there are tremendous opportunities for the discovery of new kinase inhibitors.

Protein kinases are classified into AGC, CAMK, CMGC, CK1, STE, TK, and TKL subgroups based on their phylogenetic tree [15]. The AGC protein kinase group consists of approximately 60 serine/threonine kinases related to protein kinases A, G, and C. One feature key to the regulation of AGC kinase activity is a hydrophobic region in the C-terminal that interacts with a pocket in the catalytic region. This interaction site was named the PIF, 3-phosphoinositide-dependent protein kinase–1 (PDK1)-interacting fragment, unique to the ACG family [17]. The CAMK group is the abbreviation for around 80 serine/threonine kinases related to the calcium-calmodulin–dependent protein kinases. The identification of a unique calcium/calmodulin (CaM)-binding domain is a regulatory feature found in about half of kinases in the CAMK family [18].

There are roughly 62 members of the serine/threonine kinase CMGC group that include the cyclin-dependent kinases (CDK), mitogen-activated protein kinases (MAPK), glycogen synthase kinases (GSK), and CDC-like kinases (CLK). The CK1 group, or casein kinase-1 family, is a small group of 12 serine/threonine kinases that are the most structurally distinct group of eukaryotic protein kinases. A unique aspect of the CK1 proteins is a variable C-terminal region that does not directly affect ATP catalysis but is important for regulating intracellular location and kinase functions [19, 20]. The STE kinase group, named for yeast sterile genes involved in mating signals, comprises approximately 46 serine/threonine kinases that act primarily as upstream activators of the mitogen-activated protein kinase (MAPK) proteins and include the MAP2K, MAP3K, and MAP4K proteins. The MAP2K subfamily is unique in that it is a dual specificity kinase and can phosphorylate MAPK proteins on threonine (T) and tyrosine (Y) residues within a conserved TXY motif (X is any amino acid) that regulates kinase activation. The last kinase groups consist of approximately 90 receptor and nonreceptor tyrosine kinase (TK) proteins and another 43 tyrosine kinase-like (TLK) proteins. While the TLK group shares amino acid sequence similarity to TK proteins, these proteins function as serine/threonine kinases.

The process of phosphorylation adds a negative charge to a biological molecule, which alters the molecule's structure and ultimate function in the cell. The functions of biological molecules such as proteins, nucleic acids, carbohydrates, and lipids are all regulated by phosphorylation events. Phosphorylation is a highly regulated and reversible process. Cellular functions depend on the balance between the addition of phosphates by kinases to achieve a specific cellular response and the removal of the phosphate by protein phosphatases when that cellular response is no longer needed. A consequence of disrupted balance between protein phosphorylation and dephosphorylation often results in elevated protein phosphorylation, which contributes to the development and progression of many types of cancer and inflammation-related disorders. Excess protein phosphorylation is a consequence of genetic mutations or altered expression of kinases and phosphatases. Dysregulated and constitutively active protein kinases are the primary culprits that disrupt the balance between phosphorylation and dephosphorylation. As such, inhibition of dysregulated kinase activity is a major goal in the development of safe and effective therapies for cancer, inflammatory disorders, and many other diseases.

There are currently more than 200 kinases that have been linked to various disease states and most involve proliferative disorders such as cancer [21, 22]. However, dysregulated kinase activity is also recognized to contribute to cardiovascular, metabolic, and neurodegenerative diseases [23–28]. The causes of kinase dysregulation and its role in driving disease have been studied extensively and can be narrowed down to three genetic changes. These genetic alterations consist of point mutations that change single amino acids, gene amplification, and the fusion of two different genes, all of which result in kinases with elevated or constitutive activity [21]. Further analysis of over 1000 putative cancer causing or "driver" genes, which are essential for the cells proliferative advantage, identified 91 of these genes to be protein kinases [29]. Interestingly, a remarkable 40% of the protein kinase drivers were tyrosine kinases, which is consistent with the higher emphasis on the development of tyrosine kinase inhibitors. However, despite the prevalence of clinically available tyrosine kinase inhibitors, less than half of these kinase drivers have been targeted with therapeutic agents [29].

Protein kinases serve an important function in regulating cellular responses to extracellular signals. Figure 2 shows a simplified overview of major kinase signaling pathways that respond to extracellular signals, have been found to be dysregulated in disease, and are the targets of kinase inhibitors. Extracellular cytokines and

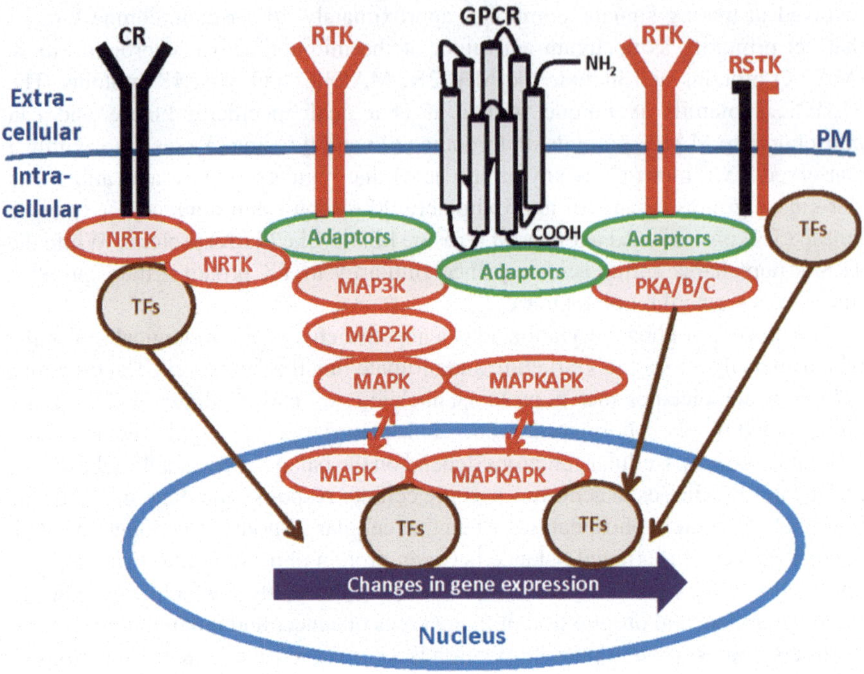

Fig. 2 Receptor-mediated kinase signaling networks. Kinases (red) target transcription factors (brown) to mediate changes in gene expression and cellular responses to extracellular signals. Adaptors (green) include G-proteins and associated proteins that couple receptors to kinase cascades. Key: *CR* cytokine receptor, *RTK* receptor tyrosine kinase, *NRTK* nonreceptor tyrosine kinase, *RSTK* receptor serine/threonine kinase, *PM* plasma membrane, *TFs* transcription factors, *MAP3K/MAP2K/MAPK* mitogen-activated protein kinase cascade, *MAPKAPK* MAP kinase-activating protein kinase, *PKA/B/C* protein kinase A, B, or C

growth factors regulate cellular responses by interacting with plasma membrane–bound receptor tyrosine kinases (RTK), G-protein coupled receptors (GPCR), cytokine receptors (CR), and receptor serine/threonine kinases (RSTK). Engagement of the extracellular ligands induces receptor conformational changes that result in the dimerization and activation of monomeric receptor proteins and the recruitment of intracellular nonreceptor tyrosine kinases (NRTK) and other adapter proteins. The recruitment of intracellular adaptor proteins to the activated receptors led to the activation of kinase cascades and regulation of specific transcription factors and gene expression. However, kinases can regulate many other nongenomic processes by phosphorylating cytoplasmic substrates that affect the size or shape of the cell and its ability to migrate and interact with other cells. To add to the complexity, there are several examples of protein kinases regulating other proteins and biological outcomes through catalytic-independent functions [30]. In most of the cases where there is no phosphate transfer, the physical interaction between a kinase and a particular protein is sufficient to modulate the protein's function and a subsequent biological outcome.

The mitogen-activated protein kinase (MAPK) and protein kinase B (Akt) signaling cascades are classic examples of RTK and GPCR-mediated signaling pathways that regulate cellular functions [31–36]. In the case of receptor serine/threonine kinases (RSTK), transcription factor activation is coupled directly to the ligand-activated receptor. The transforming growth factor-β (TGF-β) family is an example of secreted extracellular proteins that activate receptors with primarily serine/threonine kinase activity to modulate the cellular responses in many physiological systems [37]. Membrane-bound receptors, directly or through adaptor proteins, activate intracellular kinases, which in turn regulate a variety of substrates including transcription factors to alter gene expression and cellular responses. Dimerization of RTK monomers following ligand engagement facilitates inherent kinase activity of these receptors. In contrast, the ligand-activated cytokine receptors lack kinase activity and engage associated nonreceptor tyrosine kinases to initiate downstream signaling. In the case of the receptor serine-threonine kinases, only one of the monomers has kinase activity that directly phosphorylates transcription factors after receptor dimerization following ligand engagement. Several comprehensive reviews of these receptor-mediated kinase-signaling pathways are available [38, 39]. In addition, a more detailed description of specific kinase-signaling networks will be presented in later chapters.

Overview of Protein Kinase Structural Features

The typical eukaryote protein kinase has a conserved bilobed 3-D structure consisting of amino- (N) and carboxy-(C) terminal lobes that are coordinated in their movement in relation to each other depending on kinase activity. Most protein kinases contain a conserved ATP-binding site, substrate interaction sites in the C-terminal lobe, and activation sites as shown in the example of protein kinase A (Fig. 3). The N-terminal lobe consists mainly of beta sheets while the C-terminal lobe contains alpha-helices. At the base of the N-terminal lobe sits the ATP-binding and catalytic site that serves the function of removing the terminal phosphate (PO_4^{3-}) from magnesium-ATP (MgATP) and catalyzing its transfer onto the hydroxyl (OH^-) group of a serine, threonine, or tyrosine residue located on the substrate protein. The Mg^{2+} helps stabilize and position the negatively charged phosphate on ATP for transfer onto the substrate. Additional coordination of ATP involves a conserved glycine rich loop and lysine residue in the N-terminal lobe. Substrate proteins interact with specific residues in the C-terminal lobe and along a cleft formed between the N- and C-terminal lobes. However, the specific kinase residues involved in recognizing most protein substrates are not known. An overview of some of the known structural features and residues involved in kinase recognition of protein substrates will be the topic of Chap. 4. This information will be important for the identification of type IV kinase inhibitors that disrupt key kinase functions.

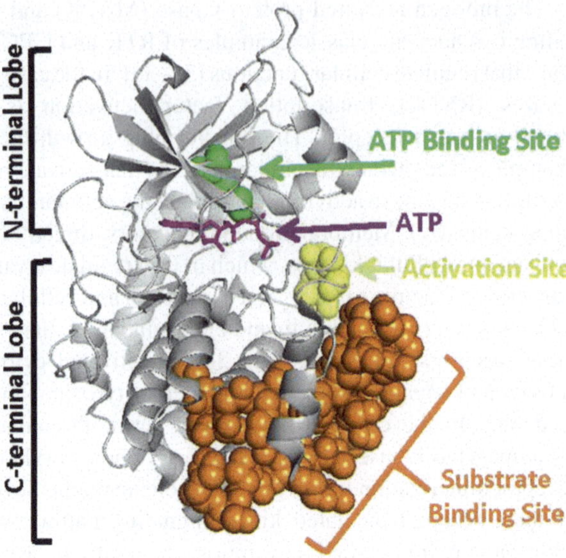

Fig. 3 General overview of protein kinase structure. A model of protein kinase A (pdb: 3FJQ) highlights the N-terminal lobe containing the ATP-binding site (conserved lysine, K73, in green) and ATP (purple). The C-terminal lobe contains the activation sites (T196 and T198 in yellow) and substrate-binding site (residues 230–260 in brown)

Human protein kinases are dynamic structures, and multiple regions distal to the catalytic site have been implicated in coordinating activity. For a more detailed analysis of the structural features involved in protein kinase regulation, the reader is directed to several intriguing studies and comprehensive reviews. For example, McClendon et al. have presented compelling molecular modeling data showing that kinases also have unique local regions, consisting of 40–60 amino acid segments that undergo unique dynamic changes that provide allosteric regulation and additional control over kinase activity and function [40]. Wang and Cole provide an excellent review of the catalytic mechanisms of protein kinases and the transfer of a phosphoryl group from ATP onto substrates [41]. This review highlights the work of many scientists who have made significant contributions to our understanding of kinase structure and catalytic mechanisms. Although protein kinases share many conserved structural features that define the core region involved in phosphoryl transfer onto protein substrates, there are regions outside of the kinase core that facilitate catalytic activity, kinase complexes, and signaling events. Gógl et al. describe the presence of intrinsically disordered regions (IDRs) in protein kinases that help fine tune kinase catalytic activity and assembly of kinases in multiprotein signaling complexes [42]. Expanding knowledge of the regulatory features of protein kinases will provide opportunities to develop new approaches to modulate protein kinase functions in disease.

References

1. Lipmann, F. A., & Levene, P. A. (1932). Serinephosphoric acid obtained by hydrolysis of vitellinic acid. *Journal of Biological Chemistry, 98*, 109–114.
2. Simoni, R. D., Hill, R. L., & Vaughan, M. (2002). Carbohydrate metabolism: Glycogen phosphorylase and the work of Carl F. and Gerty T.Cori. 1928–1943. *Journal of Biological Chemistry, 277*, 18e.
3. Burnett, G., & Kennedy, E. P. (1954). The enzymatic phosphorylation of proteins. *The Journal of Biological Chemistry, 211*, 969–980.
4. Krebs, E. G., & Fischer, E. H. (1956). The phosphorylase B to a converting enzyme of rabbit skeletal muscle. *Biochimica et Biophysica Acta, 20*, 150–157.
5. Rao, S., Du, G., Hafner, M., Subramanian, K., Sorger, P. K., & Gray, N. S. (2019). A multi-targeted probe-based strategy to identify signaling vulnerabilities in cancers. *The Journal of Biological Chemistry, 294*, 8664–8673.
6. Lydon, N. B., & Druker, B. J. (2004). Lessons learned from the development of imatinib. *Leukemia Research, 28*(Suppl 1), S29–S38.
7. Druker, B. J. (2009). Perspectives on the development of imatinib and the future of cancer research. *Nature Medicine, 15*, 1149–1152.
8. Di Felice, E., Roncaglia, F., Venturelli, F., Mangone, L., Luminari, S., Cirilli, C., Carrozzi, G., & Giorgi Rossi, P. (2018). The impact of introducing tyrosine kinase inhibitors on chronic myeloid leukemia survival: A population-based study. *BMC Cancer, 18*, 1069.
9. Roskoski, R., Jr. (2019). Properties of FDA-approved small molecule protein kinase inhibitors. *Pharmacological Research, 144*, 19–50.
10. Elgundi, Z., Reslan, M., Cruz, E., Sifniotis, V., & Kayser, V. (2017). The state-of-play and future of antibody therapeutics. *Advanced Drug Delivery Reviews, 122*, 2–19.
11. Cruz, E., & Kayser, V. (2019). Monoclonal antibody therapy of solid tumors: Clinical limitations and novel strategies to enhance treatment efficacy. *Biologics, 13*, 33–51.
12. Roskoski, R., Jr. (2016). Classification of small molecule protein kinase inhibitors based upon the structures of their drug-enzyme complexes. *Pharmacological Research, 103*, 26–48.
13. Sammons, R. M., Ghose, R., Tsai, K. Y., & Dalby, K. N. (2019). Targeting ERK beyond the boundaries of the kinase active site in melanoma. *Molecular Carcinogenesis, 58*, 1551–1570.
14. Pettersson, M., & Crews, C. M. (2019). PROteolysis TArgeting Chimeras (PROTACs)—Past, present and future. *Drug Discovery Today: Technologies, 31*, 15–27.
15. Manning, G., Whyte, D. B., Martinez, R., Hunter, T., & Sudarsanam, S. (2002). The protein kinase complement of the human genome. *Science, 298*, 1912–1934.
16. Lahiry, P., Torkamani, A., Schork, N. J., & Hegele, R. A. (2010). Kinase mutations in human disease: Interpreting genotype-phenotype relationships. *Nature Reviews Genetics, 11*, 60–74.
17. Arencibia, J. M., Pastor-Flores, D., Bauer, A. F., Schulze, J. O., & Biondi, R. M. (2013). AGC protein kinases: From structural mechanism of regulation to allosteric drug development for the treatment of human diseases. *Biochimica et Biophysica Acta, 1834*, 1302–1321.
18. Bayer, K. U., & Schulman, H. (2019). CaM kinase: Still inspiring at 40. *Neuron, 103*, 380–394.
19. Babu, P., Bryan, J. D., Panek, H. R., Jordan, S. L., Forbrich, B. M., Kelley, S. C., Colvin, R. T., & Robinson, L. C. (2002). Plasma membrane localization of the Yck2p yeast casein kinase 1 isoform requires the C-terminal extension and secretory pathway function. *Journal of Cell Science, 115*, 4957–4968.
20. Graves, P. R., & Roach, P. J. (1995). Role of COOH-terminal phosphorylation in the regulation of casein kinase I delta. *The Journal of Biological Chemistry, 270*, 21689–21694.
21. CST. (2019). *Kinase-disease associations*. Cell Signaling Technology. https://www.cellsignal.com/contents/resources-reference-tables/kinase-disease-associations/science-tables-kinase-disease.
22. Gross, S., Rahal, R., Stransky, N., Lengauer, C., & Hoeflich, K. P. (2015). Targeting cancer with kinase inhibitors. *The Journal of Clinical Investigation, 125*, 1780–1789.

23. Yarza, R., Vela, S., Solas, M., & Ramirez, M. J. (2015). c-Jun N-terminal kinase (JNK) signaling as a therapeutic target for Alzheimer's disease. *Frontiers in Pharmacology, 6*, 321.
24. Shahin, R., Shaheen, O., El-Dahiyat, F., Habash, M., & Saffour, S. (2017). Research advances in kinase enzymes and inhibitors for cardiovascular disease treatment. *Future Science OA, 3*, FSO204.
25. Maqbool, M., & Hoda, N. (2017). GSK3 inhibitors in the therapeutic development of diabetes cancer and neurodegeneration: Past, present and future. *Current Pharmaceutical Design, 23*, 4332–4350.
26. Liang, H., Nie, J., Van Skike, C. E., Valentine, J. M., & Orr, M. E. (2019). Mammalian target of Rapamycin at the crossroad between Alzheimer's disease and diabetes. *Advances in Experimental Medicine and Biology, 1128*, 185–225.
27. Nozal, V., & Martinez, A. (2019). Tau tubulin kinase 1 (TTBK1), a new player in the fight against neurodegenerative diseases. *European Journal of Medicinal Chemistry, 161*, 39–47.
28. Cuny, G. D. (2009). Kinase inhibitors as potential therapeutics for acute and chronic neurodegenerative conditions. *Current Pharmaceutical Design, 15*, 3919–3939.
29. Fleuren, E. D., Zhang, L., Wu, J., & Daly, R. J. (2016). The kinome 'at large' in cancer. *Nature Reviews Cancer, 16*, 83–98.
30. Rauch, J., Volinsky, N., Romano, D., & Kolch, W. (2011). The secret life of kinases: Functions beyond catalysis. *Cell Communication and Signaling, 9*, 23.
31. Plotnikov, A., Zehorai, E., Procaccia, S., & Seger, R. (2011). The MAPK cascades: Signaling components, nuclear roles and mechanisms of nuclear translocation. *Biochimica et Biophysica Acta, 1813*, 1619–1633.
32. Seger, R., & Krebs, E. G. (1995). The MAPK signaling cascade. *The FASEB Journal, 9*, 726–735.
33. Cargnello, M., & Roux, P. P. (2011). Activation and function of the MAPKs and their substrates, the MAPK-activated protein kinases. *Microbiology and Molecular Biology Reviews, 75*, 50–83.
34. Barnett, S. F., Bilodeau, M. T., & Lindsley, C. W. (2005). The Akt/PKB family of protein kinases: A review of small molecule inhibitors and progress towards target validation. *Current Topics in Medicinal Chemistry, 5*, 109–125.
35. Arafeh, R., & Samuels, Y. (2019). PIK3CA in cancer: The past 30 years. *Seminars in Cancer Biology, 59*, 36.
36. Rozengurt, E. (2007). Mitogenic signaling pathways induced by G protein-coupled receptors. *Journal of Cellular Physiology, 213*, 589–602.
37. Derynck, R., & Budi, E. H. (2019). Specificity, versatility, and control of TGF-beta family signaling. *Science Signaling, 12*, eaav5183.
38. Haan, C., Kreis, S., Margue, C., & Behrmann, I. (2006). Jaks and cytokine receptors—An intimate relationship. *Biochemical Pharmacology, 72*, 1538–1546.
39. Vander Ark, A., Cao, J., & Li, X. (2018). TGF-beta receptors: In and beyond TGF-beta signaling. *Cellular Signalling, 52*, 112–120.
40. McClendon, C. L., Kornev, A. P., Gilson, M. K., & Taylor, S. S. (2014). Dynamic architecture of a protein kinase. *Proceedings of the National Academy of Sciences of the United States of America, 111*, E4623–E4631.
41. Wang, Z., & Cole, P. A. (2014). Catalytic mechanisms and regulation of protein kinases. *Methods in Enzymology, 548*, 1–21.
42. Gogl, G., Kornev, A. P., Remenyi, A., & Taylor, S. S. (2019). Disordered protein kinase regions in regulation of kinase domain cores. *Trends in Biochemical Sciences, 44*, 300–311.

Overview of Current Type I/II Kinase Inhibitors

Zheng Zhao and Philip E. Bourne

Abstract Research on kinase-targeting drugs has made great strides over the last 30 years and is attracting greater attention for the treatment of yet more kinase-related diseases. Currently, 42 kinase drugs have been approved by the FDA, most of which (Wilson et al., Cancer Research 78(1):15–29, 2018) are Type I/II inhibitors. Notwithstanding these advances, it is desirable to target additional kinases for drug development as more than 200 diseases, particularly cancers, are directly associated with aberrant kinase regulation and signaling. Here, we review the extant Type I/II drugs systematically to obtain insights into the binding pocket characteristics, the associated features of Type I/II drugs, and the mechanism of action to facilitate future kinase drug design and discovery. We conclude by summarizing the main successes and limitations of targeting kinases for the development of drugs.

Keywords Type I/II kinase inhibitors · Protein kinases · Mechanisms of action · Promise and limitations

Introduction

Kinases are enzymes that phosphorylate specific substrates and in so doing play a vital role in signal transduction networks [1–3]. Clinical evidence has shown that aberrant kinase regulation and catalysis are directly associated with more than 200 diseases, especially cancer [4, 5]. Thus, exploring the therapeutic potential of the human kinome is highly desirable for the treatment of many diseases [6–9]. As of August 2018, 42 kinase-targeted drugs have been approved by the U.S. Food and

Z. Zhao
Department of Biomedical Engineering, University of Virginia, Charlottesville, VA, USA

P. E. Bourne (✉)
Department of Biomedical Engineering, University of Virginia, Charlottesville, VA, USA

Data Science Institute, University of Virginia, Charlottesville, VA, USA
e-mail: peb6a@virginia.edu

P. Shapiro (ed.), *Next Generation Kinase Inhibitors*,
https://doi.org/10.1007/978-3-030-48283-1_2

Drug Administration (FDA) [10]. Notwithstanding these advances, developing a desired kinase drug is still a challenging task due to the high similarity of the ATP-binding sites across the whole kinome thwarting selectivity [11, 12]. Here we systematically review extant kinase inhibitors, especially FDA-approved kinase drugs, to provide benchmarks and useful clues for prospective kinase drugs.

Over the last 30 years, chemically diverse kinase inhibitors with varied selectivity levels have emerged and can been classified into four types based on their binding modes: Type I, Type II, Type III, and Type IV (Fig. 1) [13–16]. Type I inhibitors, such as baricitinib (Fig. 1a), occupy the ATP-bound pocket of the kinase in the "DFG-in" conformation. Type II kinase inhibitors, such as imatinib, not only occupy the ATP-bound pocket of the kinase with the "DFG-out" inactive conformation but elongate to the adjacent allosteric pocket (Fig. 1b). Type III and Type IV inhibitors are also called allosteric inhibitors [17]. Type III inhibitors bind to the allosteric site close to the ATP-bound pocket, such as with the MEK inhibitor cobimetinib [18] (Fig. 1c). Type IV inhibitors bind to the allosteric pocket distant from the ATP-binding site, such as the allosteric pocket at the C-lobe [19] (Fig. 1d), the allosteric pockets on the surface of the kinase domain [20–22] (Fig. 1e), or the allosteric pocket at the N-lobe [23] (Fig. 1f). By numbers, the vast majority of kinase inhibitors are Type I/II inhibitors. Of the 42 FDA-approved kinase drugs, 33 are Type I inhibitors, 6 are Type II inhibitors, and 3 MEK-targeted drugs are Type III inhibitors (Table 1). Here we focus on a review of the characteristics of current Type I/II kinase inhibitors.

FDA-Approved Kinase Inhibitors: Type I and II Mechanisms of Action

Type I Binding Modes

Type I inhibitors bind at the ATP-binding pocket, which is highly conserved across the human kinome [16, 24, 25]. To achieve greater selectivity than ATP, Type I inhibitors typically not only occupy the space where the ATP adenine group binds but also extend into different proximal regions, specifically referred to as the front pocket region, the hydrophobic pocket region, the DFG motif, and the P-loop region (Fig. 2a) [26, 27]. Here we outline how inhibition occurs through the ability to combine the adenine-binding area with different proximal regions.

Gefitinib is one of the first-generation EGFR drugs for the treatment of non-small cell lung cancer (NSCLC) [28]. Gefitinib binds to EGFR by its quinazoline scaffold, which forms hydrogen bonds with the hinge region, mimicking the hydrogen bonds between the hinge region and the adenine moiety of ATP, one 4-position substitutional group extends into the hydrophobic pocket and one 6-position morpholine derivative extends into the front pocket and forms polar interactions with the adjacent residues C797 and D800 (Fig. 2a) [29]. Similarly, the other 11 kinase

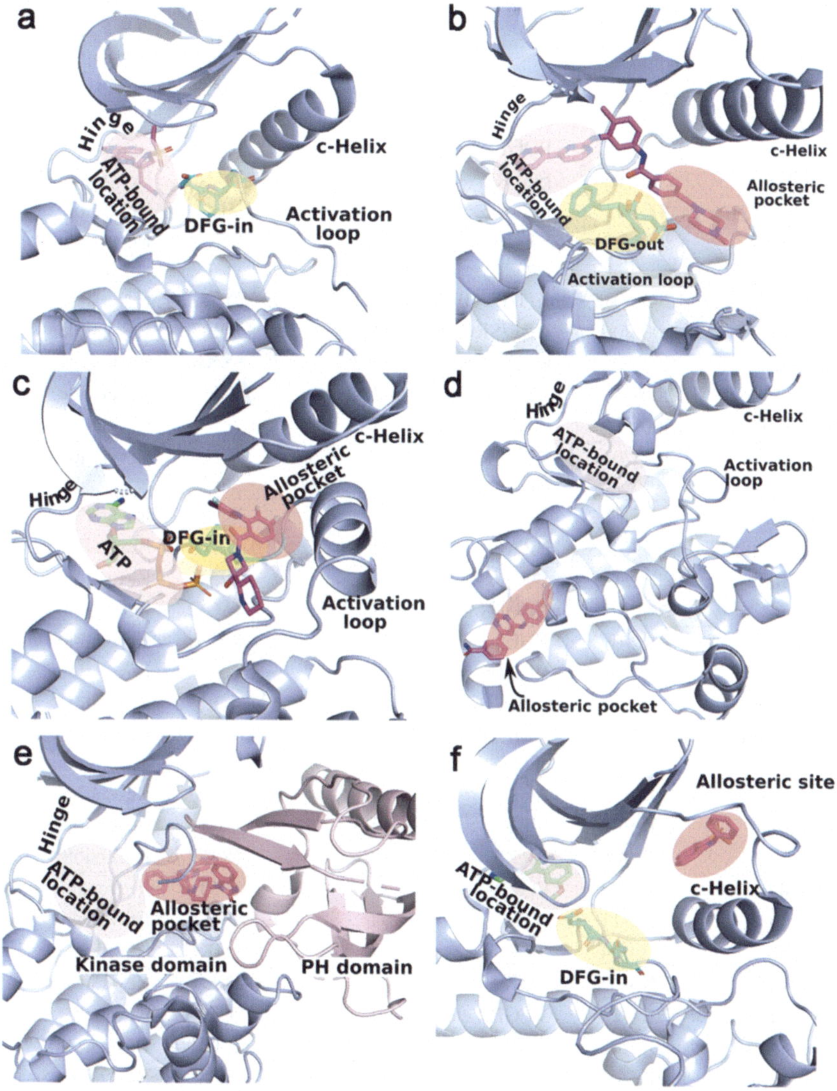

Fig. 1 The binding modes of Type I–IV inhibitors. (**a**) Type I inhibitor bound to the ATP-binding pocket (pdb 4w9x, the JAK-baricitinib complex); (**b**) Type II inhibitor occupying the ATP-binding pocket and extending into the allosteric pocket (pdb 4bkj, the ABL-imatinib complex); (**c**) Type III inhibitor bound to the allosteric pocket close to the ATP-bound pocket (pdb 4an2, the MEK-cobimetinib complex); (**d**) Type IV allosteric inhibitor bound to the allosteric pocket of the C-lobe (pdb 3k5v, the Abl-GNF-2 complex); (**e**) Type IV allosteric inhibitor bound to the allosteric pocket at the interface of the AKT1 kinase and the PH domain (pdb 3o96, the AKT1-MK-2206 complex); (**f**) Type IV allosteric inhibitor bound to the allosteric pocket at the N-lobe (pdb 3py1, the CDK2-2AN complex)

Table 1 FDA-approved kinase drugs with their associated binding modes and approval dates (as of August 2018)

Approved inhibitors	Approved date	Primary targets	Inhibitor of type	PDB entry	Reversible/ irreversible
Imatinib	2001/05	ABL/ PDGFR/c-KIT	II	1OPJ	Reversible
Gefitinib	2003/05	EGFR	I	4I22	Reversible
Erlotinib	2004/11	EGFR	I	4HJO	Reversible
Sorafenib	2005/12	VEGFR/PDGFR etc	II	4ASD	Reversible
Sunitinib	2006/01	KIT/PDGFR etc	I	2Y7J	Reversible
Dasatinib	2006/06	ABL/SRC etc	I	3QLG	Reversible
Lapatinib	2007/03	EGFR/Her2	I	1XKK	Reversible
Nilotinib	2007/10	ABL/KIT etc	II	3GP0	Reversible
Pazopanib	2009/10	c-KIT/FGFR etc	I	–	Reversible
Vandetanib	2011/04	VEGFR/EGFR etc	I	2IVU	Reversible
Crizotinib	2011/08	ALK/ROS1	I	3ZBF	Reversible
Vemurafenib	2011/08	BRAF	I	3OG7	Reversible
Ruxolitinib	2011/11	JAK1/JAK2	I	4U5J	Reversible
Axitinib	2012/01	VEGFR etc	I	4AGC	Reversible
Bosutinib	2012/09	ABL/SRC	I	4OTW	Reversible
Regorafenib	2012/09	VEGFR etc	II	–	Reversible
Tofacitinib	2012/11	JAK1/JAK3	I	3LXN	Reversible
Cabozantinib	2012/11	c-MET/VEGFR2 etc	II	–	Reversible
Ponatinib	2012/12	ABL	II	4C8B	Reversible
Trametinib	2013/05	MEK1	III	–	Reversible
Dabrafenib	2013/05	BRAF	I	4XV2	Reversible
Afatinib	2013/07	EGFR	I	4G5J	Irreversible
Ibrutinib	2013/11	BTK	I	4IFG	Irreversible
Ceritinib	2014/04	ALK	I	4MKC	Reversible
Idelalisib	2014/07	PI3Kd	I	4XE0	Reversible
Nintedanib	2014/10	VEGFR etc	I	3C7Q	Reversible
Palbociclib	2015/02	CDK4/CDK6	I	2EUF	Reversible
Lenvatinib	2015/02	VEGFR1/2/3	I	3WZD	Reversible
Cobimetinib	2015/11	MEK	III	4AN2	Reversible
Osimertinib	2015/11	EGFR	I	4ZAU	Irreversible
Alectinib	2015/12	ALK	I	5XV7	Reversible
Ribociclib	2017/03	CDK4/CDK6	I	5L2T	Reversible
Brigatinib	2017/04	ALK/EGFR	I	5J7H	Reversible
Midostaurin	2017/04	FLT3 etc	I	4NCT	Reversible
Neratinib	2017/06	EGFR/HER2	I	2JIV	Irreversible
Abemaciclib	2017/09	CDK4/CDK6	I	5L2S	Reversible
Copanlisib	2017/09	PI3Ka/PI3Kd	I	5G2N	Reversible

(continued)

Table 1 (continued)

Approved inhibitors	Approved date	Primary targets	Inhibitor of type	PDB entry	Reversible/ irreversible
Acalabrutinib	2017/10	BTK	I	–	Irreversible
Fostamatinib	2018/04	SYK	I	3FQS	Reversible
Baricitinib	2018/05	JAK1/2	I	4W9X	Reversible
Binimetinib	2018/06	MEK	III	4U7Z	Reversible
Encorafenib	2018/06	BRAF	I	–	Reversible

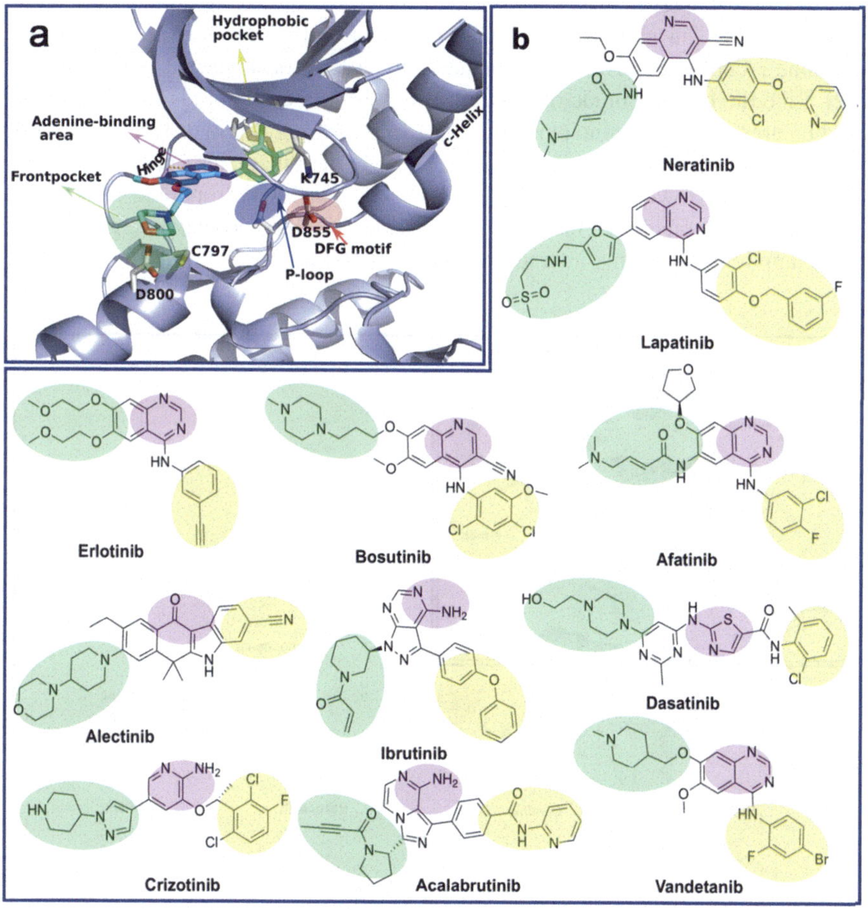

Fig. 2 Type I inhibitors that occupy the front pocket region, the adenine-binding area, and the hydrophobic pocket region. (**a**) The drug gefitinib binding to the kinase EGFR (pdb 4I22). (**b**) The other 11 drugs with the same binding features as gefitinib

drugs (Fig. 2b), although acting on different kinase targets, also share the same binding pattern as gefitinib. This class of Type I binding, which consists of binding to the adenine-binding pocket, the hydrophobic pocket region, and the front pocket region, constitutes the largest cluster of 12 FDA-approved drugs. In this class, it is worth noting that afatinib, neratinib, ibrutinib, and acalabrutinib not only contain the corresponding hydrophilic substituents elongating into the front pocket but also carry an acrylamide electrophilic group forming a covalent interaction with a nearby cysteine within the front pocket region [27, 30, 31]. The four covalent drugs together with another covalent drug osimertinib are irreversible kinase drugs, which are discussed in the chapter on irreversible inhibitors.

Ribociclib is an inhibitor of cyclin D1/CDK4 and CDK6 for the treatment of hormone receptor-positive, HER2-negative metastatic or advanced breast cancers [32]. Like the binding mode of gefitinib (Fig. 2a), ribociclib binds to the adenine-binding area via its 2-amino pyrimidine scaffold forming two hydrogen bonds with the hinge and binds to the front pocket region via the piperazine-substituent group (Fig. 3a) [33]. However, ribociclib does not occupy the hydrophobic pocket like gefitinib but interacts with the DFG-motif region via one carboxamide group. The carboxamide group forms interactions with Asp163 of the DFG motif and Lys43,

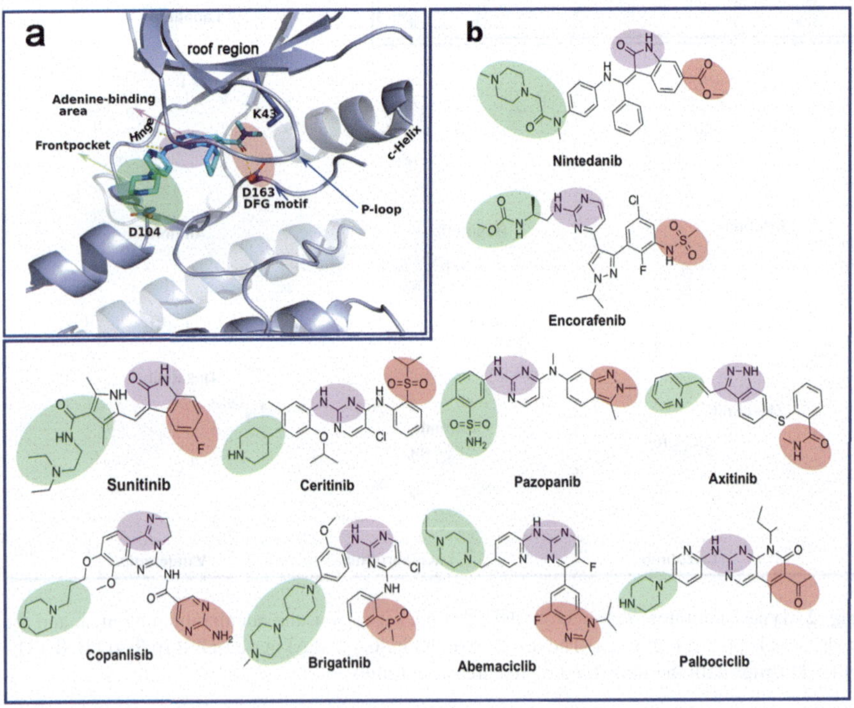

Fig. 3 Type I inhibitors bound to the front pocket region, the adenine-binding area, and the DFG-motif region. (**a**) The drug ribociclib binding to the kinase CDK6 (pdb 5l2t). (**b**) The other nine drugs with the same binding features as ribociclib

which is located on the "roof" of the ATP-binding site (Fig. 3a). The other nine drugs (Fig. 3b) share the same binding mode as that of ribociclib (i.e., occupying the front pocket region, the adenine-binding area, and the DFG-motif region) although targeting different kinases. In this class, encorafenib was approved by the FDA in combination with binimetinib for the treatment of patients in June 2018. The encorafenib/binimetinib combination has shown the best-in-class efficacy and tolerability for patients with BRAF V600E–mutant advanced unresectable or metastatic melanoma [34]. Similar drug combinations had been validated previously; dabrafenib/trametinib was approved in January 2014 and vemurafenib/cobimetinib was approved in November 2015 for the same population [35]. Using drug combinations represents an emerging kinase application strategy in clinical care owing to a more detailed understanding of the underlying kinase signaling networks.

Vemurafenib exhibits a different binding mode. Vemurafenib works specifically for melanoma patients with the BRAF V600E mutation [36] and was approved by the FDA in August 2011. Vemurafenib binds to the kinase BRAF and contains a chlorobenzene group occupying the front-pocket region, the 7-azaindole group occupies the adenine-binding area and forms hydrogen-bond interactions, the sulfonamide group interacts with the DFG-motif region, and the propyl group extends into the hydrophobic pocket region (Fig. 4a) [37]. Due to this extension of the propyl group into the hydrophobic pocket, leading to the c-Helix-out displacement, BRAF adopts a DFG-in/c-Helix-out inactive conformation [38]. The drug lenvatinib follows the same binding mode as vemurafenib (Fig. 4b) [39]. Unlike the other drugs described thus far, the binding modes of vemurafenib and lenvatinib avail themselves of additional adjacent regions to achieve selectivity, including the front-pocket region, the DFG-motif region, and the hydrophobic pocket.

Midostaurin has been found to be active against more than 100 kinases and was approved for the treatment of adult patients with fms-like tyrosine kinase 3 (FLT3)-

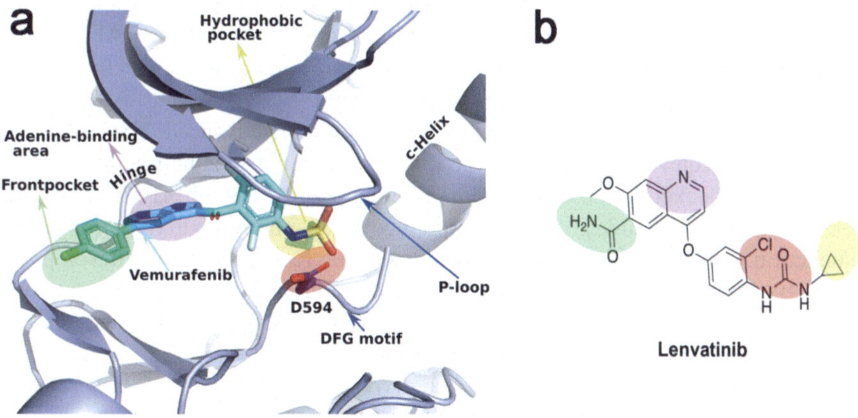

Fig. 4 Type I inhibitors bound to the front pocket region, the adenine-binding area, the hydrophobic pocket region, and the DFG-motif region. (**a**) The kinase BRAF-vemurafenib complex (pdb 3og7). (**b**) The drug lenvatinib with the same binding features as vemurafenib

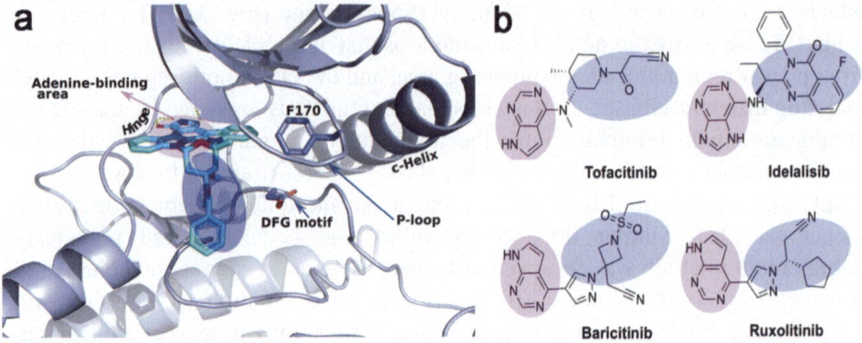

Fig. 5 Type I inhibitors bound to the adenine-binding area and the P-loop region. (**a**) The kinase DYRK1A in complex with the drug midostaurin (pdb 4nct). (**b**) The other four drugs with the same binding features as midostaurin

positive AML in combination with chemotherapy [40]. Midostaurin binds to the ATP-bound space of FLT3 (Fig. 5a). Specifically, the pyrrolidine group of midostaurin forms two hydrogen bonds with the hinge region of FLT3, and the benzamidine group and the indole group interact with the P-loop cleft. Although midostaurin is approved, common side effects result from lack of specificity and hence binding to off-targets [41]. Four other drugs (Fig. 5b), tofacitinib, idelalisib, baricitinib, and ruxolitinib, follow the same binding mode to bind to their corresponding kinase targets by also occupying the adenine-binding region and the P-loop region.

The drugs dabrafenib, osimertinib, and fostamatinib exhibit different binding modes(Fig. 6a–c). Dabrafenib is an effective drug in the treatment of advanced melanoma patients with the BRAF V600E mutation [42]. Dabrafenib binds to the front pocket region, the adenine-binding area, and the P-loop region (Fig. 6a) [43]. However, dabrafenib resistance develops in the majority of patients after approximately 6 months of treatment. To overcome this resistance, the FDA approved a combination of dabrafenib and trametinib, a MEK inhibitor [44] for BRAF V600E/K-mutant metastatic/advanced melanoma, or as an adjunct treatment for BRAF V600E advanced patients following chemotherapy [45]. Osimertinib is the third-generation EGFR T790M inhibitor to treat metastatic/advanced NSCLC [46]. Selectivity is achieved by binding to the P-loop region, the adenine-binding region, and the front pocket region of the EGFR binding pocket (Fig. 6b). To improve the selectivity, the acrylamide group is incorporated into osimeritinib to form a covalent interaction with the residue C797. In the clinic, drug resistance usually develops in about 10 months mainly due to the C797S mutation [47]. Fostamatinib is a Syk inhibitor for the treatment of chronic immune thrombocytopenia (ITP) and bears a 3,4,5-trimethoxyphenyl group at the front pocket region, a pyrimidine group occupying the adenine-binding area, a pyridine derivative occupying the P-loop region, and a phosphate group binds within the DFG-motif region (Fig. 6c).

In summary, Type I drugs bind to the common adenine scaffold region and extend into adjacent regions. Figures 2, 3, 4, 5, and 6 show that it is vital to utilize one or

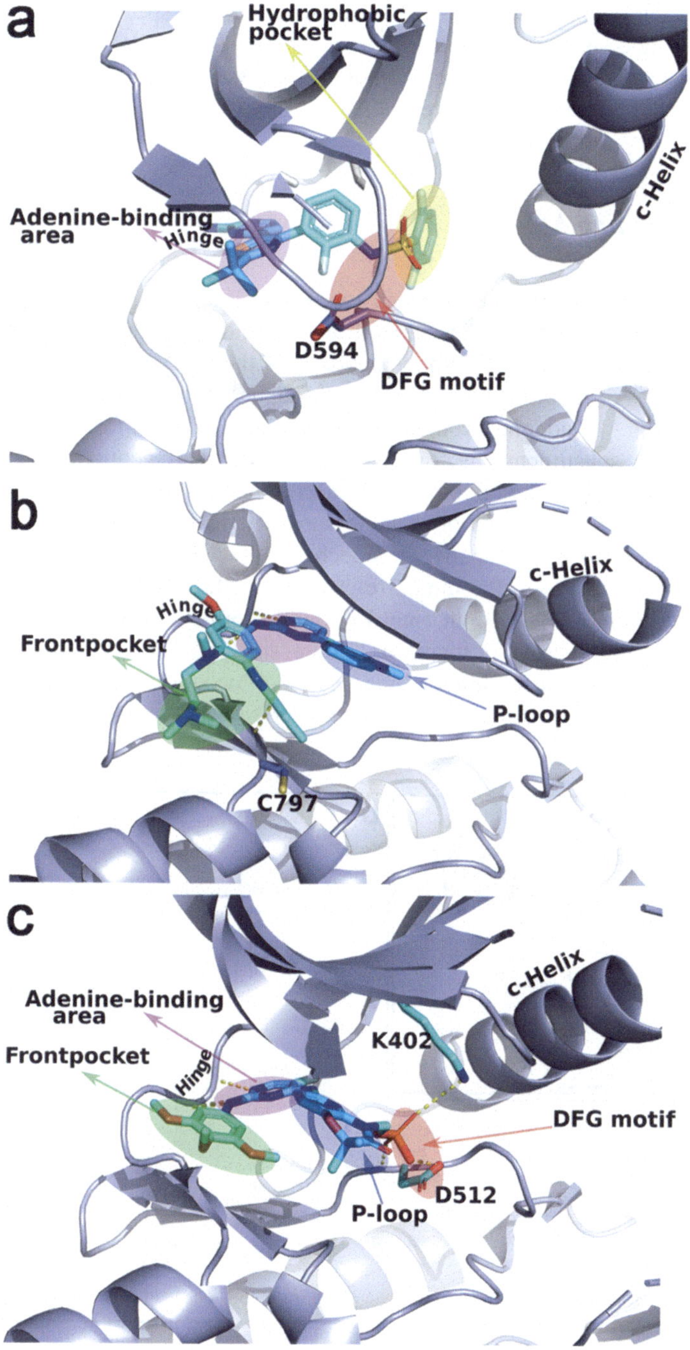

Fig. 6 Type I kinase drug-binding modes. (**a**) The drug dabrafenib bound to the adenine-binding area, the hydrophobic pocket region, and the DFG-motif region of the kinase BRAF (pdb 4xv2). (**b**) The drug osimertinib bound to the front pocket region, the adenine-binding area, and the P-loop region of the kinase EGFR (pdb 4zau). (**c**) The drug fostamatinib bound to the front pocket, the adenine-binding area, the DFG motif, and the P-loop region of the kinase Syk (pdb 3fqs)

more adjacent regions to achieve the desired selectivity for specific kinases. In Type I binding mode another common feature has the DFG motif in an "In" conformational state, which means the side chain of the aspartic acid of the DFG motif points to the hinge region of kinases, often called the "active" kinase state.

Type II Binding Modes

Kinase structure research has provided a wealth of information on conformational plasticity, a major factor to determine different binding modes [16]. The Type II binding mode was validated with the approval of the first drug, imatinib, in 2001. The cocrystal Abl-imatinib complex demonstrated that the Type II inhibitor bound not only to the ATP adenine group area but extended into the allosteric pocket with the benzamide substituent (Fig. 7a). In contrast to the aforementioned Type I binding mode required for the inhibitors to be accommodated in the "DFG-in" conformational state, the Type II inhibitor induces a dramatic displacement of the "DFG" motif (Fig. 7a) and, consequently, the sidechain of the phenylalanine of the "DFG" motif flips and points to the hinge, referred to as the "DFG-out" conformation [13]. In addition, the "DFG-out" motif normally forms a hydrogen bond interaction with the amino group of imatinib. To date, six Type II kinase drugs have been approved (Fig. 7b). Their common binding modes, occupying the adenine-binding area, the DFG-out motif region, and the allosteric pocket region, have formed the

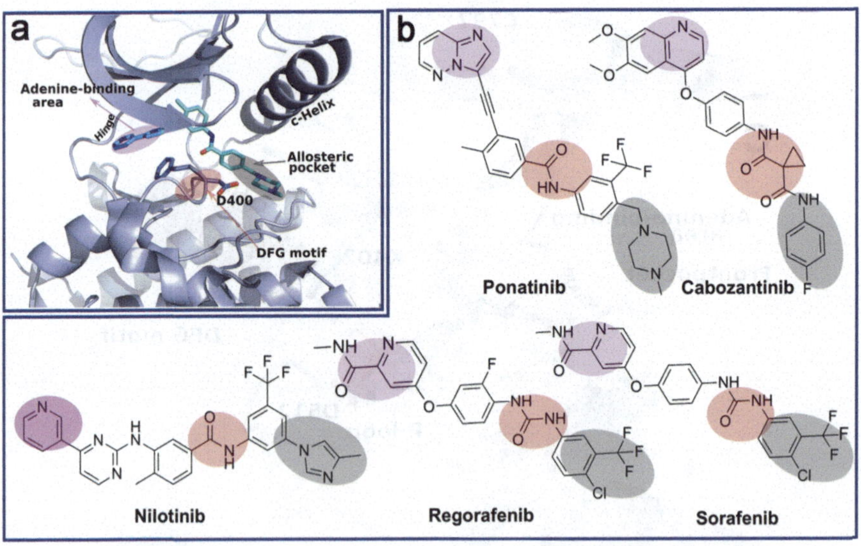

Fig. 7 Type II inhibitors bound to the adenine-binding area, the DFG motif, and the allosteric pocket region. (**a**) The Abl-imatinib cocrystal structure (pdb 1opj). (**b**) The other five drugs with the same binding features as imatinib

typical Type II binding pattern. It is worth noting that Type II inhibitors, occupying the allosteric pocket region [48], are not intrinsically more selective than Type I inhibitors [49].

Successes and Limitations

Over the last 30 years, kinase drug research has made great progress, transforming kinase targets from being "undruggable" to highly tractable. Consequently, kinase-targeted drugs have revolutionized the treatments of human cancers such as NSCLC, melanoma, thyroid cancer, breast cancer, lymphoma, and leukemia as well as rheumatoid arthritis and immune thrombocytopenia [6]. Moreover, additional promising kinase targets [8], for example, CDK7, CDK11, and DYRK1A, have been added to an expanding druggable kinome [13].

Beyond single drug–single target pharmacology lies progress in addressing multigene-driven diseases using multitarget kinase drugs. Hence, it is important to systematically verify the target spectrum of a given inhibitor across the whole kinome. Correspondingly, kinome profiling techniques, such as KinomScan and Kinativ [13], have been developed to test kinome-wide selectivity. As such, the kinome-centric view has led to a standard protocol as part of kinase drug R&D [8]. Moreover, kinase research benefits from our increased understanding of signaling networks and the pathology of human diseases, which provides support to an increasing number of combinations studies in both preclinical and clinical settings [35]. Take drug development for NSCLC as an example. Drug resistance frequently occurs after treating NSCLC with EGFR inhibitors [50]. Besides mutations in the kinase domain, notably T790M, further drug resistance arises through the dysregulation of the mesenchymal-epithelial transition factor (MET) [51]. Recently, focusing on the resistance mechanism, it was found that a drug cocktail strategy combining capmatinib (a MET inhibitor) with gefitinib (an EGFR inhibitor) is a promising treatment for patients with EGFR-mutated-MET-dysregulated, particularly MET-amplified, NSCLC [52].

Covalent drugs with reduced toxicity and favorable selectivity have rapidly emerged [31] as exemplified by the recent approval of five Type I irreversible kinase inhibitors. Kinase covalent drugs form covalent interactions with noncatalytic residues such as cysteine or lysine situated around the binding pocket [27]. This has revitalized interest in covalently targeting kinases and other protein targets in general.

Notwithstanding, side effects of applying kinase inhibitor drugs due to off-targeting still induce serious toxic effects, even end of life [6]. As such, kinase inhibitor profiling needs to be augmented to a broader spectrum of possible targets and the consequences explored both in vitro and in vivo.

A further limitation is that current kinase research focuses on approximately 40 kinases, concentrated in a few targets, which include VEGFR (eight drugs approved), EGFR (six drugs approved), ABL (five drugs approved), and ALK (four drugs approved) [10]. Yet more than 100 kinases are directly associated with over 200 diseases. Much has been done, but there is much left to do [13].

Acknowledgments Thanks to Peng Wu for useful insights and corrections when reviewing this manuscript.

References

1. Adams, J. A. (2001). Kinetic and catalytic mechanisms of protein kinases. *Chemical Reviews, 101*(8), 2271–2290.
2. Logue, J. S., & Morrison, D. K. (2012). Complexity in the signaling network: Insights from the use of targeted inhibitors in cancer therapy. *Genes and Development, 26*(7), 641–650. https://doi.org/10.1101/gad.186965.112.
3. Manning, G., Whyte, D. B., Martinez, R., Hunter, T., & Sudarsanam, S. (2002). The protein kinase complement of the human genome. *Science, 298*(5600), 1912–1934. https://doi.org/10.1126/science.1075762.
4. Cell Signaling Technology. *Kinase-disease associations*. CST. https://www.cellsignal.com/contents/resources-reference-tables/kinase-disease-associations/science-tables-kinase-disease.
5. Lahiry, P., Torkamani, A., Schork, N. J., & Hegele, R. A. (2010). Kinase mutations in human disease: Interpreting genotype-phenotype relationships. *Nature Reviews Genetics, 11*(1), 60–74. https://doi.org/10.1038/nrg2707.
6. Gharwan, H., & Groninger, H. (2016). Kinase inhibitors and monoclonal antibodies in oncology: Clinical implications. *Nature Reviews Clinical Oncology, 13*(4), 209–227. https://doi.org/10.1038/nrclinonc.2015.213.
7. Vogelstein, B., Papadopoulos, N., Velculescu, V. E., Zhou, S., Diaz, L. A., Jr., & Kinzler, K. W. (2013). Cancer genome landscapes. *Science, 339*(6127), 1546–1558. https://doi.org/10.1126/science.1235122.
8. Wilson, L. J., Linley, A., Hammond, D. E., Hood, F. E., Coulson, J. M., MacEwan, D. J., Ross, S. J., Slupsky, J. R., Smith, P. D., Eyers, P. A., & Prior, I. A. (2018). New perspectives, opportunities, and challenges in exploring the human protein kinome. *Cancer Research, 78*(1), 15–29. https://doi.org/10.1158/0008-5472.CAN-17-2291.
9. Zhang, J., Yang, P. L., & Gray, N. S. (2009). Targeting cancer with small molecule kinase inhibitors. *Nature Reviews Cancer, 9*(1), 28–39. https://doi.org/10.1038/nrc2559.
10. U.S. Food and Drug Administration. *Drugs@FDA: FDA approved drug products*. https://www.accessdata.fda.gov/scripts/cder/daf/index.cfm.
11. Knapp, S. (2018). New opportunities for kinase drug repurposing and target discovery. *British Journal of Cancer, 118*(7), 936–937. https://doi.org/10.1038/s41416-018-0045-6.
12. Muller, S., Chaikuad, A., Gray, N. S., & Knapp, S. (2015). The ins and outs of selective kinase inhibitor development. *Nature Chemical Biology, 11*(11), 818–821. https://doi.org/10.1038/nchembio.1938.
13. Ferguson, F. M., & Gray, N. S. (2018). Kinase inhibitors: The road ahead. *Nature Reviews. Drug Discovery, 17*(5), 353–377. https://doi.org/10.1038/nrd.2018.21.
14. Klaeger, S., Heinzlmeir, S., Wilhelm, M., Polzer, H., Vick, B., Koenig, P. A., Reinecke, M., Ruprecht, B., Petzoldt, S., Meng, C., Zecha, J., Reiter, K., Qiao, H., Helm, D., Koch, H., Schoof, M., Canevari, G., Casale, E., Depaolini, S. R., Feuchtinger, A., Wu, Z., Schmidt, T.,

Rueckert, L., Becker, W., Huenges, J., Garz, A. K., Gohlke, B. O., Zolg, D. P., Kayser, G., Vooder, T., Preissner, R., Hahne, H., Tonisson, N., Kramer, K., Gotze, K., Bassermann, F., Schlegl, J., Ehrlich, H. C., Aiche, S., Walch, A., Greif, P. A., Schneider, S., Felder, E. R., Ruland, J., Medard, G., Jeremias, I., Spiekermann, K., & Kuster, B. (2017). The target landscape of clinical kinase drugs. *Science, 358*(6367), eaan4368. https://doi.org/10.1126/science.aan4368.

15. Wu, P., Nielsen, T. E., & Clausen, M. H. (2015). FDA-approved small-molecule kinase inhibitors. *Trends in Pharmacological Sciences, 36*(7), 422–439. https://doi.org/10.1016/j.tips.2015.04.005.
16. Zhao, Z., Xie, L., Xie, L., & Bourne, P. E. (2016). Delineation of polypharmacology across the human structural kinome using a functional site interaction fingerprint approach. *Journal of Medicinal Chemistry, 59*(9), 4326–4341. https://doi.org/10.1021/acs.jmedchem.5b02041.
17. Wu, P., Clausen, M. H., & Nielsen, T. E. (2015). Allosteric small-molecule kinase inhibitors. *Pharmacology and Therapeutics, 156*, 59–68. https://doi.org/10.1016/j.pharmthera.2015.10.002.
18. Rice, K. D., Aay, N., Anand, N. K., Blazey, C. M., Bowles, O. J., Bussenius, J., Costanzo, S., Curtis, J. K., Defina, S. C., Dubenko, L., Engst, S., Joshi, A. A., Kennedy, A. R., Kim, A. I., Koltun, E. S., Lougheed, J. C., Manalo, J. C., Martini, J. F., Nuss, J. M., Peto, C. J., Tsang, T. H., Yu, P., & Johnston, S. (2012). Novel carboxamide-based allosteric MEK inhibitors: Discovery and optimization efforts toward XL518 (GDC-0973). *ACS Medicinal Chemistry Letters, 3*(5), 416–421. https://doi.org/10.1021/ml300049d.
19. Zhang, J., Adrián, F. J., Jahnke, W., Cowan-Jacob, S. W., Li, A. G., Iacob, R. E., Sim, T., Powers, J., Dierks, C., Sun, F., Guo, G.-R., Ding, Q., Okram, B., Choi, Y., Wojciechowski, A., Deng, X., Liu, G., Fendrich, G., Strauss, A., Vajpai, N., Grzesiek, S., Tuntland, T., Liu, Y., Bursulaya, B., Azam, M., Manley, P. W., Engen, J. R., Daley, G. Q., Warmuth, M., & Gray, N. S. (2010). Targeting Bcr–Abl by combining allosteric with ATP-binding-site inhibitors. *Nature, 463*(7280), 501–506. https://doi.org/10.1038/nature08675.
20. Hirai, H., Sootome, H., Nakatsuru, Y., Miyama, K., Taguchi, S., Tsujioka, K., Ueno, Y., Hatch, H., Majumder, P. K., Pan, B. S., & Kotani, H. (2010). MK-2206, an allosteric Akt inhibitor, enhances antitumor efficacy by standard chemotherapeutic agents or molecular targeted drugs in vitro and in vivo. *Molecular Cancer Therapeutics, 9*(7), 1956–1967. https://doi.org/10.1158/1535-7163.MCT-09-1012.
21. Wu, W. I., Voegtli, W. C., Sturgis, H. L., Dizon, F. P., Vigers, G. P., & Brandhuber, B. J. (2010). Crystal structure of human AKT1 with an allosteric inhibitor reveals a new mode of kinase inhibition. *PLoS One, 5*(9), e12913. https://doi.org/10.1371/journal.pone.0012913.
22. Zhang, X., Pickin, K. A., Bose, R., Jura, N., Cole, P. A., & Kuriyan, J. (2007). Inhibition of the EGF receptor by binding of MIG6 to an activating kinase domain interface. *Nature, 450*(7170), 741–744. https://doi.org/10.1038/nature05998.
23. Betzi, S., Alam, R., Martin, M., Lubbers, D. J., Han, H., Jakkaraj, S. R., Georg, G. I., & Schonbrunn, E. (2011). Discovery of a potential allosteric ligand binding site in CDK2. *ACS Chemical Biology, 6*(5), 492–501. https://doi.org/10.1021/cb100410m.
24. Kooistra, A. J., Kanev, G. K., van Linden, O. P. J., Leurs, R., de Esch, I. J. P., & de Graaf, C. (2016). KLIFS: A structural kinase-ligand interaction database. *Nucleic Acids Research, 44*(D1), D365–D371. https://doi.org/10.1093/nar/gkv1082.
25. van Linden, O. P., Kooistra, A. J., Leurs, R., de Esch, I. J., & de Graaf, C. (2014). KLIFS: A knowledge-based structural database to navigate kinase-ligand interaction space. *Journal of Medicinal Chemistry, 57*(2), 249–277. https://doi.org/10.1021/jm400378w.
26. Liao, J. J. (2007). Molecular recognition of protein kinase binding pockets for design of potent and selective kinase inhibitors. *Journal of Medicinal Chemistry, 50*(3), 409–424. https://doi.org/10.1021/jm0608107.
27. Zhao, Z., Liu, Q., Bliven, S., Xie, L., & Bourne, P. E. (2017). Determining cysteines available for covalent inhibition across the human kinome. *Journal of Medicinal Chemistry, 60*(7), 2879–2889. https://doi.org/10.1021/acs.jmedchem.6b01815.

28. Sordella, R., Bell, D. W., Haber, D. A., & Settleman, J. (2004). Gefitinib-sensitizing EGFR mutations in lung cancer activate anti-apoptotic pathways. *Science, 305*(5687), 1163–1167. https://doi.org/10.1126/science.1101637.
29. Gajiwala, K. S., Feng, J., Ferre, R., Ryan, K., Brodsky, O., Weinrich, S., Kath, J. C., & Stewart, A. (2013). Insights into the aberrant activity of mutant EGFR kinase domain and drug recognition. *Structure, 21*(2), 209–219. https://doi.org/10.1016/j.str.2012.11.014.
30. Chaikuad, A., Koch, P., Laufer, S. A., & Knapp, S. (2018). The cysteinome of protein kinases as a target in drug development. *Angewandte Chemie (International Ed. in English), 57*(16), 4372–4385. https://doi.org/10.1002/anie.201707875.
31. Zhao, Z., & Bourne, P. E. (2018). Progress with covalent small-molecule kinase inhibitors. *Drug Discovery Today, 23*(3), 727–735. https://doi.org/10.1016/j.drudis.2018.01.035.
32. Kim, S., Loo, A., Chopra, R., Caponigro, G., Huang, A., Vora, S., Parasuraman, S., Howard, S., Keen, N., Sellers, W., & Brain, C. (2014). Abstract PR02: LEE011: An orally bioavailable, selective small molecule inhibitor of CDK4/6-Reactivating Rb in cancer. *Molecular Cancer Therapeutics, 12*(Suppl 11), PR02. https://doi.org/10.1158/1535-7163.targ-13-pr02.
33. Chen, P., Lee, N. V., Hu, W., Xu, M., Ferre, R. A., Lam, H., Bergqvist, S., Solowiej, J., Diehl, W., He, Y. A., Yu, X., Nagata, A., VanArsdale, T., & Murray, B. W. (2016). Spectrum and degree of CDK drug interactions predicts clinical performance. *Molecular Cancer Therapeutics, 15*(10), 2273–2281. https://doi.org/10.1158/1535-7163.mct-16-0300.
34. Dummer, R., Ascierto, P. A., Gogas, H. J., Arance, A., Mandala, M., Liszkay, G., Garbe, C., Schadendorf, D., Krajsova, I., Gutzmer, R., Chiarion-Sileni, V., Dutriaux, C., de Groot, J. W. B., Yamazaki, N., Loquai, C., Moutouh-de Parseval, L. A., Pickard, M. D., Sandor, V., Robert, C., & Flaherty, K. T. (2018). Encorafenib plus binimetinib versus vemurafenib or encorafenib in patients with BRAF -mutant melanoma (COLUMBUS): A multicentre, open-label, randomised phase 3 trial. *The Lancet Oncology, 19*(5), 603–615. https://doi.org/10.1016/s1470-2045(18)30142-6.
35. Corcoran, R. B., Andre, T., Atreya, C. E., Schellens, J. H. M., Yoshino, T., Bendell, J. C., Hollebecque, A., McRee, A. J., Siena, S., Middleton, G., Muro, K., Gordon, M. S., Tabernero, J., Yaeger, R., O'Dwyer, P. J., Humblet, Y., De Vos, F., Jung, A. S., Brase, J. C., Jaeger, S., Bettinger, S., Mookerjee, B., Rangwala, F., & Van Cutsem, E. (2018). Combined BRAF, EGFR, and MEK inhibition in patients with BRAF(V600E)-mutant colorectal cancer. *Cancer Discovery, 8*(4), 428–443. https://doi.org/10.1158/2159-8290.CD-17-1226.
36. Maverakis, E., Cornelius, L., Bowen, G., Phan, T., Patel, F., Fitzmaurice, S., He, Y., Burrall, B., Duong, C., Kloxin, A., Sultani, H., Wilken, R., Martinez, S., & Patel, F. (2015). Metastatic melanoma—A review of current and future treatment options. *Acta Dermato Venereologica, 95*(5), 516–524. https://doi.org/10.2340/00015555-2035.
37. Bollag, G., Hirth, P., Tsai, J., Zhang, J., Ibrahim, P. N., Cho, H., Spevak, W., Zhang, C., Zhang, Y., Habets, G., Burton, E. A., Wong, B., Tsang, G., West, B. L., Powell, B., Shellooe, R., Marimuthu, A., Nguyen, H., Zhang, K. Y., Artis, D. R., Schlessinger, J., Su, F., Higgins, B., Iyer, R., D'Andrea, K., Koehler, A., Stumm, M., Lin, P. S., Lee, R. J., Grippo, J., Puzanov, I., Kim, K. B., Ribas, A., McArthur, G. A., Sosman, J. A., Chapman, P. B., Flaherty, K. T., Xu, X., Nathanson, K. L., & Nolop, K. (2010). Clinical efficacy of a RAF inhibitor needs broad target blockade in BRAF-mutant melanoma. *Nature, 467*(7315), 596–599. https://doi.org/10.1038/nature09454.
38. Tsai, J., Lee, J. T., Wang, W., Zhang, J., Cho, H., Mamo, S., Bremer, R., Gillette, S., Kong, J., Haass, N. K., Sproesser, K., Li, L., Smalley, K. S. M., Fong, D., Zhu, Y. L., Marimuthu, A., Nguyen, H., Lam, B., Liu, J., Cheung, I., Rice, J., Suzuki, Y., Luu, C., Settachatgul, C., Shellooe, R., Cantwell, J., Kim, S. H., Schlessinger, J., Zhang, K. Y. J., West, B. L., Powell, B., Habets, G., Zhang, C., Ibrahim, P. N., Hirth, P., Artis, D. R., Herlyn, M., & Bollag, G. (2008). Discovery of a selective inhibitor of oncogenic B-Raf kinase with potent antimelanoma activity. *Proceedings of the National Academy of Sciences of the United States of America, 105*(8), 3041–3046. https://doi.org/10.1073/pnas.0711741105.

39. Okamoto, K., Ikemori-Kawada, M., Jestel, A., von Konig, K., Funahashi, Y., Matsushima, T., Tsuruoka, A., Inoue, A., & Matsui, J. (2015). Distinct binding mode of multikinase inhibitor lenvatinib revealed by biochemical characterization. *ACS Medicinal Chemistry Letters, 6*(1), 89–94. https://doi.org/10.1021/ml500394m.
40. Weisberg, E., Boulton, C., Kelly, L. M., Manley, P., Fabbro, D., Meyer, T., Gilliland, D. G., & Griffin, J. D. (2002). Inhibition of mutant FLT3 receptors in leukemia cells by the small molecule tyrosine kinase inhibitor PKC412. *Cancer Cell, 1*(5), 433–443. https://doi.org/10.1016/s1535-6108(02)00069-7.
41. Gotlib, J., Kluin-Nelemans, H. C., George, T. I., Akin, C., Sotlar, K., Hermine, O., Awan, F. T., Hexner, E., Mauro, M. J., Sternberg, D. W., Villeneuve, M., Huntsman Labed, A., Stanek, E. J., Hartmann, K., Horny, H. P., Valent, P., & Reiter, A. (2016). Efficacy and safety of midostaurin in advanced systemic mastocytosis. *The New England Journal of Medicine, 374*(26), 2530–2541. https://doi.org/10.1056/NEJMoa1513098.
42. Gibney, G. T., & Zager, J. S. (2013). Clinical development of dabrafenib in BRAF mutant melanoma and other malignancies. *Expert Opinion on Drug Metabolism and Toxicology, 9*(7), 893–899. https://doi.org/10.1517/17425255.2013.794220.
43. Zhang, C., Spevak, W., Zhang, Y., Burton, E. A., Ma, Y., Habets, G., Zhang, J., Lin, J., Ewing, T., Matusow, B., Tsang, G., Marimuthu, A., Cho, H., Wu, G., Wang, W., Fong, D., Nguyen, H., Shi, S., Womack, P., Nespi, M., Shellooe, R., Carias, H., Powell, B., Light, E., Sanftner, L., Walters, J., Tsai, J., West, B. L., Visor, G., Rezaei, H., Lin, P. S., Nolop, K., Ibrahim, P. N., Hirth, P., & Bollag, G. (2015). RAF inhibitors that evade paradoxical MAPK pathway activation. *Nature, 526*(7574), 583–586. https://doi.org/10.1038/nature14982.
44. Zhao, Z., Xie, L., & Bourne, P. E. (2017). Insights into the binding mode of MEK type-III inhibitors. A step towards discovering and designing allosteric kinase inhibitors across the human kinome. *PLoS One, 12*(6), e0179936. https://doi.org/10.1371/journal.pone.0179936.
45. Long, G. V., Hauschild, A., Santinami, M., Atkinson, V., Mandalà, M., Chiarion-Sileni, V., Larkin, J., Nyakas, M., Dutriaux, C., Haydon, A., Robert, C., Mortier, L., Schachter, J., Schadendorf, D., Lesimple, T., Plummer, R., Ji, R., Zhang, P., Mookerjee, B., Legos, J., Kefford, R., Dummer, R., & Kirkwood, J. M. (2017). Adjuvant dabrafenib plus trametinib in stage III BRAF-mutated melanoma. *New England Journal of Medicine, 377*(19), 1813–1823. https://doi.org/10.1056/NEJMoa1708539.
46. Ayeni, D., Politi, K., & Goldberg, S. B. (2015). Emerging agents and new mutations in EGFR-mutant lung cancer. *Clinical Cancer Research, 21*(17), 3818–3820. https://doi.org/10.1158/1078-0432.CCR-15-1211.
47. Patel, H., Pawara, R., Ansari, A., & Surana, S. (2017). Recent updates on third generation EGFR inhibitors and emergence of fourth generation EGFR inhibitors to combat C797S resistance. *European Journal of Medicinal Chemistry, 142*, 32–47. https://doi.org/10.1016/j.ejmech.2017.05.027.
48. Jia, Y., Yun, C. H., Park, E., Ercan, D., Manuia, M., Juarez, J., Xu, C., Rhee, K., Chen, T., Zhang, H., Palakurthi, S., Jang, J., Lelais, G., DiDonato, M., Bursulaya, B., Michellys, P. Y., Epple, R., Marsilje, T. H., McNeill, M., Lu, W., Harris, J., Bender, S., Wong, K. K., Janne, P. A., & Eck, M. J. (2016). Overcoming EGFR(T790M) and EGFR(C797S) resistance with mutant-selective allosteric inhibitors. *Nature, 534*(7605), 129–132. https://doi.org/10.1038/nature17960.
49. Zhao, Z., Wu, H., Wang, L., Liu, Y., Knapp, S., Liu, Q., & Gray, N. S. (2014). Exploration of type II binding mode: A privileged approach for kinase inhibitor focused drug discovery? *ACS Chemical Biology, 9*(6), 1230–1241. https://doi.org/10.1021/cb500129t.
50. Juchum, M., Gunther, M., & Laufer, S. A. (2015). Fighting cancer drug resistance: Opportunities and challenges for mutation-specific EGFR inhibitors. *Drug Resistance Updates, 20*, 12–28. https://doi.org/10.1016/j.drup.2015.05.002.
51. Bean, J., Brennan, C., Shih, J. Y., Riely, G., Viale, A., Wang, L., Chitale, D., Motoi, N., Szoke, J., Broderick, S., Balak, M., Chang, W. C., Yu, C. J., Gazdar, A., Pass, H., Rusch, V., Gerald, W., Huang, S. F., Yang, P. C., Miller, V., Ladanyi, M., Yang, C. H., & Pao, W. (2007). MET ampli-

fication occurs with or without T790M mutations in EGFR mutant lung tumors with acquired resistance to gefitinib or erlotinib. *Proceedings of the National Academy of Sciences of the United States of America, 104*(52), 20932–20937. https://doi.org/10.1073/pnas.0710370104.

52. Wu, Y. L., Zhang, L., Kim, D. W., Liu, X., Lee, D. H., Yang, J. C., Ahn, M. J., Vansteenkiste, J. F., Su, W. C., Felip, E., Chia, V., Glaser, S., Pultar, P., Zhao, S., Peng, B., Akimov, M., & Tan, D. S. W. (2018). Phase Ib/II study of capmatinib (INC280) plus gefitinib after failure of endothelial growth factor receptor (EGFR) inhibitor therapy in patients with EGFR-mutated, MET factor-dysregulated non-small-cell lung cancer. *Journal of Clinical Oncology, 36*(31), 3101–3109. https://doi.org/10.1200/JCO.2018.77.7326.

Avoiding or Co-Opting ATP Inhibition: Overview of Type III, IV, V, and VI Kinase Inhibitors

Ramon Martinez III, Amy Defnet, and Paul Shapiro

Abstract As described in the previous chapter, most kinase inhibitors that have been developed for use in the clinic act by blocking ATP binding; however, there is growing interest in identifying compounds that target kinase activities and functions without interfering with the conserved features of the ATP-binding site. This chapter will highlight alternative approaches that exploit unique kinase structural features that are being targeted to identify more selective and potent inhibitors. The figure below, adapted from (Sammons et al., Molecular Carcinogenesis 58:1551–1570, 2019), provides a graphical description of the various approaches to manipulate kinase activity. In addition to the type I and II inhibitors, type III kinase inhibitors have been identified to target sites adjacent to the ATP-binding site in the catalytic domain. New information on kinase structure and substrate-binding sites has enabled the identification of type IV kinase inhibitor compounds that target regions outside the catalytic domain. The combination of targeting unique allosteric sites outside the catalytic domain with ATP-targeted compounds has yielded a number of novel bivalent type V kinase inhibitors. Finally, emerging interest in the development of irreversible compounds that form selective covalent interactions with key amino acids involved in kinase functions comprise the class of type VI kinase inhibitors.

Keywords Allosteric · Docking domains · Protein-protein interactions · Bivalent · Irreversible inhibitors

R. Martinez III · A. Defnet · P. Shapiro (✉)
Department of Pharmaceutical Sciences, University of Maryland School of Pharmacy, Baltimore, MD, USA
e-mail: rmartinez@umaryland.edu; amy.defnet@umaryland.edu; pshapiro@rx.umaryland.edu

P. Shapiro (ed.), *Next Generation Kinase Inhibitors*,
https://doi.org/10.1007/978-3-030-48283-1_3

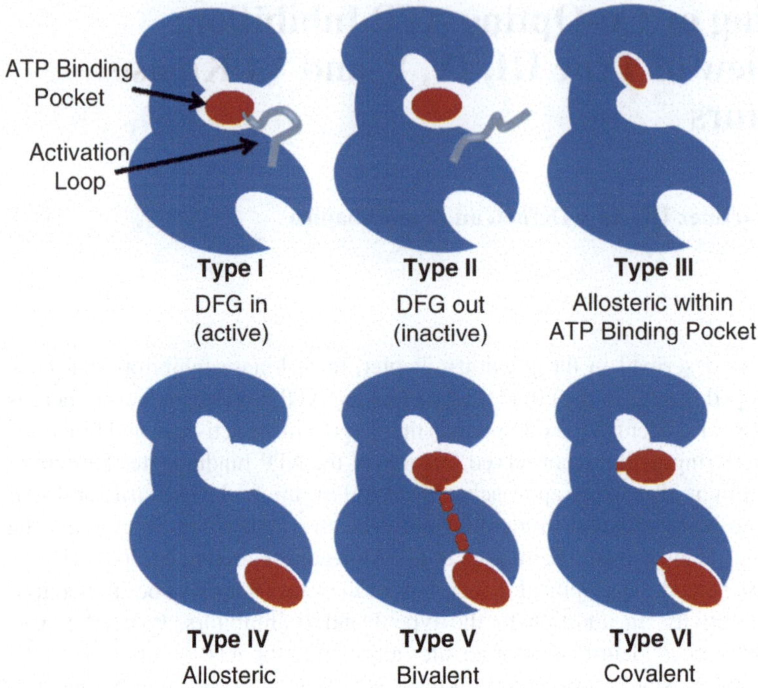

Part A: Type III Kinase Inhibitors

The identification of new details about the structural features of kinases, their role in enzyme activity, and their functions in regulating substrate recognition and phosphorylation have prompted research endeavors to develop kinase inhibitors that do not interfere with the highly conserved ATP-binding site. For example, type III kinase inhibitors are compounds that interact with specific structural features in the catalytic site that are adjacent to the ATP-binding pocket. These sorts of innovations are aimed at identifying drugs with reduced promiscuity and associated toxicities as well as avoiding the development of ATP-binding site gatekeeper mutations that are commonly observed to be responsible for acquired resistance to type I and II kinase inhibitors [1].

Type III MEK1/2 inhibitors. The most studied type III kinase inhibitors have been developed against the *M*AP or *E*RK *K*inase-1/2 (MEK1/2) proteins, which are primary mediators of constitutively active extracellular signal-regulated kinase (ERK1/2) signaling that is observed in many cancers and proliferative disorders. In the early 1990s, researchers, at what was then Parke-Davis & Company, screened a library of small molecules using an in vitro kinase assay consisting of MEK1, ERK2, and the generic substrate myelin basic protein (MBP) [2]. This screen identified the compound PD98059 to inhibit MEK1 activation of ERK2, to inhibit subsequent phosphorylation of MBP in an in vitro assay, and to block ERK activation in cells. PD98059, which turned out to be ~10 fold more selective for MEK1 than MEK2, was the first non-ATP-competitive inhibitor that paved the way for the development of additional type III MEK1/2 inhibitors. In the early 2000s, the orally bioavailable MEK1/2 inhibitor, PD184352 (CI-1040), was the first type III kinase inhibitor to enter clinical trials [3].

The first structural description of the allosteric-binding pocket on MEK1/2 [4] laid the groundwork for the discovery of additional type III MEK1/2 inhibitors, including selumetinib, cobimetinib, and trametinib that are currently being used to treat several types of cancer. As single agents, the type III MEK1/2 inhibitors have not had the anticipated clinical success [5]. However, the use of the type III MEK1/2 inhibitors in combination with other kinase inhibitors has provided clinical benefits in treating cancer, especially in the context of inhibitors of mutated BRaf where a single amino acid change from a valine to glutamate in the catalytic site causes constitutive activation of the kinase [6]. For example, progression-free survival was greatly improved in melanoma patients receiving cobimetinib (GDC-0973) in combination with the type I BRaf inhibitor vemurafenib to treat mutated BRaf expressing melanoma [7]. Similarly, the MEK1/2 inhibitor trametinib is used in combination with the type I BRaf inhibitor dabrafenib to treat mutant BRaf expressing metastatic melanoma, thyroid cancer, and non-small cell lung cancer [8–10].

The unique structural features adjacent to the ATP-binding site of MEK1/2 have been used to identify compounds that inhibit MEK1/2 activity and may have applications targeting other kinases. Zhao et al. have presented an excellent review of the type III kinase inhibitor-binding mode with a focus on interactions with MEK1/2 proteins [11]. These studies provide evidence that unique structural features in catalytic/kinase domains can be exploited to design more selective kinase inhibitors. The authors compared 29 known structures of MEK1 with type III kinase inhibitors and identified three different allosteric regions in the catalytic site that represent structural targets for inhibitor development (Fig. 1). The first region is a hydrophobic pocket that interacts with hydrophobic groups of inhibitor compounds. The second

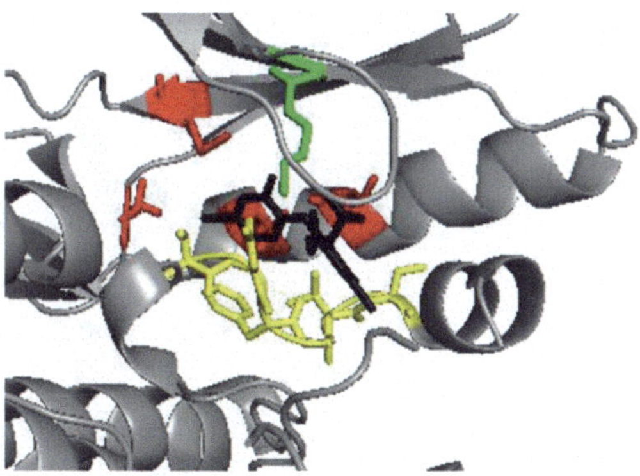

Fig. 1 Structure of MEK1 and allosteric regions near ATP-binding site. Shown is the structure of MEK1 (pdb:1S9J) and three regions, (1) a hydrophobic pocket (L115, L118, V127, and M143) in red, (2) lysine (K97) in green, and (3) residues in the activation loop ($C^{207}DFGVS^{212}$, I215, M219) in yellow, involved in allosteric drug binding. The type III inhibitor, PD318088, is shown in black lines

region is a key lysine involved in enzyme catalysis. The third region includes the DFG motif and parts of the activation loop. The activation loop of the MEK1/2 proteins is unique in that it forms a short helix that allows specific interactions with type III inhibitors [4]. While the activation loop is typically disordered in kinases where structural information is available, other kinases including p38α MAP kinase and B-Raf kinase, along with MEK1/2, have been reported to adopt these short helix structures in the activation loop [11]. Thus, this unique structural feature could be used to develop type III inhibitors for other kinases. Computational modeling further supports the formation of unique helix structures in the activation loop of other kinases and the potential for selective drug targeting [11].

The structure of cobimetinib bound to MEK1, highlighted in Chap. 2, demonstrates key features that determine the efficacy of type III MEK inhibitors in blocking MEK1/2 in cancers driven by mutations in Ras or BRaf. Previous studies indicate that wild-type and mutant BRaf proteins have differences in their mechanism of MEK1/2 activation [12]. Wild-type BRaf is dependent on the upstream Ras-G proteins whereas mutant BRaf signals through the MEK-ERK pathway in a Ras-independent manner. Based on these differences in BRaf-mediated signaling, the efficacy of MEK1/2 inhibitors in blocking mutant Ras or BRaf cancer cell lines was shown to have qualitative differences [13].

These studies went on to provide evidence that the strength of the type III MEK1/2 inhibitor's interactions with serine 212 (S212, numbering according to MEK1) in the activation loop helix determined the compound's potency in cancers with different ERK pathway driving mutations [13]. For example, the MEK inhibitors that had strong interactions with S212 resulted in stabilized Raf-MEK complexes in the context of wild-type BRaf but not with mutant BRaf. This suggests that the stabilization disrupted the ability of wild-type BRaf to access and phosphorylate MEK in cancer cells expressing mutant Ras. Alternatively, weaker interactions with S212, as is the case with cobimetinib, were more effective against cancer cells with activating BRaf mutations due to the compound's preferential binding to the activated form of MEK1. The structure of MEK1 with cobimetinib highlights the proximity of the drug with S212 (Fig. 2). These findings provide a novel example where

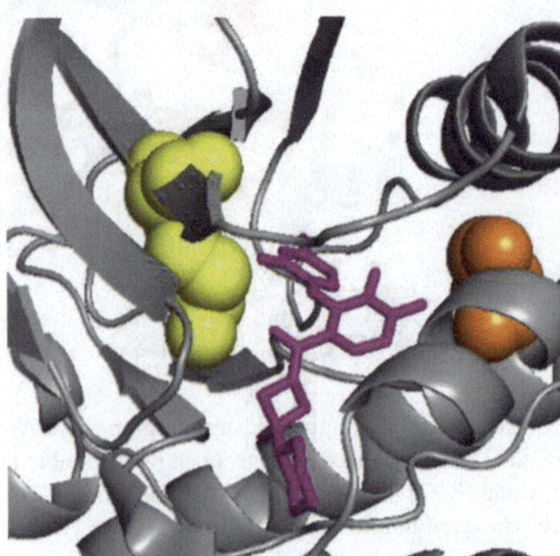

Fig. 2 Structure of MEK1 and cobimetinib. The strength of MEK1 binding to S212 is implicated in affecting the efficacy of MEK inhibitors in mutant BRaf or Ras-driven cancers. The ribbon structure of MEK1 (pdb:4LMN) is shown in complex with cobimetinib (magenta) and S212 (orange). The conserved catalytic lysine (K97) is in yellow

information on kinase regulation, structural features, and chemical synthesis can be combined to design type III inhibitors with optimal efficacy depending on the genetic mutation.

Type III PI3K and Akt inhibitors. Significant effort has gone into identifying compounds that block the *p*hospho*i*nositide-*3*-*k*inase (PI3K) or downstream Akt effector proteins, which are frequently dysregulated and active in many cancer types [14]. Constitutively active PI3K signaling provides cancer cells with survival advantages including inhibiting apoptosis signals and promoting the expression of proteins that promote proliferation [14, 15]. One of the major targets of Akt in protecting cancer cell survival is the *m*ammalian/mechanistic *t*arget *o*f *r*apamycin (mTOR) protein complex. Although there have been a number of research programs aimed at the development of ATP-competitive inhibitors of PI3K or Akt, compounds identified have shown limited clinical efficacy or cause unacceptable toxicity [14]. Nonetheless, several ATP-competitive PI3K inhibitors are in development and at least three (idelalisib, copanlisib, and alpelisib) have been approved for clinical use in treating types of lymphoma/leukemia and breast cancer [16]. However, as with other ATP-competitive protein kinase inhibitors, acquired drug resistance is a common feature preventing sustained clinical responses.

In addition to type I/II kinase inhibitors, Akt proteins have been the focus of type III kinase inhibitor development. A unique structural feature of Akt proteins is a *p*leckstrin *h*omology (PH) domain that interacts with the phosphoinositides on the intracellular side of the plasma membrane and regulates Akt activation. Based on the structural differences between a pocket formed by the PH and kinase domains in the inactive versus the active membrane bound Akt protein, a compound called Inhibitor VIII was identified and found to promote Akt1 adoption of an inactive state [17]. The crystal structure reveals key interactions with a tryptophan in the PH domain and residues in the kinase domain that are selective for the Akt1 isoform (Fig. 3). One key finding was the formation of a hydrogen bond between Inhibitor VIII and serine 205, which is not conserved amongst Akt isoforms, and could be used to design Akt1-selective inhibitors [17]. A similar allosteric inhibitor scaffold, referred to as compound Akt-I-1, that was dependent on the PH domain, was also reported to be a selective inhibitor of the Akt1 isoform [18].

Additional type III compounds with similar structures and mechanism of action, in targeting allosteric sites near the PH and kinase domains of Akt proteins, have entered clinical trials, including MK-2206 [19], BAY1125976 [20], and ARQ 092/Miransertib [21]. Given the significance of other Akt isoforms (e.g. Akt2 and 3) in mediating mTOR signaling and survival advantages in cancer cells, ARQ 092 was engineered to potently inhibit Akt1, -2, and -3 proteins. Structural studies between ARQ 092 and Akt1 revealed key interactions with W80 and T82 in the PH domain as well as Y272 and D274 in the kinase domain (Fig. 4). These residues are conserved in all Akt isoforms, which may explain the similar potencies of ARQ 092 against these proteins. Phase 1/2 clinical trials with ARQ 092 was recently reported to show beneficial effects in treating patients with diseases containing constitutively

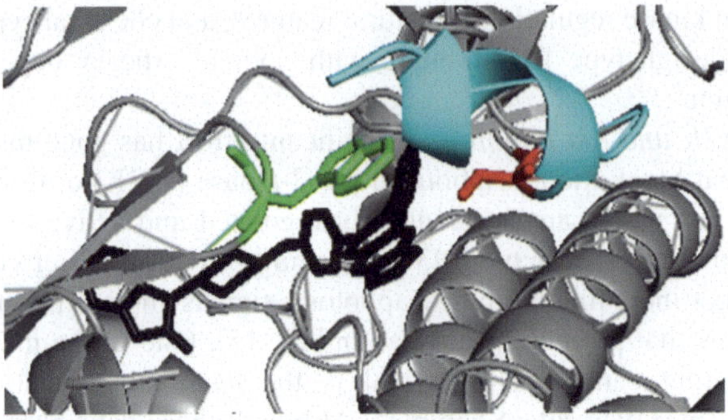

Fig. 3 Interactions between Akt1 and a type III inhibitor. Akt1 (pdb:3O96) is shown in complex with Inhibitor VIII (black lines) interacting with a tryptophan (W80) in the PH domain (red), and residues 189–198 of the αC-helix in the kinase domain (cyan), and S205 (green)

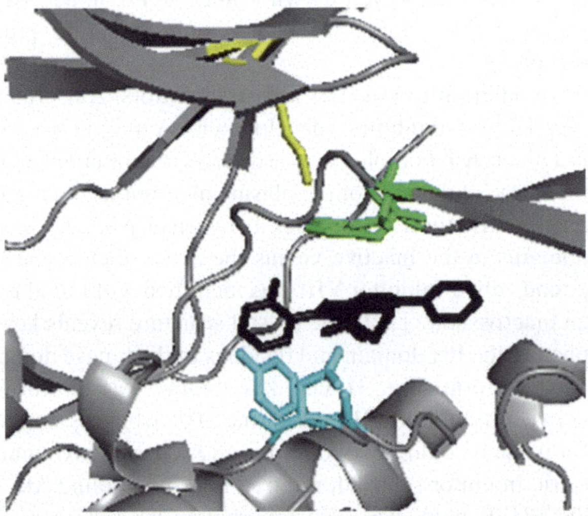

Fig. 4 Interactions between Akt1 and ARQ 092. Akt1 (pdb:5KCV) is shown in complex with ARQ 092 (black lines) interacting with a tryptophan and threonine (W80, T82) in the PH domain (green) and residues Y272 and D275 in the kinase domain (cyan). Lysine (K97) involved in enzyme catalysis is shown in yellow

active PI3K or Akt1 including PIK3CA-related overgrowth spectrum, Proteus syndrome, and ovarian carcinoma [22, 23].

Type III Trk inhibitors. The *t*ropomyosin *r*eceptor *k*inase (Trk) family consists of receptor tyrosine kinases that are mostly expressed in neuronal tissue and respond to neurotrophin stimuli to regulate nervous system function [24]. The discovery of elevated Trk activity, as a result overexpression or genetic fusions, in many cancer cell types has promoted the discovery of Trk inhibitors [25]. As a result, a number of broad-spectrum ATP-competitive inhibitors of Trk isoforms, such as FDA-approved larotrectinib and others compounds in clinical trials, are showing promising results for treating cancers with high Trk activity [26, 27].

The broad spectrum of functions performed by Trk proteins in regulating neuronal tissue has led to the investigation of isoform specific inhibitors. Of the TrkA/B/C isoforms, TrkA has been the primary isoform implicated to treat pain in mediating pain associated with inflammation [28]. Specifically, TrkA responds to nerve growth factor to maintain the growth and survival of sensory nerves that mediate pain sensation. Thus, TrkA-selective inhibitors are viewed to have clinical potential in treating pain associated with inflammation. However, the current type I and II Trk kinase inhibitors cannot discriminate between Trk isoforms. To overcome this obstacle, Bagal et al. used a cell-based assay to screen for TrkA-selective compounds and identified a type III TrkA kinase inhibitor [29]. Importantly, the compounds showed selectivity for peripheral nociceptor neurons due to enhanced recognition by blood-brain barrier efflux transporters, which reduced undesirable effects on TrkA signaling in the central nervous system [29]. The key features of the lead TrkA-selective inhibitor, compound 23, reveal interactions with amino acids in a pocket behind the ATP-binding site of TrkA including D668 and R673 (Fig. 5).

The characterization of unique allosteric sites adjacent to the ATP-binding site has promoted the development of selective type III inhibitors that have shown clinical benefits in cancer therapy. Type III kinase inhibitors may help overcome drug resistance to type I/II inhibitors that occurs with mutations in the ATP-binding site of kinases such as EGFR [30]. Additional examples of non-ATP-competitive type III kinase inhibitors have been reported for cyclin-dependent kinase-2 (CDK2) [31] and glycogen synthase kinase-3β (GSK3β) [32]. It is expected that the future clinical landscape will have more small-molecule protein kinase inhibitors that adopt non-ATP-competitive approaches in their mechanism of action.

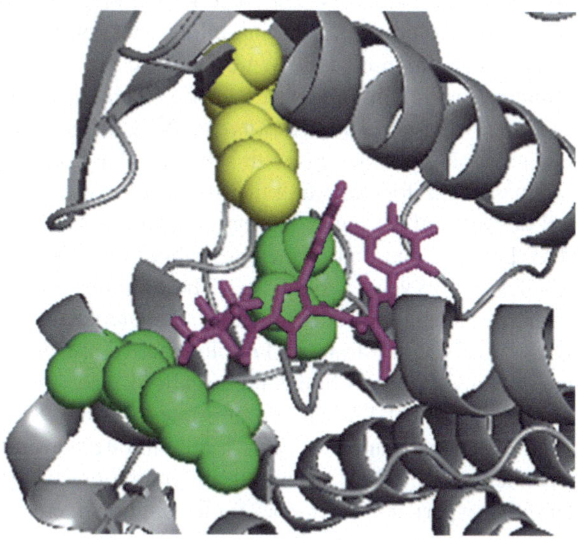

Fig. 5 Interactions between TrkA and compound 23. TrkA (pdb:6D20) are shown in complex with compound 23 (magenta lines) making key interactions with residues R673 and D668 (green). The conserved catalytic lysine (K544) near the ATP-binding site is shown in yellow

Part B: Type IV Kinase Inhibitors

A relatively new area in the development of selective kinase inhibitors has focused on targeting unique structural features outside of the ATP-binding or catalytic sites. These allosteric regions are targets of the type IV kinase inhibitor compounds and have the potential to alter enzymatic activity by disrupting the access to upstream activators or prevent the phosphorylation of select downstream substrates. As discussed in Chap. 1, most kinases have pleiotropic functions involving the phosphorylation and regulation of a variety of diverse substrates. Thus, a potential advantage of type IV kinase inhibitors is the opportunity to disrupt the phosphorylation of some but not all substrates. In other words, the type IV kinase inhibitors may enable new approaches to selectively block only the kinase functions associated with a particular disease while preserving other kinase functions that have potential benefits.

A major challenge in targeting allosteric sites outside the ATP binding/catalytic site is determining what sites are important for relevant biological functions. Chapter 4 will present information on studies that have evaluated kinase interactions with regulatory proteins or downstream substrates. This information provides a starting point to identify compounds that could disrupt these interactions. In addition, the Kinase Atlas is a publicly available resource that used FTMap computational resources to help predict potential allosteric kinase hot spots that could be targeted for the development of potential inhibitors or modulators of kinase signaling functions [33, 34]. The FTMap algorithm examined nearly 5000 kinase structures from 376 different kinases that have been deposited into the Protein Data Bank for predicted binding of small organic molecules. From this, the Kinase Atlas identified ten hot spots outside the ATP-binding/catalytic site that are predicted to contribute to binding free energy of a ligand and are potential drug targets for the development of type IV kinase inhibitors. This section will highlight some recent examples of the discovery of type IV kinase inhibitors and potential applications in modulating kinase functions in disease. Wu et al. have previously reviewed several allosteric inhibitors that fall into the type III and IV categories [35].

Type IV inhibitors of MAP kinases. New understanding of the binding sites that regulate kinase interactions with substrates has facilitated the development of type IV kinase inhibitors targeting the mitogen-activated protein (MAP) kinases. Focus will be on the three major family members of MAP kinases: ERK, JNK, and p38 MAP kinases. The first studies describing type IV inhibitors of ERK2 were published nearly 15 years ago [36, 37]. These studies used computational approaches to predict molecular structures that would interact with D-domain recruitment site (DRS)-involved substrate docking to inactive or active ERK2. Several compounds that contained a thiazolidinedione scaffold were shown to reduce ERK-mediated phosphorylation of downstream substrates such as p90 ribosomal S6 kinase (RSK-1) and the transcription factor ELK-1 and inhibited several cancer cell lines in a dose-dependent manner [36]. However, the limitations of these studies were the lack of definitive experimental evidence for the binding interactions between the compounds and ERK2 and the relative low potency of the compounds. Recent studies [38, 39] highlighting the design of new type IV inhibitors targeting the DRS on ERK2 will be the topic of discussion in Chap. 6.

Additional type IV ERK2 inhibitors have been designed to target ERK2 at the F-recruitment site (FRS), which is involved in regulating the activation of proto-oncogene transcription factors including members of the Fos family and c-Myc [40]. Bioactive compounds from these studies contained a thienyl benzenesulfonate scaffold and inhibited activator protein-1 (AP1) transcription activity and melanoma cells containing activating mutations in BRaf or NRas. The specific interactions between these compounds and ERK2 have not been experimentally determined.

Dimerization between kinase monomers may affect the activation and subcellular localization of the ERK and JNK MAP kinases [41, 42]. Although dimerization between active ERK2 monomers was initially reported to be essential for nuclear localization [42], other studies provide evidence that active ERK2 dimerization may be related to nonphysiological interactions between histidine tags used for protein purification and that untagged ERK2 exists as a monomer under physiological conditions [43]. Similarly, other studies using fluorescence imaging of live cells indicate that ERK2 dimerization is not required for nuclear entry [44]. However, active ERK2 dimers reportedly function to regulate substrate phosphorylation in the cytoplasm but not in the nucleus [45]. As such, research efforts have examined the potential to inhibit ERK2 dimerization and selectively block kinase functions in subcellular locations. Herrero et al. reported the identification of a small molecule inhibitor of ERK2 dimerization that inhibited cytoplasmic activity of ERK2 and tumor progression in mouse xenograft models [46]. Using in silico modeling, compound DEL-22379 reportedly disrupted ERK2 dimer interactions by forming contacts in a cleft near the activation loop consisting of residues D175, H176, F181, and F329. A nonhelical leucine zipper consisting of residues L333, L336, L344 and ion pairs between H176 and E343 on ERK2 monomers have been shown to be important for the formation of ERK dimers [47].

Type IV inhibitors have also been recently developed to target BRaf dimers [48]. Based on the dimerization interface, cyclized peptides were designed to disrupt BRaf dimers and activation of downstream ERK1/2 pathway signaling. Importantly, this approach may be beneficial in treating cancers with wild-type BRaf and overcome the observed paradoxical activation of ERK1/2 signaling seen with ATP-competitive BRaf inhibitors [49].

The c-*J*un *N*-terminal *k*inase (JNK) family has been implicated in a number of diseases including diabetes [50]. JNK activity is regulated through interactions with a JNK-interacting protein (JIP1), which acts as a scaffold that facilitates the interactions between JNK and its upstream kinases. Taking advantage of the structural interactions between JIP1 and JNK1, which will be highlighted in Chap. 4, new small molecules that block this interaction and inhibit JNK substrate phosphorylation were identified [51]. These studies used a fluorescence-based assay that screened compounds for their ability to disrupt the interactions between a JIP1 peptide and JNK1. Several compounds were identified to disrupt the JIP1-JNK interactions with IC_{50} values in the 500 nM range. One compound, BI-78D3, was effective at inhibiting JNK activity but was several orders of magnitude less active against related MAP kinases or unrelated kinases. While the exact binding mode of BI-78D3 with JNK1 is not known, these studies provide the basis for generating effective type IV JNK inhibitors.

Additional type IV inhibitors of JNK1 have been identified to target a unique allosteric site that sits below the activation loop [52]. These studies used mass spectrometry to screen ~500,000 compounds based on their affinity to JNK1. Of the 68 candidate JNK1 ligands identified from the screen, NMR analysis revealed compounds that bound the ATP site or allosteric sites. Figure 6 shows the interactions between JNK1 and an allosteric-binding type IV inhibitor referred to as compound 3, which contains a biaryl tetrazole scaffold. These compounds are binding to a region that has been shown to regulate interactions with substrates and regulatory proteins [53]. However, there is no evidence that compound 3 modulates kinase function through disruption of interactions with substrates. Modifications of compound 3 yielded non-ATP-competitive compounds that may stabilize JNK1 in a way that interferes with phosphorylation by the upstream MEK7 activator kinase [52].

In addition to small molecules, synthetic peptides targeting the JIP1 site on JNK have entered clinical trials to reduce ocular inflammation [54]. Brimapitide (XG-102) has completed phase II trial with 145 patients, and the effects were reported to be comparable to standard dosing with dexamethasone. Brimapitide is also being tested to reduce JNK-mediated inflammation associated with hearing loss and Alzheimer's disease [55, 56]. A phase III clinical trial at sites in Europe and Asia indicate brimapitide is effective against idiopathic sudden sensorineural hearing loss [57].

The failure of ATP-competitive p38 MAP kinase inhibitors in clinical trials for the treatment of inflammatory disorders [58] has encouraged new approaches to target p38 isoforms including the identification of novel allosteric type IV inhibitors.

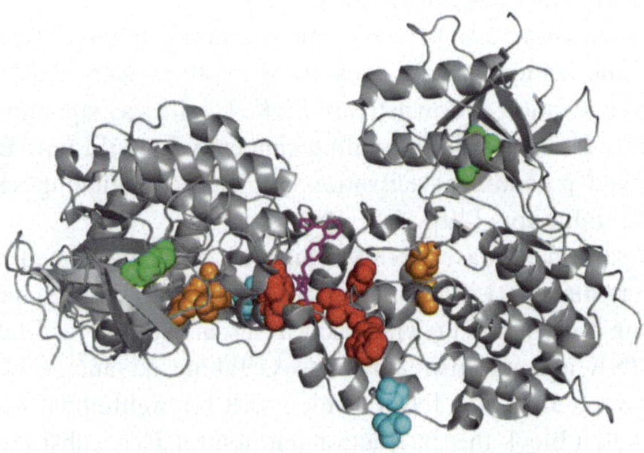

Fig. 6 Interactions between a type IV biaryl tetrazole and JNK1. Shown is a JNK1 dimer (PDB: 3O2M) with activation loop residues T183 and Y185 (red), the MAPK insert sites G242, A267 (cyan), and substrate-docking site residues Y230, I231, W234 (orange) involved in interactions with compound (magenta lines). The conserved K55 involved in ATP catalysis is shown in green

Like the previous studies identifying allosteric JNK inhibitors, Comess et al. screened for compounds that targeted allosteric sites on p38α MAP kinase [52]. An allosteric inhibitor, called compound 10, was identified and found to interact with p38α MAP kinase in a region below the activation loop similar to what was observed with the allosteric compound targeting JNK that was described in Fig. 6. Compound 10 interacted with residues below that activation site that are also adjacent to a substrate-docking site (Fig. 7). Like the JNK inhibitor compound, compound 10 is thought to cause an allosteric structural change that disrupts p38α MAP kinase activation by upstream kinases.

Shah et al. used computational approaches to identify compounds that target a pocket adjacent to the DRS of p38α MAP kinase [59]. Unique to these compounds were their isoform preference for interactions with p38α over p38β MAP kinase, which may help mitigate excess toxicity observed with the ATP-competitive inhibitors tested previously [60, 61]. Another potential advantage of these compounds is their ability to inhibit pro-inflammatory substrates involved in acute lung injury associated with acute respiratory distress syndrome (ARDS) but preserve the activation of anti-inflammatory signals that might be beneficial [62]. For example, Shah et al. describe a lead compound, UM101, that inhibited the proinflammatory substrate MAPK-activated protein kinase-2 (MAPKAPK2 or MK2) but preserved the

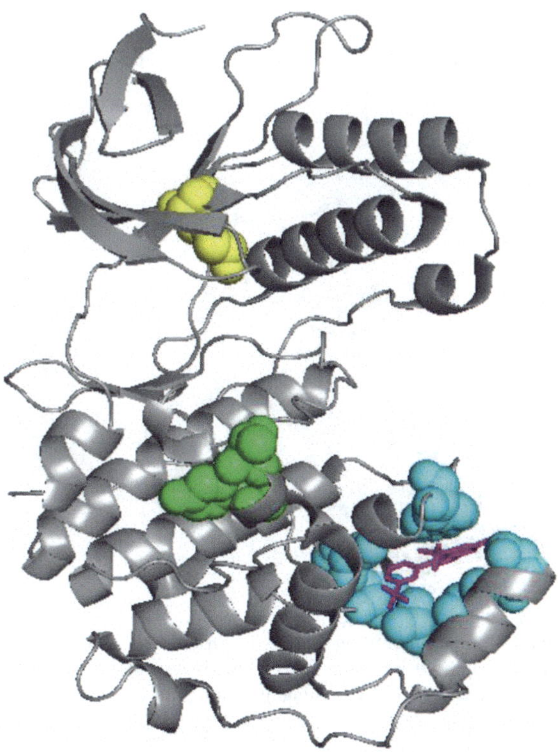

Fig. 7 Interactions between compound 10 (magenta lines) and p38α MAP kinase. (PDB: 3NEW). Interacting residues W197, S252, I250, P191, L246, L292 (cyan). Activation site resides T180 and Y182 (green). The conserved catalytic lysine (K53) is shown in yellow

activation of the antiinflammatory p38 substrates mitogen- and stress-activated protein kinase-1/2 (MSK1/2) [59]. The authors went on to demonstrate that UM101 protected against lung damage by reducing endothelial cell damage and neutrophil leakage in a mouse model of lipopolysaccharide (LPS)-induced acute lung injury. These studies provide compelling evidence that function-selective type IV p38α MAP kinase inhibitors have the potential to reduce toxicity observed with blocking all p38 MAP kinase functions while maintaining in vivo efficacy.

BCR-Abl inhibitors. Efforts to overcome resistance to ATP-competitive inhibitors in the treatment of chronic myelogenous leukemia (CML) have led to the identification of allosteric inhibitors of BCR-Abl [63, 64]. Adrian et al. designed a compound, GNF-2, that targeted the interactions between an N-terminal myristoyl group and a hydrophobic region in the C-terminus of the c-Abl kinase [65]. Myristoylation is a posttranslational modification where a fatty acid derivative of myristic acid is linked to proteins and facilitates localization to cell membranes. It is estimated that 0.5–0.8% of all eukaryotic proteins are myristoylated [66]. GNF-2 was more effective at inhibiting nonmyristoylated c-Abl than the myristoylated kinase. Similarly, GNF-2 bound to c-Abl and could be competed off with a myristoylated peptide. Furthermore, mutations in the myristoylated-binding pocket of c-Abl blocked GNF-2 inhibitory effects. NMR studies provided further evidence for GNF-2 binding to the myristoylated pocket of c-Abl [63]. GNF-2 was demonstrated to make key interactions with residues in the myristoyl-binding site (Fig. 8).

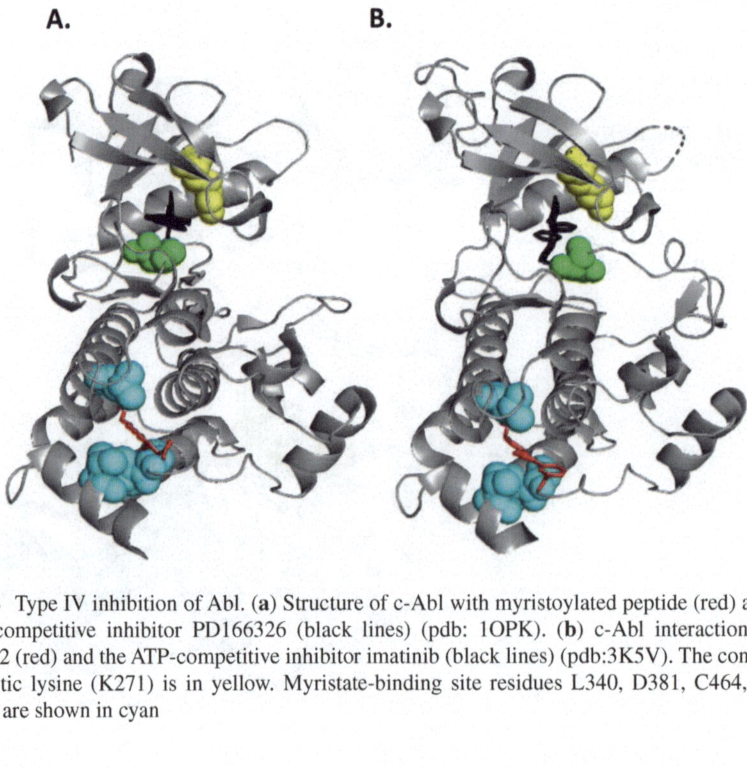

Fig. 8 Type IV inhibition of Abl. (**a**) Structure of c-Abl with myristoylated peptide (red) and the ATP-competitive inhibitor PD166326 (black lines) (pdb: 1OPK). (**b**) c-Abl interactions with GNF-2 (red) and the ATP-competitive inhibitor imatinib (black lines) (pdb:3K5V). The conserved catalytic lysine (K271) is in yellow. Myristate-binding site residues L340, D381, C464, P465, V506 are shown in cyan

Small allosteric compounds targeting the myristoyl-binding site of c-Abl have also been shown to induce conformational changes that activate kinase activity [67]. Yang and colleagues took advantage of structural studies that suggested that interactions between the myristoyl group and the myristoyl-binding site regulated c-Abl activity and identified the kinase activator DPH (5-(1,3-diaryl-1H-pyrazol-4-yl)hydantoin). In contrast to GNF-2, which locks a key α-helix (see Fig. 8) required for catalytic activity in a closed inhibited state, DPH caused an extension of this α-helix observed when c-Abl is activated [67]. While the inhibition of Abl activity is desired in the context of cancers with constitutively active BCR-Abl fusion proteins, activation of wild-type c-Abl may limit breast cancer cell proliferation and metastasis [68].

PDK1 inhibitors. An important co-activator of Akt proteins is *p*hosphoinositide-*d*ependent protein *k*inase-*1* (PDK1), which co-localizes with Akt at the plasma membrane through the PH domain. PDK1 is unique because it is required for the full activation of Akt and other members of the AGC protein kinase family [69]. PDK1 interactions with substrates occur through a PDK1 interacting fragment (PIF) pocket [70]. The PIF pocket occupies an allosteric site referred to as helix αC that regulates protein-protein interactions and kinase activity. Rettenmaier et al. identified small molecules based on a diaryl sulfonamide chemical scaffold that interact with the PIF pocket and inhibit PDK1 [71]. Structural studies revealed key interactions between their compound RS1 and residues R131 and L155 in the PIF pocket (Fig. 9). Although ATP-competitive PDK1 inhibitors had limited efficacy as a monotherapy in mice with acute myeloid leukemia xenografts [72], combining them with the PIF pocket inhibitors may provide greater inhibition of Akt signaling and subsequent tumor suppression [71].

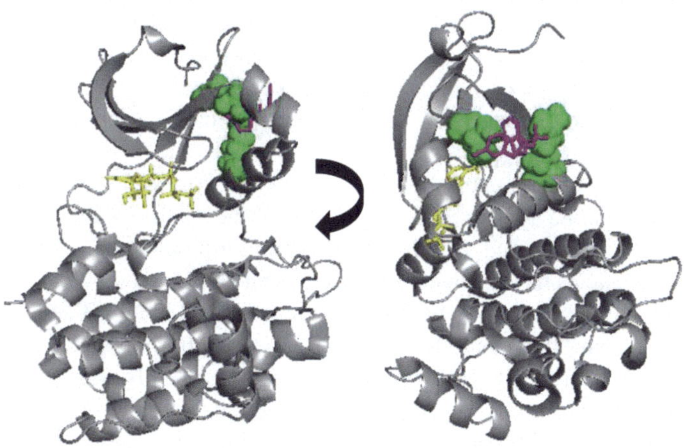

Fig. 9 Interactions between PDK1 and compound RS1. PDK1 (pdb:4RQK) is shown in complex with RS1 (magenta lines) interacting with a R131 and L155 in the PIF pocket (green). ATP is highlighted as yellow lines

Inhibitors of CDK2 interactions with cyclin A. Allosteric type IV inhibitors have been developed against cyclin-dependent kinase-2 (CDK2) [73]. Cell cycle progression depends on the activity of CDK proteins, which are regulated by association with cyclin proteins. CDK2 activity is essential for progression through G1 and S-phase of the cell cycle and requires association with cyclin A. Based on structural features of CDK2, a type IV inhibitor compound, 8-anilino-1-naphthalene sulfonate (ANS), was identified to bind an allosteric site near the DFG region and causes a structural change that disrupts interactions with cyclin A. The CDK2-ANS structure was shown previously in Chap. 2. However, ANS-binding affinity for CDK2 is relatively low (37 μM); therefore, it can be readily displaced by cyclin A [73]. To improve the binding affinity of compounds targeting CDK2 interactions with cyclin A, Rastelli et al. did a virtual screen for compounds that are predicted to interact with CDK2 in the ANS-binding site [31]. Experimental analysis of several lead compounds revealed displacement of ANS from the cyclin A–binding site, which suggested higher potency and targeting to the cyclin A–binding site. Although experimental analysis of structural interactions between these new compounds and CDK2 was not done, these studies provide the basis for targeting the activity of CDK proteins through disruption of interactions with cyclins.

Inhibitors of mTOR. Contrary to compounds that disrupt protein-protein interactions and prevent kinase activation, allosteric compounds that promote protein-protein interactions and disrupt kinase functions have been well described in the example of the mammalian target of rapamycin (mTOR) kinase. The mTOR kinase complexes (mTORC1 and mTORC2) are critical regulators of the immune system and are upregulated in many cancer cells [74, 75]. Targeted inhibition of mTOR has clinical uses as an immunosuppressant during organ transplants and as anticancer drugs [76]. The natural product rapamycin and related analogues (or rapalogs such as the FDA-approved sirolimus, temsirolimus, and everolimus) indirectly inhibit mTOR by forming a complex with FK506-binding proteins (FKBP). The rapalog-FKBP complex associates with a binding domain on mTOR that is outside the active site and involved in facilitating the activation of substrates involved in protein synthesis. In addition to their immunosuppressant roles, the mTOR inhibitors have been FDA approved to treat renal cell carcinoma, breast cancer, and neuroendocrine tumors.

IKK inhibitors. Inflammatory diseases such as arthritis, asthma, and atherosclerosis are thought to be a result of overactivation of the *N*uclear *F*actor *kappa*-light-chain-enhancer of activated *B* cells (NFκB) transcription factor [77]. As such, dozens of compounds have been identified to inhibit NFκB activity [78]. To develop more specific inhibitors, efforts to target kinases involved in NFκB activation have been pursued. The NFκB inhibitory protein, IκB, is phosphorylated by the IκB kinase (IKK), which targets IκB for degradation. Loss of IκB allows cytoplasmic NFκB to translocate into the nucleus and regulate the expression of inflammatory genes. In addition to ATP-competitive inhibitors, allosteric inhibitors of IKK have been identified [78]. Scientists at Bristol-Myers Squibb, using an in vitro kinase assay consisting of IKK isoforms and IκB to screen for compounds that inhibit IκB phosphorylation, identified the IKK inhibitor BMS-345541 that was ~10 fold more selective for IKKβ versus IKKα [79]. Although BMS-345541 does not compete with ATP binding, the exact allosteric-binding mode of this compound is currently unclear. In addition, clinical applications with this or related allosteric inhibitors of IKK have yet to be reported.

Part C: Type V Kinase Inhibitors

The conserved structure of the ATP-binding site of protein kinases makes it challenging to develop specific inhibitors that block kinases through type I or II mechanisms of action. However, developing compounds that target both the ATP-binding site and a unique structural feature found on a specific protein kinase is the basis for the development of type V or bivalent inhibitors. With the characterization of binding sites and peptide motifs that determine protein-protein interactions, highly selective and potent type V inhibitors against tyrosine and serine/threonine kinases have been identified. Gower et al. provided a relatively recent review of type V bivalent protein kinase inhibitors that have been described [80]. These compounds typically consist of a small molecule that targets the ATP-binding site coupled to a peptide representing the substrate targeted by the specific kinase. This section will describe some of these compounds and the approaches to develop selective type V protein kinase inhibitors.

Early proof of concept studies for the development of bivalent protein kinase inhibitors used the Src tyrosine kinase as a model [81]. Src and related tyrosine kinases contain an SH2 domain that recognizes phosphorylated tyrosine and surrounding amino acids on substrate proteins. Xu et al. provided the first structural information of Src describing the coordination between the SH2 and SH3 domains involved in protein-protein interactions and the catalytic site regulating kinase activity [82] (Fig. 10). Using this information, a SH2 domain–targeted peptide containing a phosphorylated tyrosine was linked to a nonphosphorylatable peptide that interacts with the Src active site through a γ-aminobutyric acid linker [81]. The key findings from these studies indicated that the targeting peptides were most potent when linked together and that the number of γ-aminobutyric acid monomers in the linker was important for maximum Src inhibition. More recent studies linked the SH2 targeting peptide with an ATP-competitive inhibitor to achieve potent bivalent c-Src inhibitors [83, 84].

Bivalent kinase inhibitors based on a protein scaffold. Bivalent protein kinase inhibitors as research tools have been developed using the DNA repair protein O^6-alkylguanine-DNA alkyltransferase (AGT) as a scaffold [85]. AGT contains a cysteine in the active site that reacts with O^6-benzylguanine (BG). This conveniently allows the coupling of an ATP-competitive inhibitor to AGT through a linkage with BG. Unique AGT fusion proteins can be expressed with a specific peptide ligand that contains the second binding moiety that determines specificity for protein recognition. This technology, referred to as SNAP-tag, provides a convenient approach

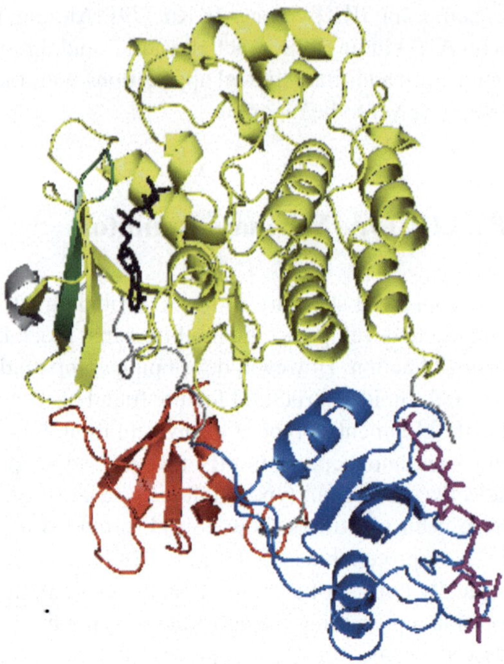

Fig. 10 Structural domains in c-Src (PDB:2SRC). The SH2 and SH3 domains are shown in blue and red, respectively. The kinase domain and ATP-binding site are shown in yellow and green, respectively. A potential peptide substrate (magenta lines) interacting with the SH-2 domain and an ATP analog (black lines) are shown

to generate and test the specificity of a variety of ligand targeting sequences and their ability to achieve kinase inhibition in combination with ATP-binding site compounds [86]. Specific AGT fusion proteins containing peptide ligands against Abl1, PIM1, p38α MAPK, c-Src, and EGFR protein kinases have been described [86–88]. Another advantage of the SNAP-tag approach is that promiscuous ATP-competitive inhibitors can be designed to be quite specific for a particular kinase [89].

Wong et al. described an analysis of three ATP-competitive inhibitors and nine SNAP-tag fusion proteins to determine the contribution of each targeting moiety to the potency of the bivalent inhibitor [90]. These studies indicated that the potency of the bivalent compound was less dependent on the affinity of the specific peptide-targeting ligand but more on the affinity of the ATP-competitive ligand. Nonetheless, even targeting peptides with low affinity can help improve selectivity and potency of bivalent kinase inhibitor compounds [90]. While the utility of these types of bivalent inhibitors will be relegated to research tools for evaluating kinase functions, these approaches provide the basis to design bivalent kinase inhibitors for clinical applications.

Small-molecule peptide bivalent Inhibitors. Several MAP kinases have been the target of bivalent inhibitors. Stebbins et al. identified compound 19 that consisted of an ATP-competitive inhibitor coupled to a short D-domain peptide, which was sufficient to displace the JIP1 protein from the D-recruitment site on JNK1, and a cell penetrating peptide [91]. Compound 19 inhibited JNK1 kinase activity in vitro and in cell-based assays at low nM and μM concentrations, respectively. This compound also improved glucose tolerance in a mouse model of type 2 diabetes, which is a potential clinical application for JNK inhibitors. A similar strategy was used to generate an ERK1/2 selective bivalent inhibitor (SBP3) consisting of an ATP-competitive inhibitor (FR180204) and a 16-amino-acid peptide corresponding to the D-domain of the ERK1/2 substrate, ribosomal S6 kinase (RSK1) [92]. Combining the targeting moieties into the bivalent compound increased the potency more than 50 times as compared to either the ATP-competitive inhibitor or the D-domain peptide alone. Figure 11 shows the reported structure of SBP3 with active ERK. As shown, SBP3 forms contacts with ERK2 through the RSK1 peptide and FR180204; however, the linker of these targeting agents does not appear to be involved in ERK2 interaction [92]. Despite the intended design for SBP3 to target ERK1/2, this compound also potently interacts with JNK and p38 MAP kinase isoforms.

A study reported the use of a cyclic decapeptide that corresponds to an extracellular region of the epidermal growth factor receptor (EGFR) regions involved in dimerization [93]. Combining two of these peptides together using a polyproline linker created a bivalent ligand that inhibited EGFR autophosphorylation presumably by preventing the two EGFR monomers from dimerizing. Ephrin type-A receptor 3 (EphA3) is another receptor tyrosine kinase targeted by bivalent compounds [94]. These studies highlight the potential of using longer linkers to couple ATP-competitive inhibitors with small peptides that target unique regions far away from the ATP-binding site. Not only did this approach enhance the potency of a weak

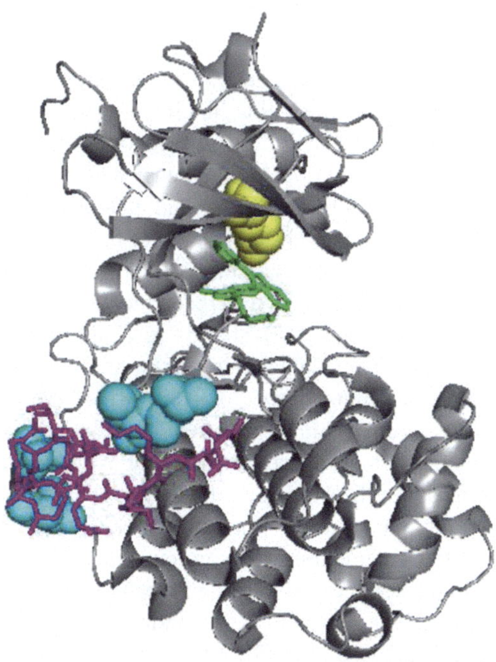

Fig. 11 Structure of bivalent compound SBP3 and ERK2 [PDB: 5V62]. SBP3 shown consisting of a RSK1 peptide (magenta lines) and the ATP-competitive compound FR180204 (green lines). D-recruitment site residues T158, T159, D316, D319 (cyan). The conserved catalytic residue (K52) is in yellow

ATP-competitive inhibitor, it supports the advantage of using structural information to design a wide range of bivalent targeting moieties.

The PIM kinases (referring to the *p*roviral *i*nsertion site in *M*oloney murine leukemia virus) are overexpressed in several cancer types and appear to exacerbate proliferative disorders [95]. Bivalent PIM kinase inhibitors have been developed using D-arginine-rich peptides (ARCs) and adenosine analogs [96]. Arginine-rich sequences are found on many substrates recognized by basophilic protein kinases found in the AGC protein kinase group. Even though PIM kinases fall in the calcium-calmodulin-dependent protein kinase (CAMK) group, Ekambaram et al. provided evidence that potent bivalent inhibitors using ARCs can be selective for PIM-1 kinase but not members of the AGC protein kinases [96].

These studies provided evidence that targeting two separate structural features on protein kinases with bivalent compounds could be an effective approach to inhibit the activity of a specific kinase. While many of the approaches to develop bivalent protein kinases inhibitors have yielded useful research tools for understanding signaling pathways and biological mechanisms, the clinical applications of these compounds in treating disease have yet to be realized. The large size of bivalent inhibitors may present barriers to their use in targeting intracellular protein kinases. The potential to design smaller peptidomimetic compounds that target specific substrate interaction sites may overcome drug delivery and bioavailability issues associated with using peptides as targeting moieties or therapeutic agents [97].

Part D: Type VI Kinase Inhibitors

There has been resurgence in the development of compounds that form covalent, and generally irreversible, interactions with protein kinases to provide sustainable inhibitory effects primarily to treat cancer. The prospect of developing covalent inhibitors faced criticism of extensive off-target effects. However, there is historical precedence for the benefits and potential risks of developing covalent-binding drugs. Probably the best example of the benefits of covalent bond–forming drugs is acetyl salicylic acid or aspirin. Although the beneficial antiinflammatory and analgesic effects of aspirin have been recognized since its discovery in the late 1890s, it was not until the 1970s that its mechanism of action was identified to involve the formation of covalent adducts on cyclooxygenase enzymes and the reduced production of inflammatory cytokines [98]. However, other drugs like acetaminophen metabolize into highly reactive species that form toxic covalent adducts with liver proteins and can cause liver damage at high doses. Despite the understandable concerns about the off-target effects of covalent-binding drugs, advances in structural and computational biology have made it feasible to develop inhibitors that form covalent interactions with protein kinase inhibitors that are selective, efficacious, and have reduced toxicity. This section will highlight some of the features of clinically relevant covalent kinase inhibitors and the potential for expanding the development and use of covalent kinase inhibitors in disease.

Recent reviews of covalent small-molecule protein kinase inhibitors provide an excellent summary of the compounds identified to target specific kinases [99, 100]. Covalent type VI protein kinase inhibitors utilize chemical features of the noncovalent type I–IV kinase inhibitors that interact with the ATP-binding or other regions near the kinase domain. What makes the type VI protein kinase inhibitors unique is the inclusion of reactive electrophilic groups or warheads that react primarily with nucleophilic cysteines although reactions with lysine, aspartic acid, and tyrosine residues can be used to form covalent interactions. Like other drug discovery approaches, type VI kinase inhibitors use structure-guided design approaches that take advantage of noncovalent interactions with the targeted kinase in order to increase specificity and position the warhead component for targeted covalent interaction that locks the inhibitor in place. The covalent adduct typically forms through a Michael addition reaction, and many of the electrophilic moieties used to develop type VI inhibitors utilize an acrylamide group that favors interactions with cysteine residues. In addition, alterations in the reactivity of the electrophile warhead may be used to create reversible covalent protein kinase inhibitors whose duration of inhibition may need tighter control [101]. For example, most protein kinase inhibitors that are used to treat cancer might be more effective by a sustained mechanism of irreversible inhibition. In contrast, shorter-acting reversible type IV inhibitors might expand the clinical applications and reduce off-target reactivity and toxicity [101, 102].

An early example of type VI covalent protein kinase inhibitors was the discovery of the mechanism of action for the fungal metabolite wortmannin [103]. Wortmannin was identified to be an irreversible inhibitor of PI3K isoforms through the formation of a covalent adduct with a conserved lysine (K802) in the catalytic site [103]. However, wortmannin is nonspecific, causing overt toxicity, which limits its use to research studies. Dalton et al. optimized reversible interactions to design compounds that covalently interacted with the analogous conserved lysine (K779) near the active site of PI3Kδ isoform [104]. PX-866 is a wortmannin analog that also forms a covalent bond with K802 that entered clinical trials but did not show promising efficacy [105]. It remains to be determined whether other type VI PI3K inhibitors will provide an advantage over the current reversible PI3K inhibitors in clinical trials [16].

The success of type VI protein kinase inhibitors has been realized with the development of EGFR- and Bruton's tyrosine kinase (BTK)-targeted compounds. Afatinib, osimertinib, dacomitinib, and neratinib are FDA-approved type VI inhibitors that target the EGFR family and are used to treat a variety of cancers [106] (Fig. 12). All these drugs form a covalent adduct with a key cysteine (C797 for EGFR) in the active site and are expected to improve treatment options especially in patients who develop drug resistance [107, 108]. While the irreversible nature of these compounds provides a more durable inhibitory response, not all type VI inhibitors may be able to overcome the development of acquired drug resistance observed with first generation type I/II reversible inhibitors [109]. Afatinib, which was designed based on the reversible inhibitor gefitinib, is not effective against the common EGFR T790M mutation that is often responsible for acquired drug resistance.

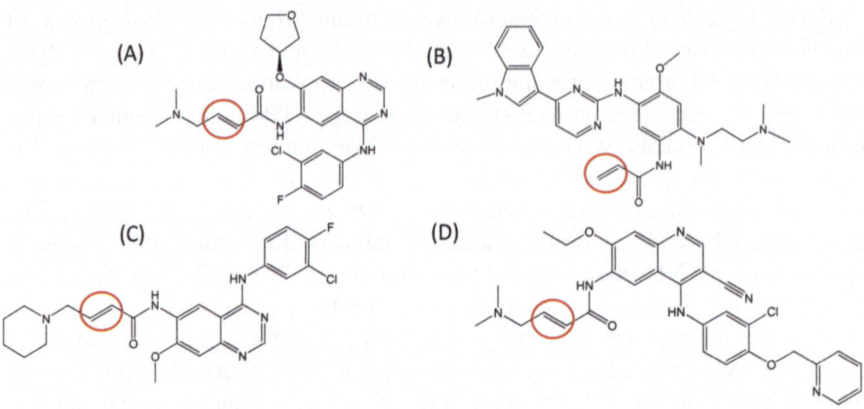

Fig. 12 The chemical structures of (**a**) afatinib, (**b**) osimertinib, (**c**) dacomitinib, and (**d**) neratinib are shown. The reactive site of the acrylamide moieties is circled in red

In addition to causing the T790M mutation, afatinib resistance mechanisms include increased expression of the c-Met receptor tyrosine kinase and V843I mutation on EGFR [110]. New structures, such as osimertinib, are less restricted by the T790M mutation and may have better treatment outcomes for patients resistant to first-line EGFR inhibitors [109].

Ibrutinib is a type VI inhibitor that forms a covalent bond on cysteine 481 (C481) in the active site of BTK and is used to treat B-cell cancers such as chronic lymphocytic leukemia (CLL) [111]. Several months after treatment, nearly 80% of relapsing patients contained a cysteine to serine (C481S) mutation that limited the efficacy of ibrutinib [112]. Alternative reversible BTK targeted compounds that tolerate the C481S mutations are showing promise in treating CLL relapses [113]. Ibrutinib has also been associated with several adverse drug events, which likely occurs due to the covalent interactions with other targets and presents a barrier for its use in some patients. Acalabrutinib is a second-generation type VI BTK inhibitor that targets C481 that reportedly causes fewer adverse events and is showing more sustained patient responses in clinical trials evaluating relapsed or refractory chronic lymphocytic leukemia [114].

The MAP kinases have been the target of several type VI inhibitors. Zhang et al. described the use of the type II kinase inhibitor imatinib to design covalent inhibitors against JNK1/2/3 isoforms [115]. The authors noted that several kinases targeted by imatinib have a potentially reactive cysteine that precedes the DFG motif of the activation loop. By attaching an electrophilic acrylamide, a compound was identified that targeted not only expected tyrosine kinases but also JNK isoforms. Further modifications identified compounds with improved JNK selectivity and potency to allow their use as reagents to examine cellular functions for the JNK pathway [115]. In a study by Ward et al., new reversible ERK1/2 inhibitors, with a pyrimidine scaffold, were identified and modified with an acrylamide functional group to make irreversible covalent inhibitors that targeted C166, which is directly adjacent to the DFG motif at the beginning of the active loop [116]. This cysteine is conserved in ERK1/2 but not in p38 or JNK MAP kinases, which is expected to provide some degree of selectivity. More recent studies have identified ERK1/2-targeted compounds that form covalent bonds with a cysteine (C159) located in the D-recruitment site (DRS) outside the ATP-binding site [39]. The lead compound, BI-78D3, appears to block interactions between ERK2 and its activator MEK1. Despite C159 being conserved in other MAP kinases, such as p38 and JNK, BI-78D3 modifications were only observed on ERK1/2 suggesting other DRS structural features facilitated selectivity [39].

New approaches for cancer therapy through targeted inhibition of transcriptional regulation by cyclin-dependent kinases (CDKs) have utilized covalent-binding compounds [117]. These studies identified a compound THZ1 that covalently binds to a cysteine (C312) that resides outside of the ATP-binding site and inhibits CDK7, and to a lesser extent CDK12 and 13, phosphorylation of RNA polymerase II. Modifications to THZ1 that improved potency and drug-like properties led to the generation of the covalent CDK7 inhibitor SY-1365, which is currently in cancer clinical trials [118]. A common problem that reduces the efficacy of THZ1 and other drugs is their efflux by the ABC transporters. Gao et al. provided evidence that upregulation of ABC transporters by THZ1 can be overcome by compounds that covalently target CDK12 and are not ABC transporter substrates [119].

Downstream of PI3K, Akt protein kinases have been targeted by covalent inhibitors [120]. Weisner et al. posited that allosteric inhibitors, such as the previously mentioned MK-2206, that targeted the PH-domain were proximal to cysteines that could be targeted to generate selective and irreversible Akt inhibitors [120]. The result of these studies is the compound borussertib, which forms a novel covalent interaction on C296 and has been shown in preclinical studies to be effective in combination with the type III MEK1/2 inhibitor trametinib for inhibiting pancreatic and colorectal cancers expressing KRas mutations [121]. The structure of borussertib in complex with Akt1 is shown in Fig. 13. Borussertib covalently binds C296 and forms hydrophobic interactions between the PH domain and the ATP-binding site.

Covalent type VI protein kinase inhibitors have provided new options for more durable responses and target selectivity. Significant benefits have been observed with type VI inhibitors, such as afatinib and ibrutinib, versus reversible type I/II inhibitors for the treatment of lung cancers [122] and lymphocytic leukemias [123]. Nonetheless, acquired drug resistance through mutations in the targeted cysteine and off-target interactions remain barriers to durable patient outcomes. Expanding the repertoire of amino acids targeted by type VI inhibitors beyond the common cysteine targets may provide advantages. For example, targeting lysine residues in the active site of protein kinases with type VI compounds may be effective at disabling enzyme activity. However, surface-exposed lysines are generally thought to be poor nucleophiles because they are protonated (pK_a ~10.5) at physiological pH [100]. Recent studies using computational predictions suggest that localized pK_a values may shift several units, allowing lysines to be amenable to reacting with

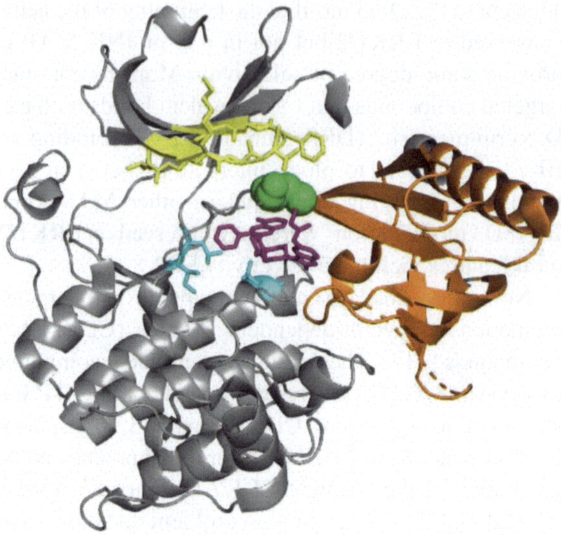

Fig. 13 Structure of borussertib in complex with Akt1 (PDB: 6HHF). Borussertib (magenta lines) interacts with C296 (green) and makes hydrophobic interactions with L210, L264, and I290 (cyan). PH domain residues 5–108 (orange), and ATP site residues 156–164 (yellow) are shown

electrophilic warheads [124]. Given the success of current covalent inhibitors targeting EGFR and BTK protein kinases, the future will likely see the development of new type VI inhibitors for treating disease.

References

1. Mancini, M., & Yarden, Y. (2016). Mutational and network level mechanisms underlying resistance to anti-cancer kinase inhibitors. *Seminars in Cell & Developmental Biology, 50*, 164–176.
2. Dudley, D. T., Pang, L., Decker, S. J., Bridges, A. J., & Saltiel, A. R. (1995). A synthetic inhibitor of the mitogen-activated protein kinase cascade. *Proceedings of the National Academy of Sciences of the United States of America, 92*, 7686–7689.
3. Sebolt-Leopold, J. S., Dudley, D. T., Herrera, R., Van Becelaere, K., Wiland, A., Gowan, R. C., Tecle, H., Barrett, S. D., Bridges, A., Przybranowski, S., Leopold, W. R., & Saltiel, A. R. (1999). Blockade of the MAP kinase pathway suppresses growth of colon tumors in vivo. *Nature Medicine, 5*, 810–816.
4. Ohren, J. F., Chen, H., Pavlovsky, A., Whitehead, C., Zhang, E., Kuffa, P., Yan, C., McConnell, P., Spessard, C., Banotai, C., Mueller, W. T., Delaney, A., Omer, C., Sebolt-Leopold, J., Dudley, D. T., Leung, I. K., Flamme, C., Warmus, J., Kaufman, M., Barrett, S., Tecle, H., & Hasemann, C. A. (2004). Structures of human MAP kinase kinase 1 (MEK1) and MEK2 describe novel noncompetitive kinase inhibition. *Nature Structural & Molecular Biology, 11*, 1192–1197.
5. Zhao, Y., & Adjei, A. A. (2014). The clinical development of MEK inhibitors. *Nature Reviews Clinical Oncology, 11*, 385–400.
6. Davies, H., Bignell, G. R., Cox, C., Stephens, P., Edkins, S., Clegg, S., Teague, J., Woffendin, H., Garnett, M. J., Bottomley, W., Davis, N., Dicks, E., Ewing, R., Floyd, Y., Gray, K., Hall,

S., Hawes, R., Hughes, J., Kosmidou, V., Menzies, A., Mould, C., Parker, A., Stevens, C., Watt, S., Hooper, S., Wilson, R., Jayatilake, H., Gusterson, B. A., Cooper, C., Shipley, J., Hargrave, D., Pritchard-Jones, K., Maitland, N., Chenevix-Trench, G., Riggins, G. J., Bigner, D. D., Palmieri, G., Cossu, A., Flanagan, A., Nicholson, A., Ho, J. W., Leung, S. Y., Yuen, S. T., Weber, B. L., Seigler, H. F., Darrow, T. L., Paterson, H., Marais, R., Marshall, C. J., Wooster, R., Stratton, M. R., & Futreal, P. A. (2002). Mutations of the BRAF gene in human cancer. *Nature, 417*, 949–954.

7. Larkin, J., Ascierto, P. A., Dreno, B., Atkinson, V., Liszkay, G., Maio, M., Mandala, M., Demidov, L., Stroyakovskiy, D., Thomas, L., de la Cruz-Merino, L., Dutriaux, C., Garbe, C., Sovak, M. A., Chang, I., Choong, N., Hack, S. P., McArthur, G. A., & Ribas, A. (2014). Combined vemurafenib and cobimetinib in BRAF-mutated melanoma. *The New England Journal of Medicine, 371*, 1867–1876.
8. Khunger, A., Khunger, M., & Velcheti, V. (2018). Dabrafenib in combination with trametinib in the treatment of patients with BRAF V600-positive advanced or metastatic non-small cell lung cancer: Clinical evidence and experience. *Therapeutic Advances in Respiratory Disease, 12*, 1753466618767611.
9. Ljubas, J., Ovesen, T., & Rusan, M. (2019). A systematic review of phase II targeted therapy clinical trials in anaplastic thyroid cancer. *Cancers (Basel), 11*(7), 943.
10. Long, G. V., Stroyakovskiy, D., Gogas, H., Levchenko, E., de Braud, F., Larkin, J., Garbe, C., Jouary, T., Hauschild, A., Grob, J. J., Chiarion-Sileni, V., Lebbe, C., Mandala, M., Millward, M., Arance, A., Bondarenko, I., Haanen, J. B., Hansson, J., Utikal, J., Ferraresi, V., Kovalenko, N., Mohr, P., Probachai, V., Schadendorf, D., Nathan, P., Robert, C., Ribas, A., DeMarini, D. J., Irani, J. G., Swann, S., Legos, J. J., Jin, F., Mookerjee, B., & Flaherty, K. (2015). Dabrafenib and trametinib versus dabrafenib and placebo for Val600 BRAF-mutant melanoma: A multicentre, double-blind, phase 3 randomised controlled trial. *Lancet, 386*, 444–451.
11. Zhao, Z., Xie, L., & Bourne, P. E. (2017). Insights into the binding mode of MEK type-III inhibitors. A step towards discovering and designing allosteric kinase inhibitors across the human kinome. *PLoS One, 12*, e0179936.
12. Garnett, M. J., Rana, S., Paterson, H., Barford, D., & Marais, R. (2005). Wild-type and mutant B-RAF activate C-RAF through distinct mechanisms involving heterodimerization. *Molecular Cell, 20*, 963–969.
13. Hatzivassiliou, G., Haling, J. R., Chen, H., Song, K., Price, S., Heald, R., Hewitt, J. F., Zak, M., Peck, A., Orr, C., Merchant, M., Hoeflich, K. P., Chan, J., Luoh, S. M., Anderson, D. J., Ludlam, M. J., Wiesmann, C., Ultsch, M., Friedman, L. S., Malek, S., & Belvin, M. (2013). Mechanism of MEK inhibition determines efficacy in mutant KRAS- versus BRAF-driven cancers. *Nature, 501*, 232–236.
14. Janku, F., Yap, T. A., & Meric-Bernstam, F. (2018). Targeting the PI3K pathway in cancer: Are we making headway? *Nature Reviews Clinical Oncology, 15*, 273–291.
15. Downward, J. (1998). Mechanisms and consequences of activation of protein kinase B/Akt. *Current Opinion in Cell Biology, 10*, 262–267.
16. Yang, J., Nie, J., Ma, X., Wei, Y., Peng, Y., & Wei, X. (2019). Targeting PI3K in cancer: Mechanisms and advances in clinical trials. *Molecular Cancer, 18*, 26.
17. Wu, W. I., Voegtli, W. C., Sturgis, H. L., Dizon, F. P., Vigers, G. P., & Brandhuber, B. J. (2010). Crystal structure of human AKT1 with an allosteric inhibitor reveals a new mode of kinase inhibition. *PLoS One, 5*, e12913.
18. Barnett, S. F., Defeo-Jones, D., Fu, S., Hancock, P. J., Haskell, K. M., Jones, R. E., Kahana, J. A., Kral, A. M., Leander, K., Lee, L. L., Malinowski, J., McAvoy, E. M., Nahas, D. D., Robinson, R. G., & Huber, H. E. (2005). Identification and characterization of pleckstrin-homology-domain-dependent and isoenzyme-specific Akt inhibitors. *The Biochemical Journal, 385*, 399–408.
19. Hirai, H., Sootome, H., Nakatsuru, Y., Miyama, K., Taguchi, S., Tsujioka, K., Ueno, Y., Hatch, H., Majumder, P. K., Pan, B. S., & Kotani, H. (2010). MK-2206, an allosteric Akt

inhibitor, enhances antitumor efficacy by standard chemotherapeutic agents or molecular targeted drugs in vitro and in vivo. *Molecular Cancer Therapeutics, 9*, 1956–1967.
20. Politz, O., Siegel, F., Barfacker, L., Bomer, U., Hagebarth, A., Scott, W. J., Michels, M., Ince, S., Neuhaus, R., Meyer, K., Fernandez-Montalvan, A. E., Liu, N., von Nussbaum, F., Mumberg, D., & Ziegelbauer, K. (2017). BAY 1125976, a selective allosteric AKT1/2 inhibitor, exhibits high efficacy on AKT signaling-dependent tumor growth in mouse models. *International Journal of Cancer, 140*, 449–459.
21. Lapierre, J. M., Eathiraj, S., Vensel, D., Liu, Y., Bull, C. O., Cornell-Kennon, S., Iimura, S., Kelleher, E. W., Kizer, D. E., Koerner, S., Makhija, S., Matsuda, A., Moussa, M., Namdev, N., Savage, R. E., Szwaya, J., Volckova, E., Westlund, N., Wu, H., & Schwartz, B. (2016). Discovery of 3-(3-(4-(1-Aminocyclobutyl)phenyl)-5-phenyl-3H-imidazo[4,5-b]pyridin-2-yl) pyridin-2-amine (ARQ 092): An orally bioavailable, selective, and potent allosteric AKT inhibitor. *Journal of Medicinal Chemistry, 59*, 6455–6469.
22. Leoni, C., Gullo, G., Resta, N., Fagotti, A., Onesimo, R., Schwartz, B., Kazakin, J., Abbadessa, G., Crown, J., Collins, C. D., Ranieri, C., Scambia, G., & Zampino, G. (2019). First evidence of a therapeutic effect of miransertib in a teenager with Proteus syndrome and ovarian carcinoma. *American Journal of Medical Genetics Part A, 179*, 1319–1324.
23. Keppler-Noreuil, K. M., Sapp, J. C., Lindhurst, M. J., Darling, T. N., Burton-Akright, J., Bagheri, M., Dombi, E., Gruber, A., Jarosinski, P. F., Martin, S., Nathan, N., Paul, S. M., Savage, R. E., Wolters, P. L., Schwartz, B., Widemann, B. C., & Biesecker, L. G. (2019). Pharmacodynamic study of miransertib in individuals with proteus syndrome. *American Journal of Human Genetics, 104*, 484–491.
24. Reichardt, L. F. (2006). Neurotrophin-regulated signalling pathways. *Philosophical Transactions of the Royal Society of London. Series B, Biological Sciences, 361*, 1545–1564.
25. Demir, I. E., Tieftrunk, E., Schorn, S., Friess, H., & Ceyhan, G. O. (2016). Nerve growth factor & TrkA as novel therapeutic targets in cancer. *Biochimica et Biophysica Acta, 1866*, 37–50.
26. Lange, A. M., & Lo, H. W. (2018). Inhibiting TRK proteins in clinical cancer therapy. *Cancers (Basel), 10*(4), 105.
27. Bhangoo, M. S., & Sigal, D. (2019). TRK inhibitors: Clinical development of larotrectinib. *Current Oncology Reports, 21*, 14.
28. Hirose, M., Kuroda, Y., & Murata, E. (2016). NGF/TrkA signaling as a therapeutic target for pain. *Pain Practice, 16*, 175–182.
29. Bagal, S. K., Omoto, K., Blakemore, D. C., Bungay, P. J., Bilsland, J. G., Clarke, P. J., Corbett, M. S., Cronin, C. N., Cui, J. J., Dias, R., Flanagan, N. J., Greasley, S. E., Grimley, R., Johnson, E., Fengas, D., Kitching, L., Kraus, M. L., McAlpine, I., Nagata, A., Waldron, G. J., & Warmus, J. S. (2019). Discovery of allosteric, potent, subtype selective, and peripherally restricted TrkA kinase inhibitors. *Journal of Medicinal Chemistry, 62*, 247–265.
30. Fasano, M., Della Corte, C. M., Califano, R., Capuano, A., Troiani, T., Martinelli, E., Ciardiello, F., & Morgillo, F. (2014). Type III or allosteric kinase inhibitors for the treatment of non-small cell lung cancer. *Expert Opinion on Investigational Drugs, 23*, 809–821.
31. Rastelli, G., Anighoro, A., Chripkova, M., Carrassa, L., & Broggini, M. (2014). Structure-based discovery of the first allosteric inhibitors of cyclin-dependent kinase 2. *Cell Cycle, 13*, 2296–2305.
32. Gao, Y., Zhang, P., Cui, A., Ye, D. Y., Xiang, M., & Chu, Y. (2018). Discovery and anti-inflammatory evaluation of benzothiazepinones (BTZs) as novel non-ATP competitive inhibitors of glycogen synthase kinase-3beta (GSK-3beta). *Bioorganic & Medicinal Chemistry, 26*, 5479–5493.
33. Yueh, C., Rettenmaier, J., Xia, B., Hall, D. R., Alekseenko, A., Porter, K. A., Barkovich, K., Keseru, G., Whitty, A., Wells, J. A., Vajda, S., & Kozakov, D. (2019). Kinase atlas: Druggability analysis of potential allosteric sites in kinases. *Journal of Medicinal Chemistry, 62*, 6512–6524.

34. Kozakov, D., Grove, L. E., Hall, D. R., Bohnuud, T., Mottarella, S. E., Luo, L., Xia, B., Beglov, D., & Vajda, S. (2015). The FTMap family of web servers for determining and characterizing ligand-binding hot spots of proteins. *Nature Protocols, 10*, 733–755.
35. Wu, P., Clausen, M. H., & Nielsen, T. E. (2015). Allosteric small-molecule kinase inhibitors. *Pharmacology & Therapeutics, 156*, 59–68.
36. Hancock, C. N., Macias, A., Lee, E. K., Yu, S. Y., Mackerell, A. D., Jr., & Shapiro, P. (2005). Identification of novel extracellular signal-regulated kinase docking domain inhibitors. *Journal of Medicinal Chemistry, 48*, 4586–4595.
37. Chen, F., Hancock, C. N., Macias, A. T., Joh, J., Still, K., Zhong, S., MacKerell, A. D., Jr., & Shapiro, P. (2006). Characterization of ATP-independent ERK inhibitors identified through in silico analysis of the active ERK2 structure. *Bioorganic & Medicinal Chemistry Letters, 16*, 6281–6287.
38. Sammons, R. M., Perry, N. A., Li, Y., Cho, E. J., Piserchio, A., Zamora-Olivares, D. P., Ghose, R., Kaoud, T. S., Debevec, G., Bartholomeusz, C., Gurevich, V. V., Iverson, T. M., Giulianotti, M., Houghten, R. A., & Dalby, K. N. (2019). A novel class of common docking domain inhibitors that prevent ERK2 activation and substrate phosphorylation. *ACS Chemical Biology, 14*, 1183–1194.
39. Kaoud, T. S., Johnson, W. H., Ebelt, N. D., Piserchio, A., Zamora-Olivares, D., Van Ravenstein, S. X., Pridgen, J. R., Edupuganti, R., Sammons, R., Cano, M., Warthaka, M., Harger, M., Tavares, C. D. J., Park, J., Radwan, M. F., Ren, P., Anslyn, E. V., Tsai, K. Y., Ghose, R., & Dalby, K. N. (2019). Modulating multi-functional ERK complexes by covalent targeting of a recruitment site in vivo. *Nature Communications, 10*, 5232.
40. Samadani, R., Zhang, J., Brophy, A., Oashi, T., Priyakumar, U. D., Raman, E. P., St John, F. J., Jung, K. Y., Fletcher, S., Pozharski, E., MacKerell, A. D., Jr., & Shapiro, P. (2015). Small-molecule inhibitors of ERK-mediated immediate early gene expression and proliferation of melanoma cells expressing mutated BRaf. *The Biochemical Journal, 467*, 425–438.
41. Nitta, R. T., Chu, A. H., & Wong, A. J. (2008). Constitutive activity of JNK2 alpha2 is dependent on a unique mechanism of MAPK activation. *The Journal of Biological Chemistry, 283*, 34935–34945.
42. Khokhlatchev, A. V., Canagarajah, B., Wilsbacher, J., Robinson, M., Atkinson, M., Goldsmith, E., & Cobb, M. H. (1998). Phosphorylation of the MAP kinase ERK2 promotes its homodimerization and nuclear translocation. *Cell, 93*, 605–615.
43. Kaoud, T. S., Devkota, A. K., Harris, R., Rana, M. S., Abramczyk, O., Warthaka, M., Lee, S., Girvin, M. E., Riggs, A. F., & Dalby, K. N. (2011). Activated ERK2 is a monomer in vitro with or without divalent cations and when complexed to the cytoplasmic scaffold PEA-15. *Biochemistry, 50*, 4568–4578.
44. Lidke, D. S., Huang, F., Post, J. N., Rieger, B., Wilsbacher, J., Thomas, J. L., Pouyssegur, J., Jovin, T. M., & Lenormand, P. (2010). ERK nuclear translocation is dimerization-independent but controlled by the rate of phosphorylation. *The Journal of Biological Chemistry, 285*, 3092–3102.
45. Casar, B., Pinto, A., & Crespo, P. (2008). Essential role of ERK dimers in the activation of cytoplasmic but not nuclear substrates by ERK-scaffold complexes. *Molecular Cell, 31*, 708–721.
46. Herrero, A., Pinto, A., Colon-Bolea, P., Casar, B., Jones, M., Agudo-Ibanez, L., Vidal, R., Tenbaum, S. P., Nuciforo, P., Valdizan, E. M., Horvath, Z., Orfi, L., Pineda-Lucena, A., Bony, E., Keri, G., Rivas, G., Pazos, A., Gozalbes, R., Palmer, H. G., Hurlstone, A., & Crespo, P. (2015). Small molecule inhibition of ERK dimerization prevents tumorigenesis by RAS-ERK pathway oncogenes. *Cancer Cell, 28*, 170–182.
47. Wilsbacher, J. L., Juang, Y. C., Khokhlatchev, A. V., Gallagher, E., Binns, D., Goldsmith, E. J., & Cobb, M. H. (2006). Characterization of mitogen-activated protein kinase (MAPK) dimers. *Biochemistry, 45*, 13175–13182.
48. Beneker, C. M., Rovoli, M., Kontopidis, G., Roring, M., Galda, S., Braun, S., Brummer, T., & McInnes, C. (2019). Design and synthesis of type-IV inhibitors of BRAF kinase that

block dimerization and overcome paradoxical MEK/ERK activation. *Journal of Medicinal Chemistry, 62*, 3886–3897.
49. Poulikakos, P. I., Zhang, C., Bollag, G., Shokat, K. M., & Rosen, N. (2010). RAF inhibitors transactivate RAF dimers and ERK signalling in cells with wild-type BRAF. *Nature, 464*, 427–430.
50. Kaneto, H. (2005). The JNK pathway as a therapeutic target for diabetes. *Expert Opinion on Therapeutic Targets, 9*, 581–592.
51. Stebbins, J. L., De, S. K., Machleidt, T., Becattini, B., Vazquez, J., Kuntzen, C., Chen, L. H., Cellitti, J. F., Riel-Mehan, M., Emdadi, A., Solinas, G., Karin, M., & Pellecchia, M. (2008). Identification of a new JNK inhibitor targeting the JNK-JIP interaction site. *Proceedings of the National Academy of Sciences of the United States of America, 105*, 16809–16813.
52. Comess, K. M., Sun, C., Abad-Zapatero, C., Goedken, E. R., Gum, R. J., Borhani, D. W., Argiriadi, M., Groebe, D. R., Jia, Y., Clampit, J. E., Haasch, D. L., Smith, H. T., Wang, S., Song, D., Coen, M. L., Cloutier, T. E., Tang, H., Cheng, X., Quinn, C., Liu, B., Xin, Z., Liu, G., Fry, E. H., Stoll, V., Ng, T. I., Banach, D., Marcotte, D., Burns, D. J., Calderwood, D. J., & Hajduk, P. J. (2011). Discovery and characterization of non-ATP site inhibitors of the mitogen activated protein (MAP) kinases. *ACS Chemical Biology, 6*, 234–244.
53. Liu, X., Zhang, C. S., Lu, C., Lin, S. C., Wu, J. W., & Wang, Z. X. (2016). A conserved motif in JNK/p38-specific MAPK phosphatases as a determinant for JNK1 recognition and inactivation. *Nature Communications, 7*, 10879.
54. Chiquet, C., Aptel, F., Creuzot-Garcher, C., Berrod, J. P., Kodjikian, L., Massin, P., Deloche, C., Perino, J., Kirwan, B. A., de Brouwer, S., Combette, J. M., & Behar-Cohen, F. (2017). Postoperative ocular inflammation: A single subconjunctival injection of XG-102 compared to dexamethasone drops in a randomized trial. *American Journal of Ophthalmology, 174*, 76–84.
55. Gourmaud, S., Thomas, P., Thomasseau, S., Tible, M., Abadie, C., Paquet, C., & Hugon, J. (2018). Brimapitide reduced neuronal stress markers and cognitive deficits in 5XFAD transgenic mice. *Journal of Alzheimer's disease, 63*, 665–674.
56. Eshraghi, A. A., Aranke, M., Salvi, R., Ding, D., Coleman, J. K. M., Jr., Ocak, E., Mittal, R., & Meyer, T. (2018). Preclinical and clinical otoprotective applications of cell-penetrating peptide D-JNKI-1 (AM-111). *Hearing Research, 368*, 86–91.
57. Staecker, H., Jokovic, G., Karpishchenko, S., Kienle-Gogolok, A., Krzyzaniak, A., Lin, C. D., Navratil, P., Tzvetkov, V., Wright, N., & Meyer, T. (2019). Efficacy and safety of AM-111 in the treatment of acute unilateral sudden deafness-a double-blind, randomized, placebo-controlled phase 3 study. *Otology & Neurotology, 40*, 584–594.
58. Xing, L. (2015). Clinical candidates of small molecule p38 MAPK inhibitors for inflammatory disease. *MAP Kinase, 4*, 24–30.
59. Shah, N. G., Tulapurkar, M. E., Ramarathnam, A., Brophy, A., Martinez, R., 3rd, Hom, K., Hodges, T., Samadani, R., Singh, I. S., MacKerell, A. D., Jr., Shapiro, P., & Hasday, J. D. (2017). Novel noncatalytic substrate-selective p38alpha-specific MAPK inhibitors with endothelial-stabilizing and anti-inflammatory activity. *Journal of Immunology, 198*, 3296–3306.
60. O'Keefe, S. J., Mudgett, J. S., Cupo, S., Parsons, J. N., Chartrain, N. A., Fitzgerald, C., Chen, S. L., Lowitz, K., Rasa, C., Visco, D., Luell, S., Carballo-Jane, E., Owens, K., & Zaller, D. M. (2007). Chemical genetics define the roles of p38alpha and p38beta in acute and chronic inflammation. *The Journal of Biological Chemistry, 282*, 34663–34671.
61. Ferrari, G., Terushkin, V., Wolff, M. J., Zhang, X., Valacca, C., Poggio, P., Pintucci, G., & Mignatti, P. (2012). TGF-beta1 induces endothelial cell apoptosis by shifting VEGF activation of p38(MAPK) from the prosurvival p38beta to proapoptotic p38alpha. *Molecular Cancer Research, 10*, 605–614.
62. Kim, C., Sano, Y., Todorova, K., Carlson, B. A., Arpa, L., Celada, A., Lawrence, T., Otsu, K., Brissette, J. L., Arthur, J. S., & Park, J. M. (2008). The kinase p38 alpha serves cell

type-specific inflammatory functions in skin injury and coordinates pro- and anti-inflammatory gene expression. *Nature Immunology, 9*, 1019–1027.
63. Zhang, J., Adrian, F. J., Jahnke, W., Cowan-Jacob, S. W., Li, A. G., Iacob, R. E., Sim, T., Powers, J., Dierks, C., Sun, F., Guo, G. R., Ding, Q., Okram, B., Choi, Y., Wojciechowski, A., Deng, X., Liu, G., Fendrich, G., Strauss, A., Vajpai, N., Grzesiek, S., Tuntland, T., Liu, Y., Bursulaya, B., Azam, M., Manley, P. W., Engen, J. R., Daley, G. Q., Warmuth, M., & Gray, N. S. (2010). Targeting Bcr-Abl by combining allosteric with ATP-binding-site inhibitors. *Nature, 463*, 501–506.
64. Adrian, F. J., Ding, Q., Sim, T., Velentza, A., Sloan, C., Liu, Y., Zhang, G., Hur, W., Ding, S., Manley, P., Mestan, J., Fabbro, D., & Gray, N. S. (2006). Allosteric inhibitors of Bcr-abl-dependent cell proliferation. *Nature Chemical Biology, 2*, 95–102.
65. Rossari, F., Minutolo, F., & Orciuolo, E. (2018). Past, present, and future of Bcr-Abl inhibitors: From chemical development to clinical efficacy. *Journal of Hematology & Oncology, 11*, 84.
66. Maurer-Stroh, S., Gouda, M., Novatchkova, M., Schleiffer, A., Schneider, G., Sirota, F. L., Wildpaner, M., Hayashi, N., & Eisenhaber, F. (2004). MYRbase: Analysis of genome-wide glycine myristoylation enlarges the functional spectrum of eukaryotic myristoylated proteins. *Genome Biology, 5*, R21.
67. Yang, J., Campobasso, N., Biju, M. P., Fisher, K., Pan, X. Q., Cottom, J., Galbraith, S., Ho, T., Zhang, H., Hong, X., Ward, P., Hofmann, G., Siegfried, B., Zappacosta, F., Washio, Y., Cao, P., Qu, J., Bertrand, S., Wang, D. Y., Head, M. S., Li, H., Moores, S., Lai, Z., Johanson, K., Burton, G., Erickson-Miller, C., Simpson, G., Tummino, P., Copeland, R. A., & Oliff, A. (2011). Discovery and characterization of a cell-permeable, small-molecule c-Abl kinase activator that binds to the myristoyl binding site. *Chemistry & Biology, 18*, 177–186.
68. Noren, N. K., Foos, G., Hauser, C. A., & Pasquale, E. B. (2006). The EphB4 receptor suppresses breast cancer cell tumorigenicity through an Abl-Crk pathway. *Nature Cell Biology, 8*, 815–825.
69. Mora, A., Komander, D., van Aalten, D. M., & Alessi, D. R. (2004). PDK1, the master regulator of AGC kinase signal transduction. *Seminars in Cell & Developmental Biology, 15*, 161–170.
70. Biondi, R. M., Kieloch, A., Currie, R. A., Deak, M., & Alessi, D. R. (2001). The PIF-binding pocket in PDK1 is essential for activation of S6K and SGK, but not PKB. *The EMBO Journal, 20*, 4380–4390.
71. Rettenmaier, T. J., Sadowsky, J. D., Thomsen, N. D., Chen, S. C., Doak, A. K., Arkin, M. R., & Wells, J. A. (2014). A small-molecule mimic of a peptide docking motif inhibits the protein kinase PDK1. *Proceedings of the National Academy of Sciences of the United States of America, 111*, 18590–18595.
72. Medina, J. R., Becker, C. J., Blackledge, C. W., Duquenne, C., Feng, Y., Grant, S. W., Heerding, D., Li, W. H., Miller, W. H., Romeril, S. P., Scherzer, D., Shu, A., Bobko, M. A., Chadderton, A. R., Dumble, M., Gardiner, C. M., Gilbert, S., Liu, Q., Rabindran, S. K., Sudakin, V., Xiang, H., Brady, P. G., Campobasso, N., Ward, P., & Axten, J. M. (2011). Structure-based design of potent and selective 3-phosphoinositide-dependent kinase-1 (PDK1) inhibitors. *Journal of Medicinal Chemistry, 54*, 1871–1895.
73. Betzi, S., Alam, R., Martin, M., Lubbers, D. J., Han, H., Jakkaraj, S. R., Georg, G. I., & Schonbrunn, E. (2011). Discovery of a potential allosteric ligand binding site in CDK2. *ACS Chemical Biology, 6*, 492–501.
74. Powell, J. D., Pollizzi, K. N., Heikamp, E. B., & Horton, M. R. (2012). Regulation of immune responses by mTOR. *Annual Review of Immunology, 30*, 39–68.
75. Li, J., Kim, S. G., & Blenis, J. (2014). Rapamycin: One drug, many effects. *Cell Metabolism, 19*, 373–379.
76. Hausch, F., Kozany, C., Theodoropoulou, M., & Fabian, A. K. (2013). FKBPs and the Akt/mTOR pathway. *Cell Cycle, 12*, 2366–2370.

77. Tak, P. P., & Firestein, G. S. (2001). NF-kappaB: A key role in inflammatory diseases. *The Journal of Clinical Investigation, 107*, 7–11.
78. Gupta, S. C., Sundaram, C., Reuter, S., & Aggarwal, B. B. (2010). Inhibiting NF-kappaB activation by small molecules as a therapeutic strategy. *Biochimica et Biophysica Acta, 1799*, 775–787.
79. Burke, J. R., Pattoli, M. A., Gregor, K. R., Brassil, P. J., MacMaster, J. F., McIntyre, K. W., Yang, X., Iotzova, V. S., Clarke, W., Strnad, J., Qiu, Y., & Zusi, F. C. (2003). BMS-345541 is a highly selective inhibitor of I kappa B kinase that binds at an allosteric site of the enzyme and blocks NF-kappa B-dependent transcription in mice. *The Journal of Biological Chemistry, 278*, 1450–1456.
80. Gower, C. M., Chang, M. E., & Maly, D. J. (2014). Bivalent inhibitors of protein kinases. *Critical Reviews in Biochemistry and Molecular Biology, 49*, 102–115.
81. Profit, A. A., Lee, T. R., & Lawrence, D. S. (1999). Bivalent inhibitors of protein tyrosine kinases. *Journal of the American Chemical Society, 121*, 280–283.
82. Xu, W., Doshi, A., Lei, M., Eck, M. J., & Harrison, S. C. (1999). Crystal structures of c-Src reveal features of its autoinhibitory mechanism. *Molecular Cell, 3*, 629–638.
83. Brandvold, K. R., Santos, S. M., Breen, M. E., Lachacz, E. J., Steffey, M. E., & Soellner, M. B. (2015). Exquisitely specific bisubstrate inhibitors of c-Src kinase. *ACS Chemical Biology, 10*, 1387–1391.
84. Johnson, T. K., & Soellner, M. B. (2016). Bivalent inhibitors of c-Src tyrosine kinase that bind a regulatory domain. *Bioconjugate Chemistry, 27*, 1745–1749.
85. Hill, Z. B., Perera, B. G., & Maly, D. J. (2009). A chemical genetic method for generating bivalent inhibitors of protein kinases. *Journal of the American Chemical Society, 131*, 6686–6688.
86. Hill, Z. B., Perera, B. G., Andrews, S. S., & Maly, D. J. (2012). Targeting diverse signaling interaction sites allows the rapid generation of bivalent kinase inhibitors. *ACS Chemical Biology, 7*, 487–495.
87. Hill, Z. B., Perera, B. G., & Maly, D. J. (2011). Bivalent inhibitors of the tyrosine kinases ABL and SRC: Determinants of potency and selectivity. *Molecular BioSystems, 7*, 447–456.
88. Tiwari, R., & Parang, K. (2009). Protein conjugates of SH3-domain ligands and ATP-competitive inhibitors as bivalent inhibitors of protein kinases. *Chembiochem, 10*, 2445–2448.
89. Gower, C. M., Thomas, J. R., Harrington, E., Murphy, J., Chang, M. E., Cornella-Taracido, I., Jain, R. K., Schirle, M., & Maly, D. J. (2016). Conversion of a single polypharmacological agent into selective bivalent inhibitors of intracellular kinase activity. *ACS Chemical Biology, 11*, 121–131.
90. Wong, M. L., Murphy, J., Harrington, E., Gower, C. M., Jain, R. K., Schirle, M., & Thomas, J. R. (2016). Examining the influence of specificity ligands and ATP-competitive ligands on the overall effectiveness of bivalent kinase inhibitors. *Proteome Science, 15*, 17.
91. Stebbins, J. L., De, S. K., Pavlickova, P., Chen, V., Machleidt, T., Chen, L. H., Kuntzen, C., Kitada, S., Karin, M., & Pellecchia, M. (2011). Design and characterization of a potent and selective dual ATP- and substrate-competitive subnanomolar bidentate c-Jun N-terminal kinase (JNK) inhibitor. *Journal of Medicinal Chemistry, 54*, 6206–6214.
92. Lechtenberg, B. C., Mace, P. D., Sessions, E. H., Williamson, R., Stalder, R., Wallez, Y., Roth, G. P., Riedl, S. J., & Pasquale, E. B. (2017). Structure-guided strategy for the development of potent bivalent ERK inhibitors. *ACS Medicinal Chemistry Letters, 8*, 726–731.
93. Toyama, K., Kobayakawa, T., Nomura, W., & Tamamura, H. (2018). Inhibition of EGFR activation by bivalent ligands based on a cyclic peptide mimicking the dimerization arm structure of EGFR. *Chemical & Pharmaceutical Bulletin, 66*, 1083–1089.
94. Kedika, S. R., & Udugamasooriya, D. G. (2018). Converting a weaker ATP-binding site inhibitor into a potent hetero-bivalent ligand by tethering to a unique peptide sequence derived from the same kinase. *Organic & Biomolecular Chemistry, 16*, 6443–6449.
95. Asati, V., Mahapatra, D. K., & Bharti, S. K. (2019). PIM kinase inhibitors: Structural and pharmacological perspectives. *European Journal of Medicinal Chemistry, 172*, 95–108.

96. Ekambaram, R., Enkvist, E., Vaasa, A., Kasari, M., Raidaru, G., Knapp, S., & Uri, A. (2013). Selective bisubstrate inhibitors with sub-nanomolar affinity for protein kinase Pim-1. *ChemMedChem, 8*, 909–913.
97. Lewis, A. L., & Richard, J. (2015). Challenges in the delivery of peptide drugs: An industry perspective. *Therapeutic Delivery, 6*, 149–163.
98. Vane, J. R., & Botting, R. M. (2003). The mechanism of action of aspirin. *Thrombosis Research, 110*, 255–258.
99. Zhao, Z., & Bourne, P. E. (2018). Progress with covalent small-molecule kinase inhibitors. *Drug Discovery Today, 23*, 727–735.
100. Gehringer, M., & Laufer, S. A. (2019). Emerging and re-emerging warheads for targeted covalent inhibitors: Applications in medicinal chemistry and chemical biology. *Journal of Medicinal Chemistry, 62*, 5673–5724.
101. Serafimova, I. M., Pufall, M. A., Krishnan, S., Duda, K., Cohen, M. S., Maglathlin, R. L., McFarland, J. M., Miller, R. M., Frodin, M., & Taunton, J. (2012). Reversible targeting of noncatalytic cysteines with chemically tuned electrophiles. *Nature Chemical Biology, 8*, 471–476.
102. Krishnan, S., Miller, R. M., Tian, B., Mullins, R. D., Jacobson, M. P., & Taunton, J. (2014). Design of reversible, cysteine-targeted Michael acceptors guided by kinetic and computational analysis. *Journal of the American Chemical Society, 136*, 12624–12630.
103. Wymann, M. P., Bulgarelli-Leva, G., Zvelebil, M. J., Pirola, L., Vanhaesebroeck, B., Waterfield, M. D., & Panayotou, G. (1996). Wortmannin inactivates phosphoinositide 3-kinase by covalent modification of Lys-802, a residue involved in the phosphate transfer reaction. *Molecular and Cellular Biology, 16*, 1722–1733.
104. Dalton, S. E., Dittus, L., Thomas, D. A., Convery, M. A., Nunes, J., Bush, J. T., Evans, J. P., Werner, T., Bantscheff, M., Murphy, J. A., & Campos, S. (2018). Selectively targeting the kinome-conserved lysine of PI3Kdelta as a general approach to covalent kinase inhibition. *Journal of the American Chemical Society, 140*, 932–939.
105. Pitz, M. W., Eisenhauer, E. A., MacNeil, M. V., Thiessen, B., Easaw, J. C., Macdonald, D. R., Eisenstat, D. D., Kakumanu, A. S., Salim, M., Chalchal, H., Squire, J., Tsao, M. S., Kamel-Reid, S., Banerji, S., Tu, D., Powers, J., Hausman, D. F., & Mason, W. P. (2015). Phase II study of PX-866 in recurrent glioblastoma. *Neuro-Oncology, 17*, 1270–1274.
106. Roskoski, R., Jr. (2019). Small molecule inhibitors targeting the EGFR/ErbB family of protein-tyrosine kinases in human cancers. *Pharmacological Research, 139*, 395–411.
107. Tomassi, S., Lategahn, J., Engel, J., Keul, M., Tumbrink, H. L., Ketzer, J., Muhlenberg, T., Baumann, M., Schultz-Fademrecht, C., Bauer, S., & Rauh, D. (2017). Indazole-based covalent inhibitors to target drug-resistant epidermal growth factor receptor. *Journal of Medicinal Chemistry, 60*, 2361–2372.
108. Landi, L., & Cappuzzo, F. (2013). Irreversible EGFR-TKIs: Dreaming perfection. *Translational Lung Cancer Research, 2*, 40–49.
109. Engel, J., Lategahn, J., & Rauh, D. (2016). Hope and disappointment: Covalent inhibitors to overcome drug resistance in non-small cell lung cancer. *ACS Medicinal Chemistry Letters, 7*, 2–5.
110. van der Wekken, A. J., Saber, A., Hiltermann, T. J., Kok, K., van den Berg, A., & Groen, H. J. (2016). Resistance mechanisms after tyrosine kinase inhibitors afatinib and crizotinib in non-small cell lung cancer, a review of the literature. *Critical Reviews in Oncology/Hematology, 100*, 107–116.
111. Roskoski, R., Jr. (2016). Ibrutinib inhibition of bruton protein-tyrosine kinase (BTK) in the treatment of B cell neoplasms. *Pharmacological Research, 113*, 395–408.
112. Woyach, J. A., Ruppert, A. S., Guinn, D., Lehman, A., Blachly, J. S., Lozanski, A., Heerema, N. A., Zhao, W., Coleman, J., Jones, D., Abruzzo, L., Gordon, A., Mantel, R., Smith, L. L., McWhorter, S., Davis, M., Doong, T. J., Ny, F., Lucas, M., Chase, W., Jones, J. A., Flynn, J. M., Maddocks, K., Rogers, K., Jaglowski, S., Andritsos, L. A., Awan, F. T., Blum, K. A., Grever, M. R., Lozanski, G., Johnson, A. J., & Byrd, J. C. (2017). BTK(C481S)-mediated

resistance to ibrutinib in chronic lymphocytic leukemia. *Journal of Clinical Oncology, 35*, 1437–1443.
113. Byrd, J. C., Smith, S., Wagner-Johnston, N., Sharman, J., Chen, A. I., Advani, R., Augustson, B., Marlton, P., Renee Commerford, S., Okrah, K., Liu, L., Murray, E., Penuel, E., Ward, A. F., & Flinn, I. W. (2018). First-in-human phase 1 study of the BTK inhibitor GDC-0853 in relapsed or refractory B-cell NHL and CLL. *Oncotarget, 9*, 13023–13035.
114. Byrd, J. C., Wierda, W. G., Schuh, A., Devereux, S., Chaves, J. M., Brown, J. R., Hillmen, P., Martin, P., Awan, F. T., Stephens, D. M., Ghia, P., Barrientos, J., Pagel, J. M., Woyach, J. A., Burke, K., Covey, T., Gulrajani, M., Hamdy, A., Izumi, R., Frigault, M. M., Patel, P., Rothbaum, W., Wang, M. H., O'Brien, S., & Furman, R. R. (2020). Acalabrutinib monotherapy in patients with relapsed/refractory chronic lymphocytic leukemia: Updated phase 2 results. *Blood, 135*(15), 1204–1213.
115. Zhang, T., Inesta-Vaquera, F., Niepel, M., Zhang, J., Ficarro, S. B., Machleidt, T., Xie, T., Marto, J. A., Kim, N., Sim, T., Laughlin, J. D., Park, H., LoGrasso, P. V., Patricelli, M., Nomanbhoy, T. K., Sorger, P. K., Alessi, D. R., & Gray, N. S. (2012). Discovery of potent and selective covalent inhibitors of JNK. *Chemistry & Biology, 19*, 140–154.
116. Ward, R. A., Colclough, N., Challinor, M., Debreczeni, J. E., Eckersley, K., Fairley, G., Feron, L., Flemington, V., Graham, M. A., Greenwood, R., Hopcroft, P., Howard, T. D., James, M., Jones, C. D., Jones, C. R., Renshaw, J., Roberts, K., Snow, L., Tonge, M., & Yeung, K. (2015). Structure-guided design of highly selective and potent covalent inhibitors of ERK1/2. *Journal of Medicinal Chemistry, 58*, 4790–4801.
117. Kwiatkowski, N., Zhang, T., Rahl, P. B., Abraham, B. J., Reddy, J., Ficarro, S. B., Dastur, A., Amzallag, A., Ramaswamy, S., Tesar, B., Jenkins, C. E., Hannett, N. M., McMillin, D., Sanda, T., Sim, T., Kim, N. D., Look, T., Mitsiades, C. S., Weng, A. P., Brown, J. R., Benes, C. H., Marto, J. A., Young, R. A., & Gray, N. S. (2014). Targeting transcription regulation in cancer with a covalent CDK7 inhibitor. *Nature, 511*, 616–620.
118. Hu, S., Marineau, J. J., Rajagopal, N., Hamman, K. B., Choi, Y. J., Schmidt, D. R., Ke, N., Johannessen, L., Bradley, M. J., Orlando, D. A., Alnemy, S. R., Ren, Y., Ciblat, S., Winter, D. K., Kabro, A., Sprott, K. T., Hodgson, J. G., Fritz, C. C., Carulli, J. P., di Tomaso, E., & Olson, E. R. (2019). Discovery and characterization of SY-1365, a selective, covalent inhibitor of CDK7. *Cancer Research, 79*, 3479–3491.
119. Gao, Y., Zhang, T., Terai, H., Ficarro, S. B., Kwiatkowski, N., Hao, M. F., Sharma, B., Christensen, C. L., Chipumuro, E., Wong, K. K., Marto, J. A., Hammerman, P. S., Gray, N. S., & George, R. E. (2018). Overcoming resistance to the THZ series of covalent transcriptional CDK inhibitors. *Cell Chemical Biology, 25*, 135–142.e5.
120. Weisner, J., Gontla, R., van der Westhuizen, L., Oeck, S., Ketzer, J., Janning, P., Richters, A., Muhlenberg, T., Fang, Z., Taher, A., Jendrossek, V., Pelly, S. C., Bauer, S., van Otterlo, W. A., & Rauh, D. (2015). Covalent-allosteric kinase inhibitors. *Angewandte Chemie (International Ed. in English), 54*, 10313–10316.
121. Weisner, J., Landel, I., Reintjes, C., Uhlenbrock, N., Trajkovic-Arsic, M., Dienstbier, N., Hardick, J., Ladigan, S., Lindemann, M., Smith, S., Quambusch, L., Scheinpflug, R., Depta, L., Gontla, R., Unger, A., Muller, H., Baumann, M., Schultz-Fademrecht, C., Gunther, G., Maghnouj, A., Muller, M. P., Pohl, M., Teschendorf, C., Wolters, H., Viebahn, R., Tannapfel, A., Uhl, W., Hengstler, J. G., Hahn, S. A., Siveke, J. T., & Rauh, D. (2019). Preclinical efficacy of covalent-allosteric AKT inhibitor borussertib in combination with trametinib in KRAS-mutant pancreatic and colorectal Cancer. *Cancer Research, 79*, 2367–2378.
122. Park, K., Tan, E. H., O'Byrne, K., Zhang, L., Boyer, M., Mok, T., Hirsh, V., Yang, J. C., Lee, K. H., Lu, S., Shi, Y., Kim, S. W., Laskin, J., Kim, D. W., Arvis, C. D., Kolbeck, K., Laurie, S. A., Tsai, C. M., Shahidi, M., Kim, M., Massey, D., Zazulina, V., & Paz-Ares, L. (2016). Afatinib versus gefitinib as first-line treatment of patients with EGFR mutation-positive non-small-cell lung cancer (LUX-lung 7): A phase 2B, open-label, randomised controlled trial. *The Lancet Oncology, 17*, 577–589.

123. Burger, J. A., Barr, P. M., Robak, T., Owen, C., Ghia, P., Tedeschi, A., Bairey, O., Hillmen, P., Coutre, S. E., Devereux, S., Grosicki, S., McCarthy, H., Simpson, D., Offner, F., Moreno, C., Dai, S., Lal, I., Dean, J. P., & Kipps, T. J. (2020). Long-term efficacy and safety of first-line ibrutinib treatment for patients with CLL/SLL: 5 years of follow-up from the phase 3 RESONATE-2 study. *Leukemia, 34*(3), 787–798.
124. Liu, R., Yue, Z., Tsai, C. C., & Shen, J. (2019). Assessing lysine and cysteine reactivities for designing targeted covalent kinase inhibitors. *Journal of the American Chemical Society, 141*, 6553–6560.

Protein Kinase Interactions with Regulatory and Effector Proteins

Amy Defnet, Ramon Martinez III, and Paul Shapiro

Abstract The previous chapters discussed the general structure of protein kinases and signaling networks that kinases use to transmit extracellular signals from plasma membrane receptors through the cell to cause changes in gene expression and cellular responses. This chapter will take a closer look at the interactions between protein kinases and their substrates and interacting partners. Despite the well-conserved organization of the ATP-binding and -catalytic site, kinases have quite diverse functions depending on the substrate that is phosphorylated. Some kinases may phosphorylate and regulate only a couple of substrates whereas other kinases may phosphorylate hundreds of different substrates. The mechanisms by which kinases recognize specific substrates are still being revealed. This chapter will describe some of the structural features that determine kinase recognition of specific protein substrates. Experimental evidence that specific kinases can phosphorylate dozens of substrates will lend support to the idea that complete inhibition of specific disease-related kinases, as currently done with type I–III kinase inhibitors, may also inhibit kinase functions that have beneficial effects. The theme of this and subsequent chapters is to show the structural features that determine specific protein kinase–substrate interactions and to highlight new approaches that inhibit the kinase interactions and functions that are involved in disease while preserving kinase activities that have clinical benefits.

Keywords Protein kinase · Substrates · Protein-protein interactions · Docking domains · Function-selective inhibition

A. Defnet · R. Martinez III · P. Shapiro (✉)
Department of Pharmaceutical Sciences, University of Maryland School of Pharmacy, Baltimore, MD, USA
e-mail: amy.defnet@umaryland.edu; rmartinez@umaryland.edu; pshapiro@rx.umaryland.edu

P. Shapiro (ed.), *Next Generation Kinase Inhibitors*,
https://doi.org/10.1007/978-3-030-48283-1_4

Introduction

In 2002, significant progress in understanding kinases was made with the determination of the human kinome and the phylogenetic classification of more than 500 kinases encoded in the human genome [1]. Research over the last 30 years has revealed the pleiotropic effects of protein kinases through their ability to regulate a diverse set of substrates and cellular functions. However, the functions for many of these kinases and their substrates are still being elucidated. To facilitate the understanding of protein kinase functions, several bioinformatics tools are available that have collated current information on kinase signaling networks and are used to determine potential substrates. In addition, several computational and structural biology tools available allow experimental examination of the exquisite and unique structural features that determine how kinases interact with specific substrates. These resources provide starting points for the development of new approaches to inhibit specific protein kinase functions through targeted disruption of select substrates.

Many of these bioinformatics resources are publicly available and provide important information on known kinases and substrate phosphorylation events. The Universal Protein Resource (UniProt; www.uniprot.org; Swiss-Prot Protein Knowledgebase [2]) contains excellent information on all identified proteins, and a list of all protein kinases is available (https://www.uniprot.org/docs/pkinfam). PhosphoSitePlus is a database that was developed over 15 years ago and has compiled nearly 300,000 phosphorylation sites based on peer-reviewed publications and unpublished data using mass spectrometry [3]. This compilation of data provides extensive information on individual phosphorylation sites, their potential function in vivo and in vitro, and primary supporting references. Protein phosphorylation events and other posttranslational modifications have also been well-documented on the bioinformatics resource iPTMnet (https://research.bioinformatics.udel.edu/iptmnet/). Other publicly available databases, such as KinaseNET: Human Protein Kinase Knowledgebank (www.kinasenet.ca), have archived extensive information on specific protein kinases, their substrates, and regulation by phosphorylation [4]. In cases where phosphorylation regulation of a protein is not known, there are resources available that use computational predictions to identify phosphorylation sites and the putative kinase involved. For example, putative phosphorylation events for a select number of kinases can be evaluated using NetPhos [5] and Phosphopredict bioinformatics [6].

Docking Interactions Between Protein Kinases and Other Proteins

Despite a remarkable similarity in the three-dimensional structure, protein kinases have the unique ability to be quite selective in the substrates they target and the amino acids they phosphorylate. Parameters such as proximity within intracellular locations and protein expression levels will certainly impact the ability for proteins to interact. Additional key determinants that facilitate protein kinase recognition and phosphorylation of a unique substrate include the amino acids that surround the serine, threonine, or tyrosine phosphorylation sites and other distant structural features that coordinate protein-protein interactions. A review by Ubersax and Ferrell provides a comprehensive description of protein kinase recognition of substrates and the determinants of phosphorylation specificity [7]. As was described in previous chapters, the kinase domain is the major determinant of whether serine/threonine versus tyrosine phosphorylation will occur depending on the size of the catalytic cleft and its ability to accommodate the bulkier tyrosine residue. In addition, the consensus basic, acidic, hydrophobic, or proline residues that surround the serine, threonine, or tyrosine phosphorylation sites will determine protein kinase specificity. Several other reviews provide detailed summaries of consensus phosphorylation site sequences on substrates and the kinases that target them [7–9].

Protein kinases also coordinate with substrates through specific interactions on regions that are distal from the catalytic cleft. Miller and Turk [9] provide an excellent summary of the features that determine interactions between kinases and substrates including the phosphorylation motif and adjacent docking interactions, distal docking sites, and the coordination with adaptor proteins to help facilitate interactions. This section will focus on the *m*itogen-*a*ctivated *p*rotein *k*inases (MAPKs) as the paradigm for examples of kinase-substrate interactions. Previous chapters outlined the major MAPK signaling pathways from the plasma membrane receptor to the kinase cascade that mediates changes in gene expression and cellular functions. This chapter will summarize the general features that regulate protein-protein interactions in MAPK signaling networks. Subsequent chapters will expand upon these structural interactions and provide additional details on the critical features that determine how protein kinases regulate specific substrates. Understanding the features that regulate these protein-protein interactions will facilitate the rationale design of molecules that disrupt the interactions that are relevant in the progression of disease.

The individual MAPK proteins represent key nodes where signaling information converges on the activation of MAPK through phosphorylation of a conserved threonine-any amino acid-tyrosine (TXY) motif by selective MAP2K (MEK) proteins. The pairing of the conventional MAP2K and corresponding MAPK is shown in Table 1. While the conventional MAP2K-MAPK interactions will be the starting point for discussions on protein kinase–substrate interactions, it should be noted that there are also atypical MAPK isoforms that do not follow this mode of regulation [10]. The atypical MAPKs, including MAPK6/4/15 (ERK3/4/7/8), while structurally similar to conventional MAPK proteins, do not appear to have corresponding MAP2K activators but are regulated through autophosphorylation or other kinases [11–13].

As indicated, MAP2K isoforms phosphorylate TXY motifs to activate their respective MAPK. However, another determinant of selectivity of MAP2K-MAPK pairing is through protein-protein interactions that are distal to the site of phosphorylation. The MAP2K proteins contain unique D-domain motifs consisting of

Table 1 Typical MAP2K (MEK) isoforms and their corresponding MAPK substrates

MAP2K (MEK) isoform →	MAPK (common name) isoform target
MAP2K1/2 (MEK1/2)	MAPK1/3 (ERK1/2)
MAP2K3/6 (MEK3/6)	MAPK14/11 (p38α/β) MAPK13/12 (p38δ/γ)
MAP2K5 (MEK5)	MAPK7 (ERK5)
MAP2K4/7 (MEK4/7)	MAPK8/9/10 (JNK1/2/3)

Table 2 Sequence alignment of amino acid residues in the N-terminus of MAP2K (MEK) isoforms

```
MAP2K1 (MEK1)-----------------------------------MPKKKP--TPIQLNPA-PDGSA-VN
MAP2K2 (MEK2)----------------------------------MLARRKPVLPALTINPTIAEGPS-PT
MAP2K3 (MEK3)----------------------------------------------------------ME
MAP2K6 (MEK6)------------------------------------------------------------
MAP2K4 (MEK4)-----------------------------------MAAPSPSGGGGSGGGSGSGTPGPVG
MAP2K7 (MEK7)MAASSLEQKLSRLEAKLKQENREARRRIDLNLDISPQRPRPTLQLPLANDGGSRSP--SS

MAP2K1 (MEK1)GTSSAETN-LEALQ---KKLEELELDEQ---------------------------QRKRL
MAP2K2 (MEK2)SEGASEAN-LVDLQ---KKLEELELDEQ---------------------------QKKRL
MAP2K3 (MEK3)SPASSQPASMPQSKGKSKRKKDLRISCMS-KPPAP---NPTPP------------RNLDS
MAP2K6 (MEK6)---------MSQSKGK-KRNPGLKIPKEAFEQPQT---SSTPP------------RDLDS
MAP2K4 (MEK4)SPAPGHPA-VSSMQGK-RKALKLNFANPPFKSTARFTLNPNPTGVQNPHIERLRTHSIES
MAP2K7 (MEK7)ESSPQHP--TPPA----RPRHMLGLPSTLFTPRSM---ESIEI---DQKLQ----EIMKQ
```

Highlighted in green are the basic, linker, and underlined hydrophobic residues that contribute to the D-domain as previously described [14]. The N-terminal methionine is highlighted in red

basic residues in the N-terminal domains connected through a short linker to hydrophobic residues. Table 2 shows a sequence alignment of the major MAP2K isoforms and the sequences that have been identified to form the D-domain [14]. Except for MAP2K7, which will be discussed in more detail later, MAP2K isoforms have a single consensus D-domain sequence. The D-domain residues on MAP2K proteins selectively interact with specific sequences on MAPK proteins that form the *D*-domain *r*ecruitment *s*ite (DRS). The DRS of MAPK isoforms is made up of C-terminal acidic residues that are referred to as the *c*ommon *d*ocking (CD) domain (Table 3) and N-terminal hydrophobic and variable residues (Table 4). The variable residues on p38 MAPK isoforms include a glutamate (E) and aspartate (*D*) and are referred to as the ED domain. Although the ED residues are different on other MAPKs, the ED designation is used as a general descriptor of this site within the DRS of all MAPK sequences (Fig. 1).

A second docking domain that has been identified on MAP kinase regulatory and downstream substrate proteins is referred to as the *d*ocking site for *E*RK, *F*-X-F (DEF) motif [15, 16]. The FXF motif is typically separated from the serine or threonine phosphorylation sites by 6–20 amino acids and is found on transcription factors, scaffold proteins, and MAP kinase phosphatases [17]. The F-site *r*ecruitment *s*ite (FRS) on MAP kinases consists primarily of hydrophobic amino acids C-terminal to the activation loop (Table 5) that form specific contacts with hydrophobic phenylalanine residues in the FXF motif.

Table 3 Sequence alignment of C-terminal acidic residues (green shading) that form the common docking (CD) residues and contribute to the D-domain recruitment site (DRS) on human MAPK isoforms

MAPK1	(ERK2)	HPYLEQYYDPSDEPIAEA
MAPK3	(ERK1)	HPYLEQYYDPTDEPVAEE
MAPK14	(p38α)	HAYFAQYHDPDDEPVADP
MAPK11	(p38β)	HAYFSQYHDPEDEPEAEP
MAPK8	(JNK1)	HPYINVWYDPSEAEAPPP
MAPK9	(JNK2)	HPYITVWYDPAEAEAPPP

Table 4 Sequence alignment of amino acid residues in the N-terminus that contribute to the DRS on human MAPK isoforms

MAPK1	(ERK2)	HSANVLHRDLKPSNLLLNTTCDLKICDFGLARVADPDHDHTGFLTEY
MAPK3	(ERK1)	HSANVLHRDLKPSNLLINTTCDLKICDFGLARIADPEHDHTGFLTEY
MAPK14	(p38α)	HSADIIHRDLKPSNLAVNEDCELKILDFGLARHTDDE------MTGY
MAPK11	(p38β)	HSAGIIHRDLKPSNVAVNEDCELRILDFGLARQADEE------MTGY
MAPK8	(JNK1)	HSAGIIHRDLKPSNIVVKSDCTLKILDFGLARTAGTSF----MMTPY
MAPK9	(JNK2)	HSAGIIHRDLKPSNIVVKSDCTLKILDFGLARTACTNF----MMTPY

Hydrophobic and variable residues of the ED domain are underlined and highlighted in purple. The conserved DFG motif and activating phosphorylation sites of MAPK isoforms are shown in yellow and cyan, respectively

The spatial organization of the combined CD and ED amino acids to form the DRS and the FRS residues on the ERK2, p38α, and JNK1 MAP kinases is depicted in Fig. 2. The DRS and FRS are positioned on opposite sides of the kinase in these static models. It is also likely that other transient interactions occur that determine substrate interactions depending on the kinase activation state. For example, structural studies on ERK2 using hydrogen deuterium exchange mass spectrometry suggest that accessibility to the FRS by substrates is limited prior to activation, and it is only after phosphorylation of ERK2 at the active sites does a conformational change in the FRS facilitate the interactions with substrates containing the DEF motif [15]. The structural features of the DRS and FRS have previously been used to identify function-selective small-molecular-weight type IV inhibitors of ERK2 and p38α MAP kinases [18–21].

MAP Kinase Interactions Through the DRS

The DRS on MAP kinases provides a docking domain for specific interactions with an upstream MAP2K activator and downstream effector proteins. The number and type of substrates regulated by the specific MAP kinases can vary extensively. For example, it has been suggested that the ERK1/2, p38α/β, and JNK1/2 MAP kinases

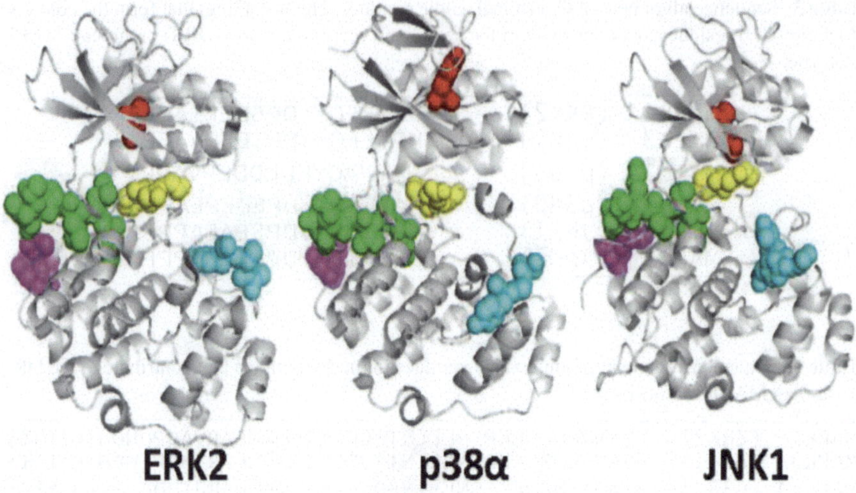

Fig. 1 The D-domain recruitment site (purple and green spheres) sits adjacent to the DFG motif (yellow) and opposite of the activation sites (blue). The conserved lysine in the ATP-binding site is shown in red. Protein Data Bank structures used for ERK2 (MAPK1), p38α (MAPK14), and JNK1 (MAPK8) were 4GT3, 5ETI, and 3O17, respectively

Table 5 Sequence alignment of the FRS between major MAPK proteins

MAPK8 (JNK1)	TPYVVTRYYRAPEVILG-MGYKENVDLWSVGCIMGEMVCHKILFPGRDYIDQW234...Y259
MAPK1 (ERK2)	TEYVATRWYRAPEIMLNSKGYTKSIDIWSVGCILAEMLSNRPIFPGKHYLDQL237...Y263
MAPK14 (p38α)	TGYVATRWYRAPEIMLNWMHYNQTVDIWSVGCIMAELLTGRTLFPGTDHIDQL232...Y258

Amino acids in the FRS are underlined and highlighted in green. The numbering of the C-terminal residues in the FRS is indicated. The conserved activating phosphorylation sites and APE motif at the end of the activation loop for major human MAPK isoforms are shown in cyan and yellow, respectively

may have more than 300, 100, and 80 substrates and binding partners, respectively [22–24]. Although some overlap exists, many of these substrates and binding partners selectively interact with their respective MAP kinase. Given the sequence similarity of the DRS across MAP kinases, the question arises as to how do MAP kinases identify and interact with their unique substrate? Earlier reports provided evidence that ED domain residues provided selectivity for substrate recognition [25, 26]. Tanoue et al. demonstrated that exchanging the ED residues between p38α and ERK2 MAP kinases could alter substrate recognition so that p38α could interact with an ERK2 substrate and vice versa [26]. This demonstrated the importance of the ED domain residues in determining substrate selectivity between structurally similar MAP protein kinases. Using D-domain peptides that represented substrates of ERK2, p38α, and JNK1 MAP kinases, Garai et al. examined structural features that determined selectivity between MAPKs and peptides representing interacting proteins [27]. These studies provided additional insight to key interactions within a docking groove that sits between the CD and ED residues and allow MAP kinases to discriminate between their substrates and binding partners.

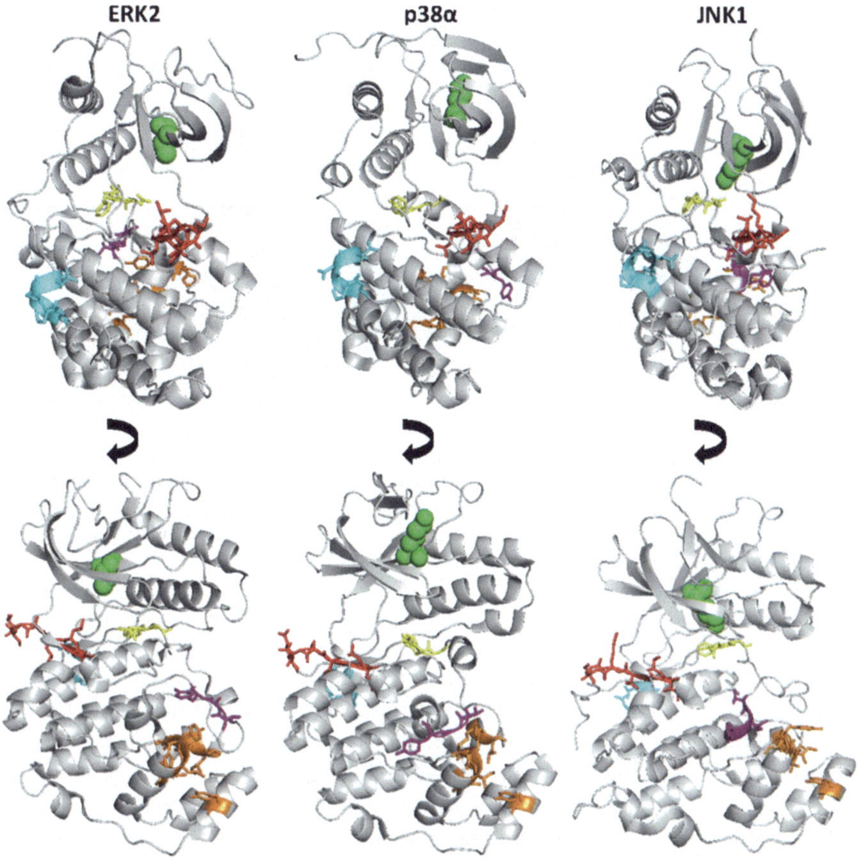

Fig. 2 Spatial organization of the DRS and FRS on MAP kinases. The ribbon structures of ERK2 (pdb:4GT3), p38α (pdb:5ETI), and JNK1 (pdb: 3O17) are shown highlighting the conserved lysine in the ATP catalytic site (green), the DFG motif (yellow), and TXY activation sites (magenta). The DRS comprising CD (cyan) and ED (red) residues and the FRS (orange) are highlighted. As shown here and in all subsequent figures, the N-terminal and C-terminal lobes of the protein kinase are positioned at the top and bottom, respectively, of each image

The following section will highlight structural studies that describe DRS interactions between the major MAP kinases and activator, effector, or regulatory proteins. Co-crystallization of the kinase with a peptide representing the interacting partner provides useful information as to how interaction with the DRS can discriminate between an activator protein and a downstream effector. Figure 3 depicts the interactions between ERK2 and peptides representing D-domain containing activator (MEK2) or p90 ribosomal S6 kinase (RSK1) effector proteins [28]. Each peptide appears to occupy the groove between the CD and ED domains. However, the interactions with a region just below the ED domain appears to show differences that could be potentially exploited to inhibit ERK1/2 activation of RSK1 while preserving ERK1/2 activation by upstream MEK proteins. Inhibition of RSK signaling

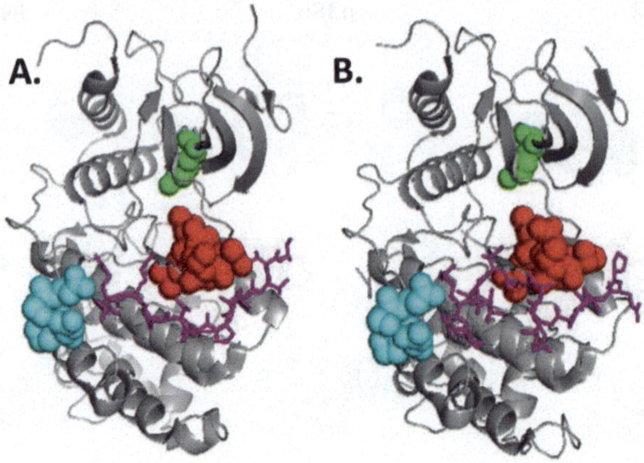

Fig. 3 Structural interactions between ERK2 and activator (MEK2) and substrate (RSK1) peptides (magenta lines). The DRS of ERK2 consists of CD (cyan) and ED (red) domain residues. The conserved lysine in the ATP catalytic site is shown in green. (**a**) MEK2 peptide (RRKPVLPALTINP) interactions with the DRS (PDB:4H3Q). (**b**) RSK1 peptide (PQLKPIESSILAQRRVRKLSPTTL) interactions with the DRS (PDB:4H3P)

may benefit the treatment of triple negative breast cancer [29], and at least one RSK-selective inhibitor, PMD-026, has entered breast cancer clinical trials as of October 2019. Additional structures of ERK2 interactions with peptides representing regulatory phosphatase proteins have been solved. The structures of ERK2 in complex with D-domain peptides of hematopoietic *p*rotein *t*yrosine *p*hosphatase (HePTP) [30] and dual-specific *M*AP *k*inase *p*hosphatase-*3* (MKP3) [31] reveal similarities and differences. In both examples, peptide interactions with the ERK2 DRS involve electrostatic interactions and hydrophobic interactions, which is also the case with p38α and JNK1 MAP kinase as discussed below. Differences that occur in the non-conserved amino acids in the DRS are thought to determine the selectivity of interacting partners with MAP kinases.

The use of peptides to determine structural interactions has limits as they do not readily form secondary structures as found in the full-length protein, and they may not reflect allosteric effects of other domains. More recently, a cocrystal structure of inactive ERK2 and the kinase domain of RSK1 was determined [32]. This structure showed similar interactions between the D-domain of RSK1 and the ERK2 DRS as to what was described previously in Fig. 3 for the RSK1 D-domain peptide, although in this case the D-domain is connected to the rest of the RSK1 kinase domain through an unstructured linker (Fig. 4). The two kinases are inverted in relation to each other with the N-terminal lobe of ERK2 facing the C-terminal lobe of the RSK1 kinase domain (Fig. 4). As suggested by this inactive complex, the threonine residue that is phosphorylated by ERK2 is positioned near the catalytic site. However, molecular dynamics simulations have suggested that structural changes occurring when ERK2 becomes activated allow positioning of the threonine close enough to the active site for phosphoryl transfer to occur [32].

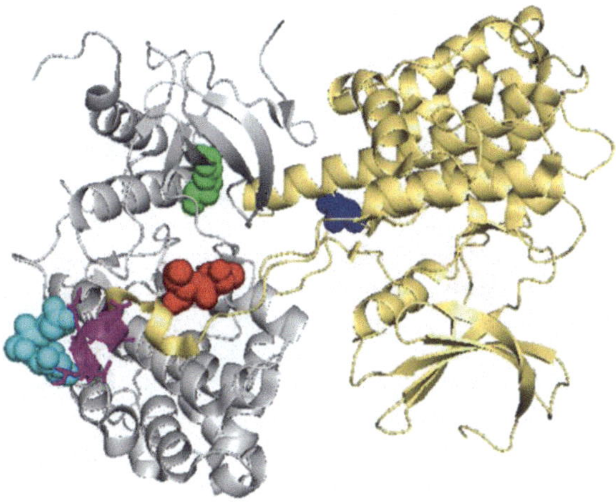

Fig. 4 Structural interactions between ERK2 and the kinase domain of RSK1. The DRS of ERK2 (MAPK1) consists of CD (cyan) and ED (red) amino acids. RSK1 (light yellow ribbon) and ERK2 (grey ribbon) are shown as a heterodimer (PDB:4NIF). The RSK1 D-domain peptide (magenta) interacts with the docking groove between the ERK2 CD and ED domains. Threonine 573 (blue) on RSK-1 is positioned for phosphorylation by ERK2. The conserved lysine in the ATP catalytic site is shown in green

The interactions of p38α MAP kinase with peptides representing activator (MEK3) and effector (MEF2A) proteins that use the DRS have been described [33]. Figure 5 shows the positioning of DRS-interacting peptides that correspond to an activator of p38α (MKK3) and a downstream transcription factor effector (MEF2). Unlike the involvement of basic residues of D-domain peptides that interact with acidic CD domain residues on ERK2, the CD domain did not appear to be involved in MEK3 and MEF2A interactions (Fig. 5) [33]. There were key differences between the interactions of MEF2A or MEK3 with p38α that could be exploited to develop a MEF2A-selective inhibitor. First, MEF2A interactions are more extensive and occupy a larger part of the groove between the CD and ED domains. Second, the common DLR sequence on both MEF2A and MEK3 peptides does not interact in the same way with the docking groove of p38α. Thus, these differences in DRS interactions could help guide the identification of inhibitors that preserve desirable p38α interactions with MEK3 and overall signaling functions but selectively block interactions between p38α and MEF2A to inhibit signaling events associated with disease [34].

To gain further insight into p38α MAP kinase interactions with downstream effector proteins, the structure of the inactive heterodimer complex of p38α and full length MAPKAPK2 (MK2) was determined [35]. MK2 is a major mediator of inflammatory signals regulated by p38 MAP kinases and targeted inhibition of MK2 could mitigate inflammatory processes involved in acute and chronic lung disease as well as rheumatoid arthritis [19, 36, 37]. The crystal structure shows a face-to-

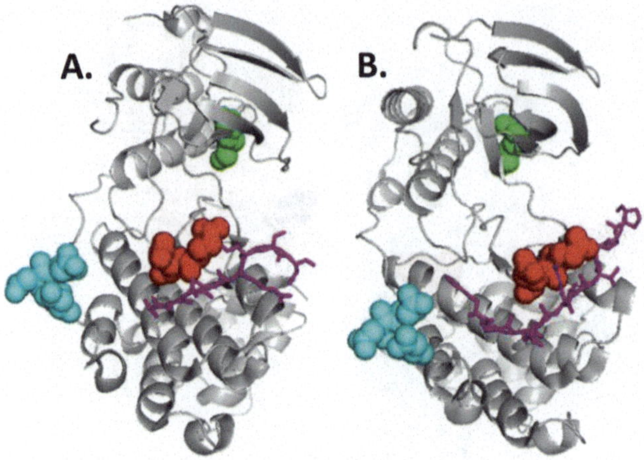

Fig. 5 Structural interactions between p38α MAPK activator (MEK3) and substrate (MEF2A) peptides. The DRS of p38α (MAPK14) consists of CD (cyan) and ED (red) amino acids. (**a**) MEK3 peptide (SKGKSKRKKDLRISCNSK) interaction with the DRS (pdb:1LEZ). (**b**) MEF2A peptide (RKPDLRVVIPPS) interaction with the DRS (pdb: 1LEW). The conserved lysines in the ATP catalytic sites are shown in green

face interaction with the ATP-binding sites of each kinase positioned adjacent to each other (Fig. 6). The MK2 C-terminal residues from 368 to 400 wrap around p38α and include the D-domain residues that form a helix that fits in the DRS docking groove, which is the major contributor of the heterodimer formation. There is also evidence to suggest some interactions between the disordered MK2 activation loop (residues 207–233 shown in black, Fig. 6) and p38α through C-terminal α helices. In this inactivated conformation, the major MK2 residues phosphorylated by p38α are spatially separated from the catalytic site (Fig. 6). However, conformational changes upon p38α activation allow ATP catalysis and phosphate transfer to these threonine residues. An interesting aspect of the MK2 D-domain residues is that they interact with p38α in a reverse order as compared to the MEF2A and MEK3 peptides shown in Fig. 5 [35]. These studies highlight subtle differences in the interactions between distinct activator and effector proteins to a common docking groove formed by the DRS of p38 MAP kinase that could be exploited in the development of inflammation-modulating agents.

Structural information on p38α MAP kinases' interactions with substrate proteins has informed the development of function-selective p38α inhibitor compounds that may mitigate tissue damage following acute myocardial infarction [38]. Stress signals associated with ischemia/reperfusion tissue injury following a heart attack result in the auto-activation of p38α though interactions with the *t*ransforming growth factor-β-*a*ctivated protein kinase 1–*b*inding protein *1* (*TAB1*) scaffold protein [39]. De Nicola et al. provided evidence that TAB1 interacts with noncanonical sites and the canonical FRS residues on p38α through hydrophobic interactions (Fig. 7a) [38]. Although the predicted interacting TAB1 hydrophobic residues were

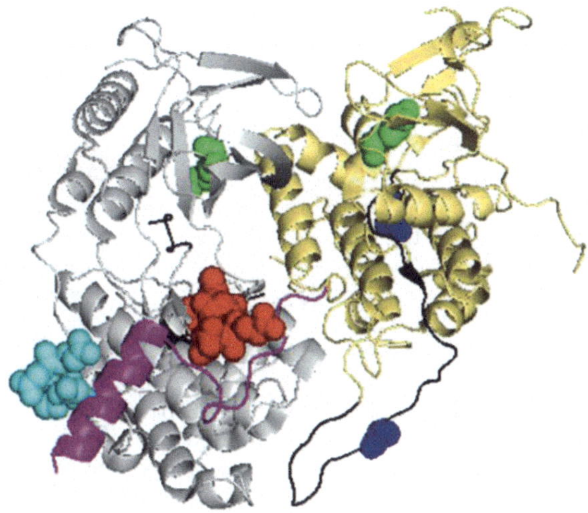

Fig. 6 Structural interactions between p38α MAP kinase and full length MK2 (pdb: 2ONL). The heterodimer structure of p38α (grey ribbon) and MK2 (light yellow ribbon) shows the C-terminal D-domain residues of MK2 (magenta) interacting with a groove between the CD (cyan) and ED (red) domains of the DRS. The activation loops of both proteins are shown in black. The conserved lysines in the ATP catalytic sites of p38α and MK2 are shown in green and MK2 sites phosphorylated by p38α (T222 in the activation loop and T334 in the C-terminus) are shown as blue spheres

disordered and not visible in the X-ray structure, mutating these residues to alanine within the putative p38α-binding site (e.g. residues V390A, Y392A, V408G, M409A) disrupted interactions with p38α and provided protection from tissue-damaging effects of myocardial infarction in a mouse model [38]. The structural information was used to identify a small molecule, 3-amino-1-adamantanol, that can interact with hydrophobic leucine residues in a noncanonical site near the FRS of p38α and inhibit interactions with TAB1 (Fig. 7b). Although this compound was not evaluated for mitigating tissue damage due to ischemia/reperfusion injury, it does provide an example of how protein structural information can inform the discovery of small molecular weight compounds that disrupt clinically relevant protein-protein interactions.

The c-*J*un-*N*-terminal *k*inases (JNK) are the other major MAP kinase family member with information on the structural interactions between activators and effector proteins. Unique to the JNK MAP kinase signaling pathway is the presence of three putative D-domains on the MEK7 activator (see Table 2) that have the potential to interact with the DRS on JNK proteins. Kragelj et al. demonstrated that all three D-domains bind with similar affinity to JNK1 suggesting that a single MEK7 protein has the potential to engage three JNK1 molecules simultaneously [40]. These studies also provided a more detailed structural analysis of the interactions between JNK1 and the second D-domain (amino acids QRPRPTLQLPLA) that suggest MEK7 may adopt different binding modes depending on the JNK1 activation state and function. One of the MEK7-binding modes shows electrostatic

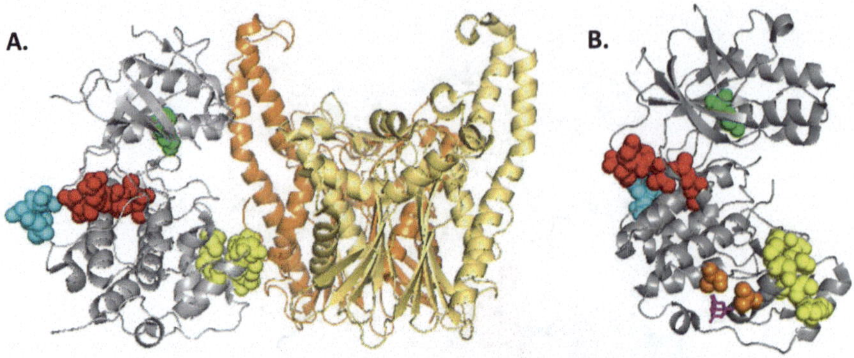

Fig. 7 Structural interactions between p38α MAP kinase, TAB1, and a TAB1 inhibitor. The CD (cyan) and ED (red) domain residues of the DRS and the conserved lysine in the ATP catalytic site (green) are shown for reference. (**a**) Heterodimer complex of p38α (gray) and TAB1 (orange/yellow) [pdb: 5NZZ]. TAB1 residues 384–412 interact with FRS residues on p38α (yellow). (**b**) Structure of p38α with the TAB1 disrupting compound, 3-amino-1-adamantanol (magenta), shown interacting with leucine residues (orange) near the FRS [pdb: 6SPL]

interaction with the CD domain along with hydrophobic interactions with D-domain peptide leucine residues (Fig. 8a).

The *J*NK-*i*nteracting *p*rotein-*1* (JIP1) scaffold protein is an important regulator of stress-induced JNK activity through interactions with DRS [41]. JIP1 is highly expressed in brain and adipose tissue and may have particularly important roles in regulating JNK activity associated with obesity, the development of type II diabetes, and neurodegenerative disorders [42]. A structure of a JIP1 D-domain peptide interacting with JNK1 has been determined [43]. Typical of other D-domain sequences, hydrophobic leucine residues contact α helices between the CD and ED domain of JNK1 (Fig. 8b). However, unlike the MEK7 peptide where prominent interactions with basic lysine residues and acidic residues on the CD domain of JNK1 are observed, this interaction was not evident from the JIP1-JNK1 structure (compare the peptide interactions with CD domain in Fig. 8a, b). The structural features of JIP1 interactions with JNK1 have helped facilitate the development of new compounds that target the JIP1 docking site and show improved management of glucose levels in animal models of diabetes [44, 45]. While these studies provide proof of principle that disruption of JIP1 interactions with JNK proteins has clinical benefits, translating these concepts to patient studies has yet to be achieved.

While many upstream activators, regulatory proteins, and substrates contain D-domains that facilitate interactions with their respective MAP kinases, few studies have examined how differences between D-domains impact protein-protein binding affinities and subsequent signaling events that control cellular responses. Laughlin et al. provided structural insight into three D-domain-containing proteins and their interactions with the DRS of JNK3 to explain differences in their binding affinities [46]. JNK3 shares a high degree of sequence identity with other JNK isoforms, including 75% sequence identity with JNK1. These studies used 11 amino

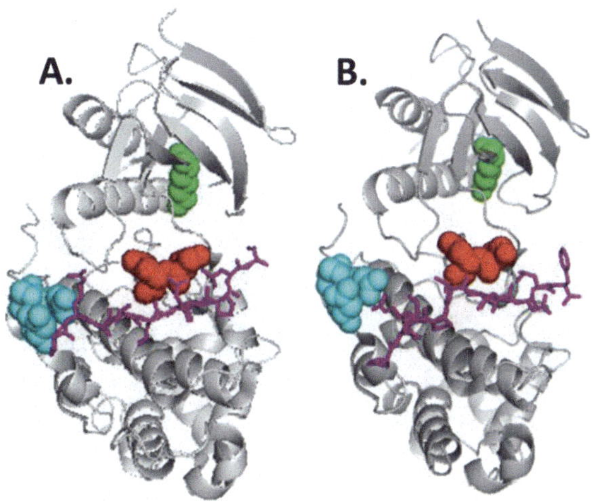

Fig. 8 Structural interactions between JNK1 and peptides representing activator (MEK7) or regulatory (JIP1) proteins. The DRS of JNK1 (MAPK8) consists of CD (cyan) and ED (red) amino acids. Lysine in the ATP catalytic site is shown in green. (**a**) MEK7 peptide (magenta) interacting with DRS (pdb:4UX9). (**b**) The JIP1 peptide (magenta) interacting with DRS (pdb:1UKI)

acid peptides representing two scaffold proteins, JIP1 and SAB (SH3-binding protein 5 or SH3BP5), or the transcription factor ATF2 to examine how each D-domain coordinated interactions with JNK3 [46]. As previously discussed, JIP1 plays several roles in regulating JNK activity, including regulation of obesity-induced insulin resistance, while SAB is localized to the mitochondria and involved in JNK-mediated *r*eactive *o*xygen *s*pecies (ROS) generation associated with acetaminophen-induced liver injury [47]. ATF2 is a member of the AP-1 transcription factor family that can heterodimerize with several other transcription factors to modulate cell survival especially in response to stress [48].

A major objective addressed by Laughlin et al. was to determine the D-domain differences that were responsible for the JIP1 peptide having ~20-fold higher JNK3-binding affinity compared to the SAB or ATF2 peptides [46]. Cocrystallization studies indicated that the SAB and ATF2 peptides caused the disordered JNK3 activation loop to coil into an inhibitory helix that interacted with the ATP-binding site (Fig. 9). These structural changes suggested a potential mechanism for a docked substrate to inhibit JNK catalytic activity prior to activation loop phosphorylation. JIP1 peptide interactions with carboxy (C)-terminal residues induced a rotation of the amino (N)-terminal lobe in agreement with previous studies describing how overexpressed JIP1 inhibits JNK activity [43]. Binding of the SAB and ATF2 peptides caused a similar allosteric rotation of the N-terminal lobe.

Several differences between the peptides were observed that could explain the higher binding affinity of JIP1 [46]. For example, the electrostatic interactions between basic residues of the D-domain and acidic residues (cyan in Fig. 9) of the DRS were ~1 Å closer with JIP1 as compared to ATF2. Another difference observed was extensive hydrogen (H)-bond interactions of the middle amino acids of the JIP1 peptide compared to fewer H-bonds with the SAB peptide. Finally, hydrophobic residues in the C-terminus of the JIP1 peptide formed additional van der Waals interactions that were not observed with the ATF2 peptide. The higher binding affin-

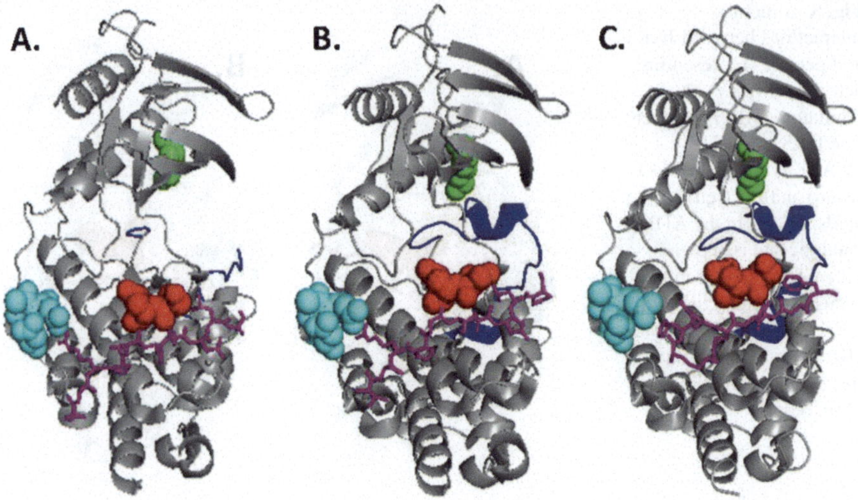

Fig. 9 Structural interactions between JNK3 and the D-domain peptides representing (**a**) JIP1 [pdb:4H39], (**b**) SAB [pdb:4H3B], and (**c**) ATF2 [4H36]. The peptides are represented as magenta lines. The CD and ED domains of the DRS are highlighted in cyan and red, respectively. The activation loop (residues 207–230) shown in blue forms a helix (**b** and **c**) that fits in the catalytic site. The conserved lysine (K93) in the catalytic site is shown in green

ity of JIP1 compared to SAB was attributed to a C-terminal proline in the SAB peptide that altered the positioning of an adjacent leucine and helped stabilize the inhibitor helix formed by the activation loop. Since all three of these DRS-interacting proteins have diverse cellular functions, these structural studies provide the basis to rationally design compounds that target select protein-protein interactions to achieve maximal therapeutic benefits.

MAP Kinase Interactions Through the FRS

The *F*-*r*ecruitment *s*ite (FRS) on MAP kinases represent another docking site that controls interactions with substrates and regulatory proteins. All MAP kinases have a putative FRS (see Fig. 2 and Table 5), and the use of X-ray crystallography and other approaches to define the structural role for this site in mediating interactions with DEF-motif containing proteins has been examined in a few examples. Other biophysical studies have provided compelling evidence that several transcription factors (e.g., Elk-1, c-Fos, and c-Myc) and phosphatases (e.g. MKP3 and MKP7) require a DEF motif to interact with MAP kinases [49–51]. In addition, some MAP kinase substrates and regulators (e.g. Elk-1, MKP3, and KSR1) have both a D-domain and DEF motif that coordinate MAP kinase interactions [52, 53]. Tzarum et al. provided biochemical evidence that the FRS of p38α is required for the efficient phosphorylation of the transcription factors Elk-1 and ATF2 [54]. As was previously described in Fig. 9, ATF2 contains a D-domain peptide but does not contain a consensus FXF sequence characteristic of the DEF motif, suggesting that the FRS on MAP kinases can adapt to other peptide motifs.

The *M*AP *k*inase *p*hosphatases (MKP) family, also referred to as the *du*al *s*pecificity *p*hosphatases (DUSP), are key DEF motif-containing regulators of MAP kinase activity through their ability to specifically dephosphorylate threonine and tyrosine residues in the activation loop. Targeted inhibition of MKP proteins may have a beneficial role in modulating the immune response and enhancing the treatments for cancer and inflammatory disorders [55, 56]. One of the few examples of structural interactions between the DEF motif and FRS of a MAP kinase has recently been described for JNK1 interactions with the catalytic domain of MKP7 in cocrystallization studies [57]. The complex reveals the expected bilobed JNK1 kinase structure consisting mostly of N-terminal β-sheets and C-terminal α-helices adjacent to the MKP7 catalytic domain, which contains the typical MKP configuration consisting of a central β-sheet that is surrounded by six α-helices (Fig. 10). Extensive hydrophobic and electrostatic interactions between the DEF motif and the FRS orient the active site of MKP7 adjacent to the phosphorylated activation loop of JNK1 (Fig. 10). Unique to these studies was the assignment of distinct roles for the phenylalanine residues in the consensus DEF motif [57]. Interactions with the first phenylalanine (F285) appeared to be important for JNK1 binding whereas the second phenylalanine (F287) was more involved in positioning the MKP7 active site for efficient dephosphorylation.

Conclusions

This chapter provided some examples of the structural determinants based on X-ray crystallography describing the interactions between protein kinases and activator, regulatory, and effector substrate proteins. Protein kinase signaling networks depend upon these protein-protein interactions to coordinate the appropriate phosphorylation events for cellular responses. The examples provided in this chapter focused on well-characterized docking sites, the DRS and FRS, found on MAP kinases that interact with D-domain and/or DEF motif regions found on interacting protein partners. There are similarities between each docking site across MAP kinases, which may explain why some substrates (e.g., Elk-1, ATF2, and c-Fos) are phosphorylated on the same site by several MAP kinase family members. However, MAP kinase members also retain selectivity in their ability to recognize unique substrates and interacting partners, which can be attributed to subtle differences in each MAP kinase docking site and the likely existence of additional contact points on MAP kinases that regulate specific protein-protein interactions. A detailed characterization of the determinants of the contact between a protein kinase and its substrate or regulatory proteins will provide opportunities to develop function-selective protein kinase inhibitors that reduce dysregulated signaling events in disease.

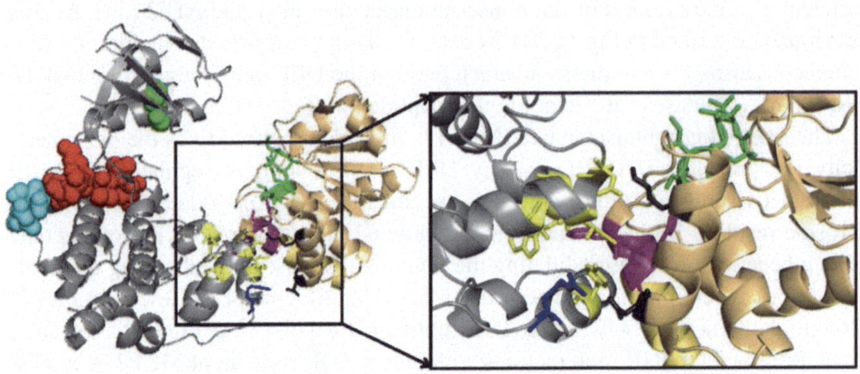

Fig. 10 Structural interactions between JNK1 and the catalytic domain of MKP7 [pdb:4YR8]. JNK1 and the catalytic domain of MKP7 are shown as grey and orange ribbons, respectively. The FRS of JNK1 (residues I197, L198, D229, Y230, I231, W234, Y259) are shown in yellow. The MKP7 active site (residues 245–250; CLAGISR) and DEF motif (residues 285–288; FNFL) are shown in green and magenta, respectively. Electrostatic interactions between MKP7 (black lines) and JNK1 (blue lines) are indicated. The DRS of JNK1 consisting of the CD (cyan spheres) and ED (red spheres) amino acids and the conserved lysine in the ATP catalytic site (green spheres) are shown for reference. Inset shows an expanded view of the DEF motif interaction with the FRS

There are several experimental approaches available for determining protein-kinase-interacting partners. As an example, specific antibodies can be used to immunoprecipitate a protein kinase from a complex protein mixture, and cointeracting proteins can be identified by mass spectrometry. This approach has been used to identify an ERK1 MAP kinase interactome in the context of neuronal cell differentiation [23]. Most of the ERK1-interacting proteins identified contained D-domains. However, variability in binding affinities and immunoprecipitation conditions may bias some protein interactions and fail to identify other interactions that occur in vivo. Other experimental approaches to identify protein kinase substrates include the *p*hosphatase *i*nhibitor and *k*inase *i*nhibitor *s*ubstrate *s*creening (PIKISS) method, which was later renamed the *ki*nase-*o*riented *s*ubstrate *s*creening (KIOSS) method to take into account the use of kinase activators and inhibitors [58]. This approach enriches phosphorylated proteins from cells or tissue following the treatment of specific kinase activators or inhibitors and then uses mass spectrometry to identify the substrates. A compilation of many protein kinase interaction networks can be found at the STRING Consortium (https://string-db.org/), which provides a database of thousands of known or predicted protein-protein interactions based on experimental evidence. While these experimental approaches and database compilations provide the basis for manipulating specific protein-protein-interactions, a detailed analysis of the structural features involved will allow the rational identification and development of compounds that modulate these interactions.

A variety of methodologies for structure-based drug design, including X-ray crystallography, nuclear magnetic resonance, and cryo-electron microscopy, have been widely used to generate structural information on protein kinases [59]. Other approaches such as hydrogen-deuterium exchange mass spectrometry can evaluate dynamic structural movements within a protein to evaluate regions of flexibility or rigidity under various conditions [60]. With new information on the structural details of protein kinases, new opportunities to develop function-selective inhibitors of protein-protein interactions involved in disease will emerge. The next chapter will describe the use of computational approaches, which consider the structural features of protein-protein interactions identified by experimental approaches to design new small-molecule inhibitors of protein kinases.

References

1. Manning, G., Whyte, D. B., Martinez, R., Hunter, T., & Sudarsanam, S. (2002). The protein kinase complement of the human genome. *Science, 298*, 1912–1934.
2. UniProt, C. (2010). The universal protein resource (UniProt) in 2010. *Nucleic Acids Research, 38*, D142–D148.
3. Hornbeck, P. V., Chabra, I., Kornhauser, J. M., Skrzypek, E., & Zhang, B. (2004). PhosphoSite: A bioinformatics resource dedicated to physiological protein phosphorylation. *Proteomics, 4*, 1551–1561.
4. Safaei, J., Manuch, J., Gupta, A., Stacho, L., & Pelech, S. (2011). Prediction of 492 human protein kinase substrate specificities. *Proteome Science, 9*(Suppl 1), S6.
5. Blom, N., Sicheritz-Ponten, T., Gupta, R., Gammeltoft, S., & Brunak, S. (2004). Prediction of post-translational glycosylation and phosphorylation of proteins from the amino acid sequence. *Proteomics, 4*, 1633–1649.
6. Song, J., Wang, H., Wang, J., Leier, A., Marquez-Lago, T., Yang, B., Zhang, Z., Akutsu, T., Webb, G. I., & Daly, R. J. (2017). PhosphoPredict: A bioinformatics tool for prediction of human kinase-specific phosphorylation substrates and sites by integrating heterogeneous feature selection. *Scientific Reports, 7*, 6862.
7. Ubersax, J. A., & Ferrell, J. E., Jr. (2007). Mechanisms of specificity in protein phosphorylation. *Nature Reviews Molecular Cell Biology, 8*, 530–541.
8. Pinna, L. A., & Ruzzene, M. (1996). How do protein kinases recognize their substrates? *Biochimica et Biophysica Acta, 1314*, 191–225.
9. Miller, C. J., & Turk, B. E. (2018). Homing in: Mechanisms of substrate targeting by protein kinases. *Trends in Biochemical Sciences, 43*, 380–394.
10. Cargnello, M., & Roux, P. P. (2011). Activation and function of the MAPKs and their substrates, the MAPK-activated protein kinases. *Microbiology and Molecular Biology Reviews, 75*, 50–83.
11. Abe, M. K., Kahle, K. T., Saelzler, M. P., Orth, K., Dixon, J. E., & Rosner, M. R. (2001). ERK7 is an autoactivated member of the MAPK family. *The Journal of Biological Chemistry, 276*, 21272–21279.
12. Deleris, P., Trost, M., Topisirovic, I., Tanguay, P. L., Borden, K. L., Thibault, P., & Meloche, S. (2011). Activation loop phosphorylation of ERK3/ERK4 by group I p21-activated kinases (PAKs) defines a novel PAK-ERK3/4-MAPK-activated protein kinase 5 signaling pathway. *The Journal of Biological Chemistry, 286*, 6470–6478.
13. Klevernic, I. V., Stafford, M. J., Morrice, N., Peggie, M., Morton, S., & Cohen, P. (2006). Characterization of the reversible phosphorylation and activation of ERK8. *The Biochemical Journal, 394*, 365–373.
14. Bardwell, A. J., Frankson, E., & Bardwell, L. (2009). Selectivity of docking sites in MAPK kinases. *The Journal of Biological Chemistry, 284*, 13165–13173.

15. Lee, T., Hoofnagle, A. N., Kabuyama, Y., Stroud, J., Min, X., Goldsmith, E. J., Chen, L., Resing, K. A., & Ahn, N. G. (2004). Docking motif interactions in MAP kinases revealed by hydrogen exchange mass spectrometry. *Molecular Cell, 14*, 43–55.
16. Jacobs, D., Glossip, D., Xing, H., Muslin, A. J., & Kornfeld, K. (1999). Multiple docking sites on substrate proteins form a modular system that mediates recognition by ERK MAP kinase. *Genes & Development, 13*, 163–175.
17. Sheridan, D. L., Kong, Y., Parker, S. A., Dalby, K. N., & Turk, B. E. (2008). Substrate discrimination among mitogen-activated protein kinases through distinct docking sequence motifs. *The Journal of Biological Chemistry, 283*, 19511–19520.
18. Hancock, C. N., Macias, A., Lee, E. K., Yu, S. Y., Mackerell, A. D., Jr., & Shapiro, P. (2005). Identification of novel extracellular signal-regulated kinase docking domain inhibitors. *Journal of Medicinal Chemistry, 48*, 4586–4595.
19. Shah, N. G., Tulapurkar, M. E., Ramarathnam, A., Brophy, A., Martinez, R., 3rd, Hom, K., Hodges, T., Samadani, R., Singh, I. S., MacKerell, A. D., Jr., Shapiro, P., & Hasday, J. D. (2017). Novel noncatalytic substrate-selective p38alpha-specific MAPK inhibitors with endothelial-stabilizing and anti-inflammatory activity. *Journal of Immunology, 198*, 3296–3306.
20. Chen, F., Hancock, C. N., Macias, A. T., Joh, J., Still, K., Zhong, S., MacKerell, A. D., Jr., & Shapiro, P. (2006). Characterization of ATP-independent ERK inhibitors identified through in silico analysis of the active ERK2 structure. *Bioorganic & Medicinal Chemistry Letters, 16*, 6281–6287.
21. Samadani, R., Zhang, J., Brophy, A., Oashi, T., Priyakumar, U. D., Raman, E. P., St John, F. J., Jung, K. Y., Fletcher, S., Pozharski, E., MacKerell, A. D., Jr., & Shapiro, P. (2015). Small-molecule inhibitors of ERK-mediated immediate early gene expression and proliferation of melanoma cells expressing mutated BRaf. *The Biochemical Journal, 467*, 425–438.
22. Trempolec, N., Dave-Coll, N., & Nebreda, A. R. (2013). SnapShot: p38 MAPK substrates. *Cell, 152*, 924–924 e1.
23. von Kriegsheim, A., Baiocchi, D., Birtwistle, M., Sumpton, D., Bienvenut, W., Morrice, N., Yamada, K., Lamond, A., Kalna, G., Orton, R., Gilbert, D., & Kolch, W. (2009). Cell fate decisions are specified by the dynamic ERK interactome. *Nature Cell Biology, 11*, 1458–1464.
24. Bogoyevitch, M. A., & Kobe, B. (2006). Uses for JNK: The many and varied substrates of the c-Jun N-terminal kinases. *Microbiology and Molecular Biology Reviews, 70*, 1061–1095.
25. Tanoue, T., Adachi, M., Moriguchi, T., & Nishida, E. (2000). A conserved docking motif in MAP kinases common to substrates, activators and regulators. *Nature Cell Biology, 2*, 110–116.
26. Tanoue, T., Maeda, R., Adachi, M., & Nishida, E. (2001). Identification of a docking groove on ERK and p38 MAP kinases that regulates the specificity of docking interactions. *The EMBO Journal, 20*, 466–479.
27. Garai, A., Zeke, A., Gogl, G., Toro, I., Fordos, F., Blankenburg, H., Barkai, T., Varga, J., Alexa, A., Emig, D., Albrecht, M., & Remenyi, A. (2012). Specificity of linear motifs that bind to a common mitogen-activated protein kinase docking groove. *Science Signaling, 5*, ra74.
28. Gogl, G., Toro, I., & Remenyi, A. (2013). Protein-peptide complex crystallization: A case study on the ERK2 mitogen-activated protein kinase. *Acta Crystallographica Section D Biological Crystallography, 69*, 486–489.
29. Ludwik, K. A., Campbell, J. P., Li, M., Li, Y., Sandusky, Z. M., Pasic, L., Sowder, M. E., Brenin, D. R., Pietenpol, J. A., O'Doherty, G. A., & Lannigan, D. A. (2016). Development of a RSK inhibitor as a novel therapy for triple-negative breast cancer. *Molecular Cancer Therapeutics, 15*, 2598–2608.
30. Zhou, T., Sun, L., Humphreys, J., & Goldsmith, E. J. (2006). Docking interactions induce exposure of activation loop in the MAP kinase ERK2. *Structure, 14*, 1011–1019.
31. Liu, S., Sun, J. P., Zhou, B., & Zhang, Z. Y. (2006). Structural basis of docking interactions between ERK2 and MAP kinase phosphatase 3. *Proceedings of the National Academy of Sciences of the United States of America, 103*, 5326–5331.

32. Alexa, A., Gogl, G., Glatz, G., Garai, A., Zeke, A., Varga, J., Dudas, E., Jeszenoi, N., Bodor, A., Hetenyi, C., & Remenyi, A. (2015). Structural assembly of the signaling competent ERK2-RSK1 heterodimeric protein kinase complex. *Proceedings of the National Academy of Sciences of the United States of America, 112*, 2711–2716.
33. Chang, C. I., Xu, B. E., Akella, R., Cobb, M. H., & Goldsmith, E. J. (2002). Crystal structures of MAP kinase p38 complexed to the docking sites on its nuclear substrate MEF2A and activator MKK3b. *Molecular Cell, 9*, 1241–1249.
34. Chen, X., Gao, B., Ponnusamy, M., Lin, Z., & Liu, J. (2017). MEF2 signaling and human diseases. *Oncotarget, 8*, 112152–112165.
35. ter Haar, E., Prabhakar, P., Liu, X., & Lepre, C. (2007). Crystal structure of the p38 alpha-MAPKAP kinase 2 heterodimer. *The Journal of Biological Chemistry, 282*, 9733–9739.
36. Singh, R. K., & Najmi, A. K. (2019). Novel therapeutic potential of mitogen-activated protein kinase activated protein kinase 2 (MK2) in chronic airway inflammatory disorders. *Current Drug Targets, 20*, 367–379.
37. Schett, G., Zwerina, J., & Firestein, G. (2008). The p38 mitogen-activated protein kinase (MAPK) pathway in rheumatoid arthritis. *Annals of the Rheumatic Diseases, 67*, 909–916.
38. De Nicola, G. F., Bassi, R., Nichols, C., Fernandez-Caggiano, M., Golforoush, P. A., Thapa, D., Anderson, R., Martin, E. D., Verma, S., Kleinjung, J., Laing, A., Hutchinson, J. P., Eaton, P., Clark, J., & Marber, M. S. (2018). The TAB1-p38alpha complex aggravates myocardial injury and can be targeted by small molecules. *JCI Insight, 3*(18), 121144.
39. Thapa, D., Nichols, C., Bassi, R., Martin, E. D., Verma, S., Conte, M. R., De Santis, V., De Nicola, G. F., & Marber, M. S. (2018). TAB1-induced autoactivation of p38alpha mitogen-activated protein kinase is crucially dependent on threonine 185. *Molecular and Cellular Biology, 38*(5), e00409–e00417.
40. Kragelj, J., Palencia, A., Nanao, M. H., Maurin, D., Bouvignies, G., Blackledge, M., & Jensen, M. R. (2015). Structure and dynamics of the MKK7-JNK signaling complex. *Proceedings of the National Academy of Sciences of the United States of America, 112*, 3409–3414.
41. Whitmarsh, A. J., Kuan, C. Y., Kennedy, N. J., Kelkar, N., Haydar, T. F., Mordes, J. P., Appel, M., Rossini, A. A., Jones, S. N., Flavell, R. A., Rakic, P., & Davis, R. J. (2001). Requirement of the JIP1 scaffold protein for stress-induced JNK activation. *Genes & Development, 15*, 2421–2432.
42. Jaeschke, A., Czech, M. P., & Davis, R. J. (2004). An essential role of the JIP1 scaffold protein for JNK activation in adipose tissue. *Genes & Development, 18*, 1976–1980.
43. Heo, Y. S., Kim, S. K., Seo, C. I., Kim, Y. K., Sung, B. J., Lee, H. S., Lee, J. I., Park, S. Y., Kim, J. H., Hwang, K. Y., Hyun, Y. L., Jeon, Y. H., Ro, S., Cho, J. M., Lee, T. G., & Yang, C. H. (2004). Structural basis for the selective inhibition of JNK1 by the scaffolding protein JIP1 and SP600125. *The EMBO Journal, 23*, 2185–2195.
44. Stebbins, J. L., De, S. K., Pavlickova, P., Chen, V., Machleidt, T., Chen, L. H., Kuntzen, C., Kitada, S., Karin, M., & Pellecchia, M. (2011). Design and characterization of a potent and selective dual ATP- and substrate-competitive subnanomolar bidentate c-Jun N-terminal kinase (JNK) inhibitor. *Journal of Medicinal Chemistry, 54*, 6206–6214.
45. Stebbins, J. L., De, S. K., Machleidt, T., Becattini, B., Vazquez, J., Kuntzen, C., Chen, L. H., Cellitti, J. F., Riel-Mehan, M., Emdadi, A., Solinas, G., Karin, M., & Pellecchia, M. (2008). Identification of a new JNK inhibitor targeting the JNK-JIP interaction site. *Proceedings of the National Academy of Sciences of the United States of America, 105*, 16809–16813.
46. Laughlin, J. D., Nwachukwu, J. C., Figuera-Losada, M., Cherry, L., Nettles, K. W., & LoGrasso, P. V. (2012). Structural mechanisms of allostery and autoinhibition in JNK family kinases. *Structure, 20*, 2174–2184.
47. Win, S., Than, T. A., Han, D., Petrovic, L. M., & Kaplowitz, N. (2011). c-Jun N-terminal kinase (JNK)-dependent acute liver injury from acetaminophen or tumor necrosis factor (TNF) requires mitochondrial Sab protein expression in mice. *The Journal of Biological Chemistry, 286*, 35071–35078.

48. Watson, G., Ronai, Z. A., & Lau, E. (2017). ATF2, a paradigm of the multifaceted regulation of transcription factors in biology and disease. *Pharmacological Research, 119*, 347–357.
49. Burkhard, K. A., Chen, F., & Shapiro, P. (2011). Quantitative analysis of ERK2 interactions with substrate proteins: Roles for kinase docking domains and activity in determining binding affinity. *The Journal of Biological Chemistry, 286*, 2477–2485.
50. Dimitri, C. A., Dowdle, W., MacKeigan, J. P., Blenis, J., & Murphy, L. O. (2005). Spatially separate docking sites on ERK2 regulate distinct signaling events in vivo. *Current Biology, 15*, 1319–1324.
51. Zhou, B., Zhang, J., Liu, S., Reddy, S., Wang, F., & Zhang, Z. Y. (2006). Mapping ERK2-MKP3 binding interfaces by hydrogen/deuterium exchange mass spectrometry. *The Journal of Biological Chemistry, 281*, 38834–38844.
52. Zhang, J., Zhou, B., Zheng, C. F., & Zhang, Z. Y. (2003). A bipartite mechanism for ERK2 recognition by its cognate regulators and substrates. *The Journal of Biological Chemistry, 278*, 29901–29912.
53. Fantz, D. A., Jacobs, D., Glossip, D., & Kornfeld, K. (2001). Docking sites on substrate proteins direct extracellular signal-regulated kinase to phosphorylate specific residues. *The Journal of Biological Chemistry, 276*, 27256–27265.
54. Tzarum, N., Komornik, N., Ben Chetrit, D., Engelberg, D., & Livnah, O. (2013). DEF pocket in p38alpha facilitates substrate selectivity and mediates autophosphorylation. *The Journal of Biological Chemistry, 288*, 19537–19547.
55. Jeffrey, K. L., Camps, M., Rommel, C., & Mackay, C. R. (2007). Targeting dual-specificity phosphatases: Manipulating MAP kinase signalling and immune responses. *Nature Reviews Drug Discovery, 6*, 391–403.
56. Keyse, S. M. (2008). Dual-specificity MAP kinase phosphatases (MKPs) and cancer. *Cancer Metastasis Reviews, 27*, 253–261.
57. Liu, X., Zhang, C. S., Lu, C., Lin, S. C., Wu, J. W., & Wang, Z. X. (2016). A conserved motif in JNK/p38-specific MAPK phosphatases as a determinant for JNK1 recognition and inactivation. *Nature Communications, 7*, 10879.
58. Nishioka, T., Amano, M., Funahashi, Y., Tsuboi, D., Yamahashi, Y., & Kaibuchi, K. (2019). In vivo identification of protein kinase substrates by kinase-oriented substrate screening (KIOSS). *Current Protocal in Chemical Biology, 11*, e60.
59. Batool, M., Ahmad, B., & Choi, S. (2019). A structure-based drug discovery paradigm. *International Journal of Molecular Sciences, 20*, 2783.
60. Masson, G. R., Jenkins, M. L., & Burke, J. E. (2017). An overview of hydrogen deuterium exchange mass spectrometry (HDX-MS) in drug discovery. *Expert Opinion on Drug Discovery, 12*, 981–994.

Developing Kinase Inhibitors Using Computer-Aided Drug Design Approaches

Wenbo Yu, David J. Weber, Paul Shapiro, and Alexander D. MacKerell Jr

Abstract Computational methods are useful tools to assist and interact with experiment techniques to expedite the drug design process in general. Provided here is an introduction of well-established and newly developed computer-aided drug design (CADD) approaches that are regularly being used in the development of kinase inhibitors. This includes methods from the two major CADD categories: structure-based drug design (SBDD) and ligand-based drug design (LBDD). With known three-dimensional structure of the target, SBDD approaches help to identify key structural and interaction features that are responsible for specific biological functions of the target. Such information can be utilized to design inhibitors via a number

W. Yu (✉)
Department of Pharmaceutical Sciences, School of Pharmacy, University of Maryland, Baltimore, MD, USA

Institute for Bioscience and Biotechnology Research (IBBR), Rockville, MD, USA

Center for Biomolecular Therapeutics (CBT), School of Medicine, University of Maryland, Baltimore, MD, USA
e-mail: wenbo@outerbanks.umaryland.edu

D. J. Weber
Institute for Bioscience and Biotechnology Research (IBBR), Rockville, MD, USA

Center for Biomolecular Therapeutics (CBT), School of Medicine, University of Maryland, Baltimore, MD, USA

P. Shapiro
Department of Pharmaceutical Sciences, University of Maryland School of Pharmacy, Baltimore, MD, USA

A. D. MacKerell Jr (✉)
Department of Pharmaceutical Sciences, School of Pharmacy, University of Maryland, Baltimore, MD, USA

Institute for Bioscience and Biotechnology Research (IBBR), Rockville, MD, USA

Center for Biomolecular Therapeutics (CBT), School of Medicine, University of Maryland, Baltimore, MD, USA

SilcsBio LLC, Baltimore, MD, USA
e-mail: alex@outerbanks.umaryland.edu

P. Shapiro (ed.), *Next Generation Kinase Inhibitors*,
https://doi.org/10.1007/978-3-030-48283-1_5

of approaches including database screening, fragment-based drug design, and ligand optimization. LBDD methods focus on known inhibitors for a target to establish a relationship between their intrinsic properties with experimental activities, termed structure-activity relationship, information that can be used for optimization of known inhibitors in order to improve their activities. In this chapter, CADD protocols from both SBDD and LBDD will be presented along with real-life examples of successful applications of these methods for kinase inhibitor discovery in our laboratory.

Keywords Computer-aided drug design · SILCS · Molecular dynamics · ERK kinase · P38 map kinase · P56 Lck kinase

Introduction

Serving as the phosphate group transportation mediator, kinases together with phosphatases modulate a wide range of physiological activities, associated with the more than 500 kinases encoded in the human genome [1]. Since almost all signal transductions are related to phosphate group transportation, protein kinases regulate most of the signal transductions in eukaryotic cells. Thus, protein kinases are identified as promising therapeutic targets in cancers which are caused by aberrations in their signaling network [1, 2]. In addition, observations about the important role of deregulation of kinase function in inflammatory, immunological, and degenerative diseases make kinases attractive targets for these conditions [3, 4] Accordingly, dozens of kinase inhibitors have been approved thus far, targeting a wide range of kinases including MEK, JAK, CDK, and EGFR, and even more drugs are in clinical trials [5].

Despite the established druggability profile of kinases, challenges still remain in the drug discovery of kinase inhibitors [6]. This includes but is not limited to overcoming drug resistance, enhancing target selectivity to reduce off-target toxicity, and identifying new targetable binding sites for kinase inhibitors. Toward these goals, computer-aided drug design (CADD) approaches can be extensively utilized together with wet-lab techniques to expedite the discovery progress. CADD methods apply mathematical models to describe the behavior of both target macromolecules and small drug molecules and link them to experimental observations often in a predictive manner. Benefiting from the fast growth of computer power and advances in the development of new algorithms, CADD methods are both economically efficient and of appropriate accuracy to facilitate the drug discovery process [7, 8] and help to address existing challenges to the development of new kinase inhibitors. In this chapter we present an introduction to CADD methods, focusing on those used in the drug design studying kinases. This is followed by more detailed information on CADD studies on kinases with emphasis on studies performed in our laboratories. In particular we present our successful efforts to overcome challenges associated with the development of specific kinase inhibitors by targeting the regions of the protein involved in protein-protein interactions with substrate proteins [9–13].

Basic Concepts of CADD and Typical CADD Methods

Figure 1 illustrates a typical CADD workflow including both SBDD and LBDD methods that can be interactively used with experimental techniques for drug discovery [14–16]. CADD methods can be separated into structure-based (SBDD) and ligand-based (LBDD) approaches. Once the therapeutic target on biological pathway gets identified, CADD approaches can be utilized with wet-lab techniques to promote the whole drug design process. With target structure being solved either by crystallography or nuclear magnetic resonance (NMR) [17], SBDD methods can be used to explore important contributors to drug binding at the atomic level and help to design new drugs from scratch or optimize known drugs [7, 8]. Sometimes, even without an experimentally solved target structure, SBDD methods can build computational structure models based on sequence information alone using techniques such as homology modeling [18] even though the models' accuracy usually depends on the sequence identity of the target with template structures being used to build the models. Typical SBDD methods include molecular dynamics (MD)-based techniques such as various free-energy prediction methods [19–21] and virtual screening techniques such as docking [22, 23] and receptor-based pharmacophore methods [24, 25].

Once one or several hit molecules get identified even without a known target structure, LBDD methods can be used to start new hit searches usually through chemical-fingerprint-based similarity searches [26, 27] or hit optimization usually by building structure-activity relationships (SAR) [28–30] using experimental activity data. Similarity search has the ability to locate more hit compounds based on the assumption that chemically similar compounds should have similar activities while SAR models have the power to prioritize new designs and interact with bioassay tests to refine the hits and find better binders. Another type of a typical LBDD method is the ligand-based pharmacophore method, which is different from receptor-based pharmacophore methods in that the pharmacophore models are built from known ligands without using receptor information [31, 32]. There is no dividing line between the two type of CADD methods, and at the later stage of drug discovery when abundant information about both the receptor and ligand is available, SBDD and LBDD methods are frequently used together with experimental techniques to facilitate the drug design process.

A central feature of computational modeling of biological systems is to build mathematical relationships between structures and energies of the studied systems and then relate calculated observables to biological data for explanations of biological phenomenon. In terms of drug design, CADD methods [7, 8] are mathematical tools to manipulate and quantify the properties of potential drug candidates and study their interactions with macromolecular receptors such as proteins as described

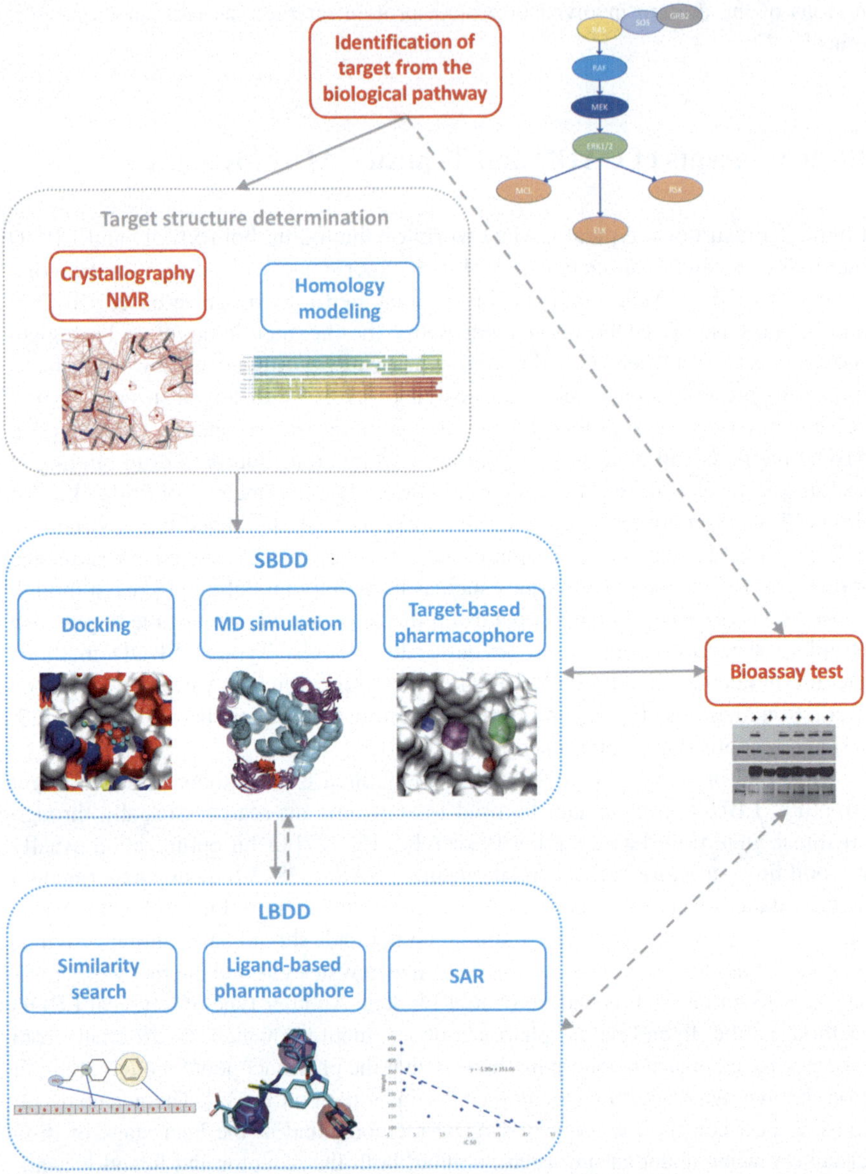

Fig. 1 General workflow of CADD involved in drug discovery. Experimental and computational techniques are colored in red and blue, respectively. Double-headed arrow indicates the two techniques can be used interactively. SBDD methods usually follow the steps indicated by solid arrows and LBDD methods follow dashed arrows. Different methods can be used together and exchange information between each other, e.g., MD simulation can provide conformations for other SBDD methods

by the equilibrium in eq. (1) where receptor and ligand are in their free states on the left of the equation while they form a complex on the right:

$$\text{Receptor} + \text{Ligand} \leftrightarrow \text{Receptor} - \text{Ligand} \quad (1)$$

To physically describe the strength of such ligand-receptor interactions, the free energy change, ΔG, upon binding is used and this physical term can be separated into enthalpy (H) and entropy (S) terms as defined in eq. (2), where T is the system temperature:

$$\Delta G = \Delta H - T\Delta S \quad (2)$$

Here enthalpy can be calculated using defined energy terms while entropy can be estimated from motions occurring in the drug, receptor, and surrounding solvent environment, referred to as the conformational properties. And since the drug design process is to identify, optimize, and develop drug molecules that tightly bind to their receptors, drug-receptor interaction strengths need to be modeled. Thus, the ability to calculate energies related to enthalpy and conformational properties related to entropy are the two most basic yet important capabilities being used throughout all CADD methods. Accordingly, one of the major differences in CADD methods is the level of approximations being made to calculate energy and conformation. The approximations include the level of detail used to describe the energy of a molecule, which describe the conformation of a molecule rigidly or dynamically. It is this level of detail that determines the accuracy and speed of the modeling. Obviously, accuracy and computational cost are correlated and usually people make compromises between the two according to their simulation needs.

Considering the energy of a molecule, a physical way to describe the potential energy of a molecule is achieved by using a force field [33–38]. A force field has an energy functional form and associated parameters used to fit into the function in order to calculate energy and forces. The energy function includes both bonded terms for description of bonded atoms in a molecule and nonbonded terms for electrostatic and van der Waals interactions that occur between atoms and molecules. For an all-atom force field, parameters for every type of atom in a system are provided and were optimized to reproduce experimental and quantum mechanics data. Commonly used force fields include the CHARMM [33–36] and AMBER [37, 38] families. The approaches based on all-atom force fields include energy minimizations and MD simulations of proteins with ligands including an explicit representation of the solvent environment.

Alternative are virtual screening methods that can be applied to large numbers of ligands binding to a protein. To rapidly predict binding energy in virtual screening that includes millions of chemical compounds, a simplified empirical scoring function is frequently used to dock molecules into a binding pocket on the protein. These empirical scoring functions [39–42], such as GlideScore, [39] only incorporate several energy terms and, typically, include lipophilic, hydrogen bonding, and solvation terms with weighting factors and are typically fitted to a training set of receptor-ligand complexes with known experimental binding data.

As an extreme version of scoring function, VS pharmacophore methods [24, 25, 31, 32] further simplify the energetic details into a pharmacophore model which contains spatially distributed chemical features that are essential for specific ligand-receptor binding. And virtual screening is conducted by examining the compliance of a ligand conformation with pharmacophore features usually in a root-mean-square deviation term. Thus, the binding of ligand is quantified through a qualitative way so that its computational cost is the least compared to other interaction energy evaluation methods.

With the rapid growth of artificial intelligence, new machine learning techniques are empowering the CADD field. Unlike force fields or empirical energy functions, machine-learning-based scoring schemes do not have a predetermined energy function but are inferred directly from the data instead [43–45]. Trained using big data sets, machine-learning-based scoring protocols, such as RF-Score-VS [45], have been indicated to achieve a higher accuracy level compared to traditional energy calculation schemes. However, to date that success has been limited to the chemical space of the ligands and the proteins in the data set used to train the machine learning model [46].

With respect to conformational properties, MD simulation is a good physical approach to generate meaningful conformational ensembles for both the receptor and ligand molecules [47]. The structure of a biological molecule is highly related to its biological function, and thus finding biological meaningful conformations of a studied system is a key step in predicting its biological activity [48]. When a small ligand binds to a macromolecular receptor, both molecules change their conformation to a varying extent in order to maximize the complementary interactions between the two. Accordingly, taking conformational flexibility into account is quite important to maximize the prediction accuracy [49, 50]. MD simulations are performed by integrating the molecular system forward in time according to Newton's equations of motion. Thus, MD simulations can capture conformational changes that happen on the simulation time scale, which is typically in the range of up to microseconds, though longer simulations have been reported. To treat longer time scale conformational changes, enhanced MD techniques such as replica exchange (REMD) [51] and targeted MD (TMD) [52] can be used while only consuming a relatively short simulation time.

For virtual docking to consider ligand conformational flexibility, various sampling algorithms may be employed [53]. The incremental construction method adopted by the docking software DOCK [54] put a rigid central portion of the ligand as the anchor at the binding site, and the rest of the ligand is incrementally grown to sample different conformations. Another docking code, AutoDock [55], uses a Lamarckian genetic algorithm to generate ligand conformations on the fly during docking. These approaches are designed to obtain biologically meaningful conformations of the ligands though they are often performed in conjunction with a rigid protein structure.

During different stages of a drug discovery, different levels of CADD methods can be used to satisfy different needs [7, 8]. In the hit identification stage of drug discovery, since no or limited drug information is available, usually million times of energy evaluations need to be done in a fast fashion. Efficient and low computation demanding methods such as VS approaches are needed with a tolerance of sacrificing some extent of accuracy. When it comes to the lead optimization stage of CADD, more accurate methods that require heavy computational costs are needed to capture subtle balances between various contributors to the drug-receptor interaction. This level of detail is required to finely tune a lead molecule to enhance its binding affinity. As this stage, more sophisticated methods such as MD-based free energy perturbation (FEP) methods [20, 21, 56] can be used. FEP methods calculate free energy difference between two states by summation over ensemble averages of Hamiltonian differences between neighboring intermediate states along the pathway connecting the two end states [20, 21]. Thus, such methods require more conformational samplings and energy evaluations and come at high computational costs but can enhance the predictability of CADD models.

Researchers are continually developing and implementing new CADD techniques to pursue higher levels of accuracy and faster speed, and many new methods are emerging to make better balance between the two aspects. To overcome the high computational costs associated with FEP and related techniques, our lab developed an end state method to evaluate relative binding free energy difference between two ligands with small functional group modifications based on a single-step free energy perturbation (SSFEP) formula [57]. The SSFEP method uses existing MD simulation data of a ligand in a given environment and postprocesses the data to estimate the alchemical free energy change of chemically modifying the ligand. Thus, compared to normal FEP calculations, SSFEP can be orders of magnitude faster during drug optimization stage since it allows data from a single ligand receptor complex simulation to be rapidly postprocessed to evaluate tens to hundreds of possible modifications.

Another novel CADD protocol developed in our lab is the site-identification by ligand competitive saturation (SILCS) method [58–60]. SILCS uses all-atom explicit-solvent MD simulations that include small organic solutes, such as benzene, propane, methanol and others, to identify 3D functional-group binding patterns on the target. Probe molecules being used in SILCS can represent various chemical functional types involved in interactions with the target that includes apolar, hydrogen bonding and charged interactions. Such binding information can be used qualitatively to direct ligand design when converted to fragment occupancy maps termed FragMaps or can be used quantitatively to estimate the relative binding affinities of ligands free energies when converted into grid free energy (GFE) terms based on Boltzmann transformation [60]. Precomputed FragMaps can be used to perform fast binding affinity predictions with minimal computational costs once the FragMaps have been calculated. The current applications of FragMaps include docking protocol using SILCS-MC [60, 61] and pharmacophore modeling using SILCS-Pharm [62, 63]. And the related methods can benefit from the free energy context of the FragMaps which take both conformational flexibility and desolvation effect into account intrinsically along with ligand-protein interactions.

In SILCS-MC, the ligand is thoroughly sampled using the MC technique in the GFE FragMaps that come from SILCS simulation [60, 61]. During the sampling, each atom in the ligand positioned within a voxel of FragMap of the same type will be assigned the voxel GFE value, and the docking score named ligand GFE (LGFE) is the sum of GFEs contributed from all atoms in the ligand. Since FragMaps comes from explicit solvent full MD-based SILCS simulations, receptor flexibility is implicitly considered in the maps. Similar to the technique as used by AutoDock [55], using GFE grid maps has the benefit to efficiently evaluate docking poses. But different from the AutoDock docking grids, the GFE values from the FragMap grids contain abundant energy information that directly comes from our SILCS free energy binding assay. Thus, the SILCS-MC protocol presents a way to efficiently use free energy information from MD in a docking manner to balance both accuracy and efficiency. A recent study even shows it outperforms traditional FEP methods in the estimation of relative binding free energies of inhibitors targeting two kinase systems, ACK1 and p38 MAP kinase [57].

In the pharmacophore modeling application, SILCS-Pharm converts the spatial distributions of FragMaps of a specific type into pharmacophore features of the same type, and an importance score defined as feature GFE (FGFE) is assigned to each feature automatically [62, 63]. Volume constraints, which are derived by using SILCS exclusion maps, are also included in a pharmacophore model to represent for the forbidden region of small molecules. Based on the tests performed on eight protein targets from the DUD database [64], better performances of SILCS-Pharm are seen when compared to some typical target-based pharmacophore methods and docking methods [62, 63]. Unlike the other receptor-based pharmacophore modeling method, which mostly uses both rigid receptor structure and rigid probe molecules [24, 25], SILCS-Pharm extracts features based on FragMaps that intrinsically contain flexibility consideration for both receptor and probe molecules. And it also benefits from using the GFE score that contains free energy like information with desolvation effects to prioritize important features.

The above fully described methods are mainly SBDD methods while LBDD methods are also very useful. The similarity search method [26, 27] requires the least inputs among all CADD methods since it only requires one lead compound and can help to quickly accumulate more hit compounds for other CADD methods to perform further analysis. The philosophy behind the similarity search method is that structural similar chemicals are likely to have similar activities. And so, this approach may be used to potentially identify compounds with improved activities and develop SAR for each series of compounds that may be used to direct further ligand design. To calculate the similarity between two compounds, fingerprint, which is a collection of structural or physiochemical properties about a molecule, is usually used. Chemical fingerprints such as BIT-MACCS [65] encode information such as the presence of specific types of atoms, bonds, or scaffolds in the molecule into bits in a string and can be used to identify compounds that are structurally similar to the lead. Physiochemical fingerprints such as MP-MFP [66] encode properties such as molecular weight, polarity, and free energy of solvation, which can be used to locate compounds with similar physiochemical properties, but dissimilar structures and may help to identify new hits with new scaffolds. More details about typical LBDD methods can be found in a previous review from our laboratory [67].

Applications of CADD Methods for Kinase Inhibitor Development

CADD methods were regularly utilized by researchers to help with the development of kinase inhibitors. A major challenge to the development of kinase inhibitors is drug resistance. Resistance to kinases can be caused by different mechanisms such as amplification of the oncogenic protein kinase gene [68] but, most frequently, is caused by inherent or acquired missense mutations in the targeted kinase [69]. Understanding the atomic-level mechanism behind the kinase inhibitor resistance helps in the design of new generation kinase inhibitors to overcome the resistance.

Tanneeru et al. studied the molecular mechanism of native and mutant breakpoint cluster region-Abelson (BCR-ABL) kinases inhibition by Ponatinib at the atomic level using molecular dynamics (MD) simulations [70]. BCR-ABL is the cytoplasmic fusion oncoprotein with constitutive tyrosine kinase activity that is related to chronic myeloid leukemia [71]. Well-established kinase inhibitors such as imatinib are effective but are resistant to some BCR-ABL mutations including the T315I mutation while the new generation ABL inhibitor ponatinib is able to inhibit both wild-type and most of the clinically relevant mutants [72]. In the study, MD simulations were performed on 14 mutant ABL kinase-ponatinib complexes and ponatinib binding free energies were calculated. Residues that are responsible for ponatinib binding were identified and their conformational changes upon mutations analyzed to obtain insights that would be helpful in the design of new ABL inhibitors that can inhibit a wide range of mutants and overcome the mutational resistance [70].

In another study conducted by Hauser et al., resistance of 8 kinase inhibitors across 144 clinically identified ABL mutations were predicted using alchemical free energy calculations [73]. The ability for free energy calculations to predict how kinase mutations modulate inhibitor affinities to ABL was examined, and high accuracy of the applied modeling protocol was observed. This study established the potential of using computational modeling to reliably predict drug resistance to kinase mutations in an automated fashion.

The majority of kinase inhibitors target the ATP-binding site located between two lobes of the kinase. Since the ATP-binding site has conserved motifs across most kinases, it is a challenge to design selective kinase inhibitors [74]. To address this, Huang et al. presented a bioinformatics study on kinase selectivity using network analysis [75]. They identified ATP-binding site residues for most human kinases using structure- and sequence-based approaches. Based on known strategies for developing selective kinase inhibitors, key residues were recognized which were encoded into fingerprints and analyzed by a network approach to yield kinase selectivity potential networks. Such networks can help to propose systematic guidelines to develop selective kinase inhibitors.

In another study, using the WaterMap protocol [76], Robinson et al. studied kinase inhibitor selectivity for four kinase systems [77]. Comparisons of the locations and energetics of ATP-binding site water molecules from MD simulations were made, and differences in water structures and energetics were used to qualitatively explain the observed variations in activity. Such a computational technique may help to examine selectivity of designed inhibitors and suggest priority for testing during the development of selective kinase inhibitors.

Going beyond the ATP-binding site and finding alternative binding sites for kinase inhibitors is another approach to overcome kinase selectivity and resistance issues. Using CADD approaches, our laboratory together with experimentalists designed new extracellular-signal-regulated kinase (ERK) inhibitors targeting the substrate docking domains that have the potential to develop selective inhibitors for specific substrates involved in pathological conditions while preserving interactions involved in normal cellular processes [9–13]. In silico database screening was conducted to search for small-molecular-weight compounds, and several bioassay confirmed compounds were verified by experimental studies to inhibit ERK-specific phosphorylation of ribosomal S6 kinase-1 (Rsk-1) and the ternary complex factor Elk-1 (TCF/Elk-1), which are involved in promoting cell proliferation. Lead compounds being identified in these studies set the road toward the development of novel non-ATP-dependent inhibitors selective for ERK and its interactions with substrates involved in cancer cell proliferation.

In this section, an overview of research works from our laboratory employing CADD methods targeting kinase systems is presented. These examples put various CADD methods in a practical context to help the reader better understand how CADD methods can interact with experimental techniques to expedite the development of kinase inhibitors.

Extracellular-Signal-Regulated Kinases (ERK)

The extracellular-signal-regulated kinases (ERK) are members of the mitogen-activated protein (MAP) kinase family that play an integral role in signaling events that regulate cell growth, proliferation, differentiation, inflammatory responses, and programmed cell death [78, 79]. The ERK proteins consist of two isoforms, ERK1 and ERK2. Activation of ERK proteins is tightly regulated by direct phosphorylation of residues Thr183 and Tyr185 (according to ERK2 and is shown by stick representation in Fig. 2a), and resulted movement of the ATP-binding site (as shown by pink spheres in Fig. 2a) in the N-terminal lobe in proximity with the C-terminal lobe allows phosphorylation of many substrate proteins [80, 81]. Unregulated activation

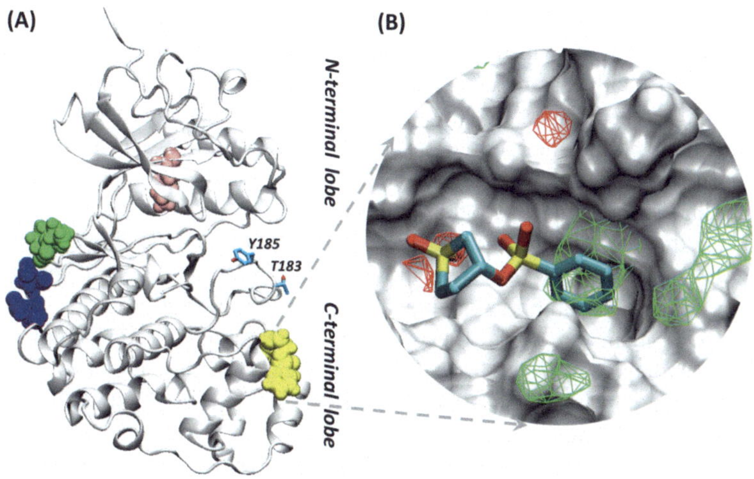

Fig. 2 (**a**) Binding sites on ERK2 protein. ERK2 structure contains N-terminal and C-terminal lobes. ATP-binding site is indicated by residue K52 in VDW representation as shown by pink spheres. CD site residues D316 and D319 are shown by blue spheres while ED site residues T157 and T158 are shown by green spheres. Phosphorylation site residues T183 and Y185 are shown in stick representations. Binding response identified site 5 at the FRS site is indicated by yellow spheres. (**b**) Enlarged view of crystal binding pose of compound 2.3.2 at the FRS-binding site and overlaid FragMaps around it. Favorable apolar and hydrogen bond acceptor FragMaps are shown by green and red frames, respectively. FragMaps on the ligand-binding orientation reproduce important binding patterns while those surround the binding pose indicate additional binding information that can be utilized to optimize the current lead

of ERK1/2 signaling has been found in a variety of cancers [82]. Thus, ERK1/2 serve as promising cancer-related drug targets.

Structural studies show conservation of the catalytic domain that includes the ATP-binding site among MAP kinase proteins, and many early kinase inhibitors were developed to target this region for competition of ATP binding [83]. However, such designed inhibitors lack specificity. Thus, researchers were looking for a way to target beyond the ATP-binding site in order to develop more selective inhibitors. This effort in our laboratories focused on the identification of compounds that can interrupt interactions between ERK1/2 and specific substrates involved in disease processes such as cancer cell proliferation or inflammatory responses while preserving ERK-mediated regulation of substrates involved in normal cell functions.

A number of experimental studies identified two docking domains on ERK1/2 that are involved in interactions with substrates leading to their phosphorylation. The first-identified such docking domain is the common docking (CD) domain, which is located on the opposite side to the MAP kinase activation lip and consists of aspartate residues 316 and 319 in ERK2 as shown by blue spheres in Fig. 2a [84]. The CD domain of ERK2 was shown to facilitate interactions with the upstream activating proteins [84], and mutagenesis study indicated its interaction with the D domain on substrate proteins [81]. Another docking site that is adjacent to the CD domain is referred to as the ED domain, which consists of threonine residues 157 and 158 in ERK2 as shown by green spheres in Fig. 2a, and was shown to confer specificity [85]. Studies using deuterium exchange and mass spectrometry to measure solvent protection revealed hydrophobic regions near the activation lip of ERK2 identified a third site referred to as the F-site recruitment site (FRS) [86]. The FRS site consists of residues L198, Y231, L232, L235 and Y261 and was shown to interact with F domain on substrate proteins [86].

To reach the goal of substrate-specific ERK1/2 inhibitors, the above-mentioned docking domains were targeted to search for small-molecular-weight ligands that bind to these sites and inhibit interactions with selected substrate proteins. Since the ED and CD domains are close to each other, CADD methods were employed to target this region [9–11]. In our first attempt [9], the crystal structure of ERK2 in the unphosphorylated inactive state (PDB ID: 1ERK) [87] was used with SBDD methods. To search for putative binding sites, complimentary probe spheres that occupy concave sites on the protein were generated on the solvent accessible surface (SAS) of the protein. The SAS was generated using the program DMS [88], and spheres were calculated with the SPHGEN code [89] associated with the program DOCK [54]. Spheres that were within both 10 Å of the CD domain and 12 Å of the ED domain were selected, yielding a sphere cluster of 11 spheres located in a groove between the CD and ED domains. This sphere set served as the target site for in silico docking studies performed using the program DOCK [54].

An in-house database containing more than 800,000 commercially available compounds was screened in the VS study. During the docking, ligands were treated as flexible based on the anchored search method and a two-step fashion docking algorithm [9]. At the primary docking step, the applied anchored search method involved separating each compound into rigid segments and those with more than five heavy atoms were used as anchors. Anchors were docked into the binding site in 250 orientations based on overlap with the sphere set defining the site and then energy minimized. The other parts of the molecule were then built around the anchor by adding them in a layer-by-layer manner based on segments connected through rotatable bonds. At each step, the dihedral around the rotatable bond was sampled in increments of 10°, and the lowest conformation was reserved. Each rotatable bond was minimized as it was created without re-minimizing the other bonds. The top 20,000 hit compounds from the primary docking step were selected based on their normalized van der Waals (VDW) interaction energy to minimize the bias toward the selection of highly polar compounds. The use of the VDW interaction energy leads to compound selection being focused on the molecule-target site shape complementarity. In addition, to maximize the hit compound druglikeness, a size normalization approach [90] was applied to lead to the selection of lower-molecular-weight compounds. In the secondary docking step of the selected 20,000 compounds, additional minimization of all rotatable bonds simultaneously was performed during the anchor-based VS approach used in the primary docking in order to treat ligand flexibility in a more rigorous way. The normalized total interaction energy was used to select the top 500 hit compounds for further diversity analysis.

To maximize the chemical diversity of selected compounds for bioassay testing, the top 500 compounds from the docking VS were subjected to chemical similarity clustering. Clustering used the Jarvis-Patrick algorithm [91] implemented in the MOE program [92] with the BIT-MACCS fingerprint to describe each molecule, and the similarity between fingerprints of two molecules were evaluated using the Tanimoto coefficient [93]. From this effort, approximately 100 clusters of various sizes were obtained with the compounds in each cluster being similar. One or more compounds per cluster were chosen with emphasis on druglikeness according to Lipinski's rule of 5 (RO5) [94]. A total of 86 compounds were selected from which 80 were purchased from commercial vendors for experimental testing. Several compounds from this CADD effort were shown to inhibit the phosphorylation of two ERK substrates, ribosomal S6 kinase-1 (Rsk-1) and transcription factor Elk-1. Direct binding of the compounds to ERK2 was confirmed via fluorescence spectroscopy. Active compounds also showed dose-dependent inhibition of proliferation in several cancer cell lines. These compounds serve as the first ATP-independent inhibitors of ERK [9].

Following the initial VS effort, a similar CADD VS was performed targeting the active phosphorylated ERK2 structure (PDB ID: 2ERK) [95]. The second screen, which applied the same CADD protocol, was motivated by the fact that the activated ERK proteins are likely to be more biologically relevant in the context of proliferating cancer cells [10]. As only small conformational changes between inactive and active ERK2 structures are presented in the region of the ED and CD domains, the VS hit compounds had significant overlap with the initial VS study. However, there were still 45 new compounds identified which appeared to be associated with the subtle structural change around the CD domain. And 4 out of the 13 tested compounds were shown to have strong inhibition against ERK-mediated phosphorylation of Rsk-1 and Elk-1 [10].

Once compounds that inhibit the binding of substrate proteins to ERK were identified, the LBDD method was applied to identify additional active compounds [12]. This involved the use of the similarity search method to identify compounds that are structurally similar to the active compounds. The similarity search was conducted using the BIT-MACCS fingerprint with the Tanimoto similarity index against a virtual database of over one million commercially available compounds. From this effort, 5 and 10 compounds similar to the lead compounds 17 and 76, respectively, were selected and tested for inhibition of cell proliferation. One compound 76.3 was found to have higher potency than the lead compound 76. In addition, compounds 76.2 and 76.4 had similar potencies and biological effects. Cell-based and in vitro kinase assays indicated that compounds 76.3 and 76.4 directly inhibited ERK-mediated phosphorylation of caspase-9 and the p90Rsk-1 kinase, which phosphorylates and inhibits Bad, more effectively than the lead compound 76. Thus, the LBDD method was able to locate more potent inhibitors and accumulate more selective molecules that can help with future development of more chemotherapeutic agents with improved efficacy to disable some of ERK1/2 protein functions [12].

Besides CD and ED sites, we have also used CADD methods to target the FRS site, which has been shown to be involved in ERK-substrate interactions [13]. To identify putative binding sites around FRS site region, MD simulations were conducted to generate biologically meaningful conformations on both phosphorylated and unphosphorylated ERK2 structures. In addition, SILCS simulations were conducted with probe molecules to explore possible conformational changes that would allow for ligand-binding pockets not evident in the crystal structures, nor observed in the standard MD simulations, to be identified [96]. The protein conformations from the three simulations were collected and clustered to yield 18 representative conformations that used in the following binding site analyses focusing on the FRS region based on the binding response (BR) protocol developed in our lab [97]. BR involved docking a preselected batch of representative drug molecules to each conformation of the protein. The geometric fitness of drug molecules to the binding site and their DOCK interaction energies with binding site residues are calculated with putative binding sites ranked based on a combination of the favorable binding energies and geometric fitness. The method has been tested against a number of known protein-ligand complexes and shown to identify the experimental binding sites to a high level of accuracy [97].

From the BR calculations, a docking site named site 5 at the FRS site was identified as shown by yellow colored spheres in Fig. 2 and was targeted in VS. The two-step fashion docking protocol used for ED and CD site studies was used to screen an in-house database composed of 1.5 million commercial compounds. To consider conformational flexibility of ERK2, representative protein conformations from MD simulations were used in the docking studies, and each compound was docked to all conformations with the best scored docking pose across all conformations being retained for each ligand for use in the final ligand ranking. The top 1000 compounds from the two-step docking were clustered based on their similarities, and seven chemically diverse compounds were selected for the bioassay involving their effects on ERK1/2-mediated phosphorylation and signaling events. Several hit compounds were shown to inhibit ERK1/2-mediated phosphorylation of the transcription factor Elk-1 with compound 2.3.2 being the best one [13].

Of the active compounds, further optimization was undertaken on compound 2.3.2. This involved use of the SILCS FragMaps obtained from SILCS simulations using benzene and propane in aqueous solution. As shown in Fig. 2b, apolar FragMaps identified a putative binding pose of the phenyl group of 2.3.2, and the hydrogen bond acceptor FragMap captured the binding mode of sulfonyl oxygens. This indicates the ability of SILCS FragMaps to capture important binding patterns at the FRS site of ERK2. Notably, additional apolar FragMaps were seen near the 2.3.2 binding location as shown in Fig. 2b. The presence of such maps suggests that additional hydrophobic groups added to 2.3.2 might lead to improved affinity of ligands for the FRS site. Following this observation, three compounds with additional hydrophobic groups including methyl, biphenyl, and naphthyl moieties were designed, and their binding affinity changes related to the parent compound 2.3.2 were evaluated using LGFE scores which indicated that the modification would increase affinity for the binding pocket. These compounds were then realized by chemical syntheses, and the following bioassay tests verified these LGFE scored designs. Furthermore, the 2.3.2 analogs were shown to inhibit the expression of

F-site containing immediate early genes (IEGs) of the Fos family, including c-Fos and Fra1, and transcriptional regulation of the activator protein-1 (AP-1) complex. Moreover, this class of compounds was shown to selectively induce apoptosis in melanoma cells containing mutated BRaf and constitutively active ERK1/2 signaling, including melanoma cells that are inherently resistant to clinically relevant kinase inhibitors. Thus, the SILCS-based SBDD method successfully helped to optimize the lead compound, yielding a novel class of compounds that inhibit ERK1/2 signaling functions [13].

Structure-related biological mechanisms can also be studied using SBDD methods. As introduced previously, ERK1/2 can be activated by phosphorylation of two conserved residues on the activation lip mediated by MAP/ERK kinases. In addition, it had been found that certain mutations can activate ERK2 through an autoactivation mechanism [98]. This involves the gatekeeper residue Q103 and adjacent hydrophobic residues I84 and L73, and mutation of these hydrophobic residues to smaller residues led to enhanced autophosphorylation and kinase activity. We conducted a series of MD simulations of ERK1 and ERK2 in various stages of activation and the constitutively active mutants to investigate such an autoactivation mechanism [99]. The crystal structures of inactive and active ERK2 and monophosphorylated ERK1 as well as modeled structures of ERK2 mutants L73P, I84A, Q103A, R65S, K162M, and G83A were used to initialize the study. The MD simulations were performed in the NPT ensemble using the CHARMM program [100] with the CHARMM all-atom force fields [33–36]. MD simulations using the original [52] and restricted perturbation targeted MD methods [101] with the CHARMM [100] and NAMD [102] programs were conducted to identify transition pathways from the inactive to the active state of unphosphorylated ERK2.

Analyses on the MD trajectories showed that domain closure between N domain and C domain was observed in all states except for the inactive kinase, and such closure happened early in the simulation prior to folding of the activation lip and of L16 loop. Quasi-harmonic analyses of both the inactive and active states, a method used to identify global conformational changes in proteins and macromolecules [103], showed that hinge-type compression over the substrate-binding site and ED motif was a dominant motion for activation. Variance-covariance matrices analyses, which provide information about the extent of correlation of the motions of residues [104], showed that the correlations in the active and inactive states are generally equal in sign but different in magnitude. In particular, the various binding sites were much more strongly coupled in the inactive state.

Structure analyses further showed that the second phosphorylation event on T183 disrupts hydrogen bonding involving residue D334, thereby allowing the kinase to lock into the active conformation. Different effects brought by different mutations can be summarized from the simulation as follows. The G83A mutation was predicted to impede activation while Q64C was hypothesized to stop folding of loop L16, thereby perturbing the homodimerization interface. All these results extracted from MD simulations provide additional information to give a better understanding on functions of ERK proteins and may help with the design of new ERK specific inhibitors [99].

P38 MAP Kinase

P38 MAP kinases are also members of the MAP kinase family. The p38 MAP kinases contribute to the pathogenesis of many human diseases including cancer [105] and inflammatory bowel disease [106]. P38 MAP kinases–mediated regulation of endothelial and epithelial barrier function and leukocyte trafficking are central to the pathogenesis of acute and chronic inflammatory disorders [107]. Thus, preclinical studies strongly support the pharmacologic targeting of p38 as a treatment for inflammatory diseases.

The P38 MAP kinase family is composed of several isoforms, and genetic and pharmacologic studies have identified p38α as the proinflammatory isoform [108] whereas other studies showed that p38β signaling to be cytoprotective [109]. However, most of the existing p38 inhibitors are short of selectivity between isoforms and are active against both p38α and p38β [110]. In addition, these inhibitors lack efficacy and showed toxicity, and they have had very limited success in clinical testing [111]. Finally, the majority of the inhibitors are targeting the p38α catalytic site so that all p38α signaling events will be blocked among which some are essential for reestablishing and maintaining homeostasis.

To overcome the above limitations, we took a strategy similar to that was done with ERK to go beyond the ATP-binding site and obtain for p38α specific small-molecule inhibitors [112]. The CADD effort targeted the substrate-binding groove of p38α, which stretches between two acidic patches, the common docking (CD) and glutamate-aspartate (ED) domains. The crystal structure of mouse p38α (PDB ID: 1P38) [113] was used to initialize the study. The NAMD program [102] with the CHARMM force field [33–36] was used to conduct a MD simulation in order to generate multiple protein conformations. Protein structures from MD trajectory were subjected to clustering to identify 20 representative protein conformations that were used in the BR method to identify potential binding sites. Out of this effort, a pocket near the ED site comprising of ten amino acid residues was identified and, importantly, only seven residues in this pocket are shared between p38α and p38β, indicating the specificity that can be pursued. Overlay of structures of unphosphorylated and dual-phosphorylated p38α revealed near-superposition of the targeted pocket in the two forms, which indicates the preserved conformation of this site even when being activated. Thus, ligands binding to this site inhibit interactions with substrates for both activated and nonactivated forms.

A similar two-step docking protocol used for ERK [9] was employed. An in-house database of commercially available compounds from the Maybridge [114] was used in the screening. At the first step of docking, compounds were ranked based on their VDW energies with size-based score normalization, and 50,000 compounds were selected for a second step of docking with additional minimization of the small molecules. Then, the top 1000 compounds were selected based on the total interaction energy including size-based normalization from the second step of docking. Chemical-fingerprint-based cluster analysis was performed to identify chemically diverse compounds, and the final list of hit compounds were selected based on our scalar 4-dimensional bioavailability (4DBA) metric [115] to account for drug-likeness. The 4DBA descriptor was developed in our lab to address the first four criteria in RO5 in order to judge the druglikeness of a compound based on a scalar metric and thus facilitate the VS hit selection in an automatic fashion [115]. A panel of 150 diverse compounds was selected for biological testing from which 20 of these structurally dissimilar compounds were obtained for functional analysis.

Testing of the 20 compounds yielded an active compound, UM101. Experiments showed this compound to be at least as effective as one existing inhibitor, SB203580 [116], targeting the catalytic site in stabilizing endothelial barrier function, reducing inflammation, and mitigating LPS-induced mouse lung injury. Specificity of UM101 on binding to p38α but not p38β was verified by differential scanning fluorimetry and saturation transfer difference-nuclear magnetic resonance. RNA sequencing analysis revealed that UM101 inhibited more genes and transcription factors than the catalytic inhibitor SB203580 but spared the antiinflammatory p38α substrate and the mitogen- and stress-activated kinase (MSK) 1/2 pathway.

The MD-based SBDD method can also help with the optimization of p38 small molecule binders that target the catalytic site. In a validation study of the SILCS method that included p38 [60], it was shown that FragMaps from SILCS can correctly reproduce the crystal binding modes of important function groups in six known p38 ligands as indicated by overlaps between the SILCS FragMaps and ligand functional groups of the same types. Analyses were also done for correlations between experimental affinities computed from experimental IC_{50} data and LGFE scores calculated from different conformational ensembles including those from minimization, single dynamics, multidynamics, and SILCS-MC samplings. High correlation was seen for the p38 system using the SILCS-MC approach. This earlier study verified that SILCS can be used both qualitatively and quantitatively for drug design on the p38 MAP kinase protein.

In another study [117], we tested the ability of the SSFEP and SILCS-MC approaches to estimate relative binding affinities of known p38 MAP kinase inhibitors and compared their performances with the traditional FEP method. Fifteen chemical transformations with experimental relative binding affinity data for p38 MAP kinase were evaluated using the FEP, SSFEP, and SILCS-MC methods. The GROMACS program [118] with the CHARMM force field was used to conduct all MD simulations. FEP calculations were set up in solution and determined in the protein environment for all evaluated transformations. For SSFEP, MD simulation on each reference ligand was performed, and postprocessing of MD simulation data of the reference ligand system was conducted to calculate free energy changes for all transformations related to the reference ligand. For SILCS, simulations were setup according to the GCMC/MD protocol [119, 120]. After the FragMaps was generated, SILCS-MC samplings of each ligand in the presence of GFE grids were performed to predict binding strength using either the lowest LGFE from the best predicted binding mode or the average LGFE of all predicted binding modes. From this study, better correlations between prediction and experimental data were observed for SSFEP and SILCS-MC results with removal of one outlier when compared with FEP for p38, and results using the minimum LGFE from SILCS-MC being the best.

In this study, we also tested the performance of SILCS-MC on a larger dataset for p38 from the literature [121], which was also studied by Wang et al. using the more expensive FEP+ method [122]. A similar level of correlation between prediction and experimental data was seen for SILCS-MC when compared with the FEP+ method. However, SILCS-MC predictions yielded a larger number of correct results with respect to the sign of the relative binding free energy changes than the FEP+ method. While both the SSFEP and SILCS-MC approaches require a significant upfront computational investment, they offer a 1000-fold computational savings over FEP for calculating the relative affinities of ligand modifications once those precomputations are complete. The competitive results of SSFEP and SILCS-MC indicate their ability to facilitate the drug optimization stage by screening many possible chemical modifications at cheap computational costs. As a proof-of-concept, in this study we also applied SSFEP and SILCS-MC to the simulation data for the p38 ligand L11, and relative free energy predictions on 147 chemical modifications at 15 sites on the molecule were conducted in a matter of hours, yielding results on a time scale that can lead the drug optimization process [117].

In a most recent study, the SILCS-MC method was extensively validated on several protein systems including p38 [61]. Optimization of the SILCS-MC protocol using a number of different scoring schemes and MC sampling protocols was undertaken to further improve the predictive capability of the method. For the p38 system, inclusion of an ether-containing probe in SILCS and the resulting ether FragMaps yield an increase in the predictability of the model since the entire set of ligands contains ether oxygen-type atoms [121]. Another piece of knowledge gained from this study is that the machine learning technique [123] can be used to further optimize the scaling factors of individual contributing GFE energy terms in the LGFE score. Once a set of lead compounds got confirmed, the FragMap weighting factors can be trained to improve the predictive capability of the model and helps with the design of new binders.

The p38 MAP kinase system was also used to validate the SILCS-Pharm method [62, 63]. From the SILCS FragMaps of p38, pharmacophore features were deduced within the catalytic-binding site. Pharmacophore features were then ranked based on their FGFE scores, which is a sum over GFEs of all voxels composing the feature. For a given number of features, a pharmacophore model which contains the highly ranked features was built and used in VS to check its performance. A pharmacophore model for p38 that contains one hydrogen bond donor feature and two hydrophobic features was found to outperform other docking results with a high enrichment. This study proved the ability of the SILCS-Pharm method to guide SBDD and its utility in rational drug design to identify binders when no known compounds are available using a pharmacophore-based VS approach.

P56 T Cell Tyrosine Kinase (Lck)

P56 T cell tyrosine kinase (Lck) is a kinase predominantly expressed in T lymphocytes where it plays a critical role in T-cell-mediated immune response [124]. It is responsible for the phosphorylation of conserved tyrosine residues of the CD3 receptor called immunoreceptor tyrosine-based activation motifs (ITAMs), and such phosphorylation serves as the first step required for T cell activation signaling cascades leading to the expression of IL2 and the proliferation of T cells [125]. Thus, interruption of Lck-ITAM interaction offers the potential of suppressing immune response and may help to find a therapeutic way for the treatment of T cell leukemias and autoimmune diseases such as rheumatoid arthritis [124].

Lck participates in phosphotyrosine (pY) dependent protein-protein interactions through its modular binding units, called Src homology-2 (SH2) domains [126]. And the most obvious feature to target is the pY binding pocket on the SH2 domain. However, small compound binders targeting the pY pocket may lack specificity since a large number of signaling proteins contain this motif. A previous study conducted a phosphopeptide library screen and identified a preferred pY-containing peptide binding sequence Ac-pY-E-E-I for the Lck SH2 domain [127]. Structural analysis of the crystal structure revealed that the pY and Ile residues are bound to two well-defined cavities that are referred as pY and pY+3 binding sites. Site mutation studies of residues in the pY+3 binding site showed switched binding specificity, indicating the pY+3 pocket is important for specific binding [128]. Thus, this site represents a good candidate to target for identifying specific inhibitors of the p56 Lck SH2 domain.

Accordingly, our lab performed CADD screening to identify small molecular binders targeting the pY+3 site of the Lck SH2 domain [129]. Ligand identification was targeted at an in-house database composed of two million commercially available compounds. Sphere sets, as required for the initial placement of the ligand during docking using the DOCK program [54], were generated, and only spheres within 6 Å of the pY+3 binding site and within 3 Å of the crystal location of the Ile residue were selected for the VS. A phenolphosphate with assigned neutral charge was maintained in the pY-binding site of the SH2 domain during the screening to avoid docked compounds interacting with the pY pocket.

Docking again involved two steps going from two million to 25,000 in the first round of screening, with compounds selected based on molecular-weight-normalized VDW interaction energy, to two sets of 1000 compounds in the second round of screening, which were based on the total interaction energy and the molecular–weight-normalized total interaction energy, respectively. Both sets of selected compounds were subjected to similarity-based clustering followed by selection of compounds for bioassay tests from individual clusters according to the Lipinski's RO5. From this effort, 196 available compounds were purchased from commercial vendors and were tested for their ability to inhibit p56 Lck SH2 domain association with phosphotyrosine containing C-terminal ITAM2 peptide in an affinity precipitation assay. Thirty-four compounds were shown to have activity in this assay, and 13 compounds were further verified to have inhibitory activity in a mixed lymphocyte culture assay. Fluorescence titration experiments on four of these active compounds verified their direct binding to the SH2 domain [129].

Based on this effort, our lab then conducted similarity searches on 12 lead compounds against a database containing 1,300,000 commercially available compounds to develop SAR and potentially identify compounds with improved activity [130]. The inhibitory activity of the selected compounds was assessed using enzyme immunoassay (EIA). In general, the most active parent compounds yield the most active similar compound even though there were cases that low activity parent compounds yielded multiple similar compounds with high activities. This observation emphasized the importance of introduction of diversity when selecting compounds for the first round of the bioassay test. For lead compound 276, based on structural analysis of identified similar compounds that showed activity, it was concluded that the heterocycle-amide-phenyl core moiety is important for the binding of compounds from this series. And the presence of a furan ring linked to benzoic acid moiety also facilitates activity, and an alternate functional group with acceptor moieties can also help to enhance the inhibition. And based on docked binding orientations of 276 series of compounds, protein residues K179, K182, and R184 of the Lck SH2 domain were identified as important for inhibitor binding. All the information obtained using CADD methods will be useful for further exploration and optimization of Lck SH2 domain inhibitors [130].

Summary

In this chapter, basic concepts and typical methods for CADD are introduced with real-life examples on how CADD methods can interact with experimental techniques to help identify novel kinase inhibitors. With the development on both hardware, e.g., more powerful computers equipped with enhanced graphic processing units, and software, e.g., advanced artificial intelligence techniques, CADD techniques are anticipated to be further enhanced with improved accuracy and efficiency in the future to be better incorporated with experiments to expedite the drug design process targeting kinase systems.

Acknowledgments This work was supported by GM131710 to ADM, Jr., University of Maryland Center for Biomolecular Therapeutics, Samuel Waxman Cancer Research Foundation, and the Computer-Aided Drug Design (CADD) Center at the University of Maryland, Baltimore.

Conflict of interest: A.D.M. is cofounder and CSO of SilcsBio LLC.

References

1. Manning, G., Whyte, D. B., Martinez, R., Hunter, T., & Sudarsanam, S. (2002). The protein kinase complement of the human genome. *Science, 298*, 1912–1934.
2. Ferguson, F. M., & Gray, N. S. (2018). Kinase inhibitors: The road ahead. *Nature Reviews Drug Discovery, 17*, 353–376.
3. Levitzki, A. (2003). Protein kinase inhibitors as a therapeutic modality. *Accounts of Chemical Research, 36*, 462–469.
4. Muller, S., Chaikuad, A., Gray, N. S., & Knapp, S. (2015). The ins and outs of selective kinase inhibitor development. *Nature Chemical Biology, 11*, 818–821.
5. Wu, P., Nielsen, T. E., & Clausen, M. H. (2015). FDA-approved small-molecule kinase inhibitors. *Trends in Pharmacological Sciences, 36*, 422–439.
6. Cohen, P., & Alessi, D. R. (2013). Kinase drug discovery—What's next in the field? *ACS Chemical Biology, 8*, 96–104.
7. Yu, W., Guvench, O., & MacKerell, A. D. (2013). Computational approaches for the design of protein–protein interaction inhibitors. In G. Zinzalla (Ed.), *Understanding and exploiting protein–protein interactions as drug targets* (pp. 99–102). London: Future Science Ltd..
8. Yu, W., & MacKerell, A. D. (2017). Computer-aided drug design methods. In P. Sass (Ed.), *Antibiotics. Methods in molecular biology* (Vol. 1520, pp. 85–106). New York: Humana Press.
9. Hancock, C. N., Macias, A., Lee, E. K., Yu, S. Y., MacKerell, A. D., & Shapiro, P. (2005). Identification of novel extracellular signal-regulated kinase docking domain inhibitors. *Journal of Medicinal Chemistry, 48*, 4586–4595.
10. Chen, F., Hancock, C. N., Macias, A., Joh, J., Still, K., Zhong, S., MacKerell, A. D., & Shapiro, P. (2006). Characterization of ATP-independent ERK inhibitors identified through in silico analysis of the active ERK2 structure. *Bioorganic & Medicinal Chemistry Letters, 16*, 6281–6287.
11. Burkhard, K., Smith, S., Deshmukh, R., MacKerell, A. D., & Shapiro, P. (2009). Development of extracellular signal-regulated kinase inhibitors. *Current Topics in Medicinal Chemistry, 9*, 678–689.
12. Boston, S. R., Deshmukh, R., Strome, S., Priyakumar, U. D., MacKerell, A. D., & Shapiro, P. (2011). Characterization of ERK docking domain inhibitors that induce apoptosis by targeting Rsk-1 and caspase-9. *BMC Cancer, 11*, 7.
13. Samadani, R., Zhang, J., Brophy, A., Oashi, T., Priyakumar, U. D., Raman, E. P., St John, F. J., Jung, K., Fletcher, S., Pozharski, E., MacKerell, A. D., & Shapiro, P. (2015). Small-molecule inhibitors of ERK-mediated immediate early gene expression and proliferation of melanoma cells expressing mutated BRaf. *The Biochemical Journal, 467*, 425–438.
14. Van Drie, J. (2007). Computer-aided drug design: The next 20 years. *Journal of Computer-Aided Molecular Design, 21*, 591–601.
15. Sliwoski, G., Kothiwale, S., Meiler, J., & Lowe, E. W. (2014). Computational methods in drug discovery. *Pharmacological Reviews, 66*, 334–395.
16. Cavasotto, C. N. (Ed.). (2015). *In silico drug discovery and design: Theory, methods, challenges, and applications*. Boca Raton: CRC Press.
17. MacArthur, M. W., Driscoll, P. C., & Thornton, J. M. (1994). NMR and crystallography complementary approaches to structure determination. *Trends in Biotechnology, 12*, 149–153.
18. Cavasotto, C. N., & Phatak, S. S. (2009). Homology modeling in drug discovery: Current trends and applications. *Drug Discovery Today, 14*, 676–683.
19. Simonson, T., Archontis, G., & Karplus, M. (2002). Free energy simulations come of age: Protein–ligand recognition. *Accounts of Chemical Research, 35*, 430–437.
20. Lee, M. S., & Olson, M. A. (2006). Calculation of absolute protein-ligand binding affinity using path and endpoint approaches. *Biophysical Journal, 90*, 864–877.

21. Shivakumar, D., Williams, J., Wu, Y., Damm, W., Shelley, J., & Sherman, W. (2010). Prediction of absolute solvation free energies using molecular dynamics free energy perturbation and the OPLS force field. *Journal of Chemical Theory and Computation, 6*, 1509–1519.
22. Kitchen, D. B., Decornez, H., Furr, J. R., & Bajorath, J. (2004). Docking and scoring in virtual screening for drug discovery: Methods and applications. *Nature Reviews Drug Discovery, 3*, 935–949.
23. Sousa, S. F., Fernandes, P. A., & Ramos, M. J. (2006). Protein–ligand docking: Current status and future challenges. *Proteins: Structure, FUnction, and Bioinformatics, 65*, 15–26.
24. Yang, S. (2010). Pharmacophore modeling and applications in drug discovery: Challenges and recent advances. *Drug Discovery Today, 15*, 444–450.
25. Pirhadi, S., Shiri, F., & Ghasemi, J. B. (2013). Methods and applications of structure based pharmacophores in drug discovery. *Current Topics in Medicinal Chemistry, 13*, 1036–1047.
26. Willett, P. (2006). Similarity-based virtual screening using 2D fingerprints. *Drug Discovery Today, 11*, 1046–1053.
27. Cereto-Massague, A., Ojeda, M. J., Valls, C., Mulero, M., Garcia-Vallve, S., & Pujadas, G. (2015). Molecular fingerprint similarity search in virtual screening. *Methods, 71*, 58–63.
28. Gedeck, P., Kramer, C., & Ertl, P. (2010). 4—computational analysis of structure-activity relationships. In G. Lawton & D. R. Witty (Eds.), *Progress in medicinal chemistry* (pp. 113–160). Amsterdam: Elsevier.
29. Cherkasov, A., Muratov, E. N., Fourches, D., Varnek, A., Baskin, I., Cronin, M., Dearden, J., Gramatica, P., Martin, Y. C., Todeschini, R., Consonni, V., Kuzmin, V. E., Cramer, R., Benigni, R., Yang, C., Rathman, J., Terfloth, L., Gasteiger, J., Richard, A., & Tropsha, A. (2014). QSAR modeling: Where have you been? Where are you going to? *Journal of Medicinal Chemistry, 57*, 4977–5010.
30. Verma, J., Khedkar, V. M., & Coutinho, E. C. (2010). 3D-QSAR in drug design—A review. *Current Topics in Medicinal Chemistry, 10*, 95–115.
31. Leach, A. R., Gillet, V. J., Lewis, R. A., & Taylor, R. (2010). Three-dimensional pharmacophore methods in drug discovery. *Journal of Medicinal Chemistry, 53*, 539–558.
32. Wolber, G., Seidel, T., Bendix, F., & Langer, T. (2008). Molecule-pharmacophore superpositioning and pattern matching in computational drug design. *Drug Discovery Today, 13*, 23–29.
33. MacKerell, A. D., Bashford, D., Bellott, M., Dunbrack, R. L., Evanseck, J. D., Field, M. J., Fischer, S., Gao, J., Guo, H., Ha, S., Joseph-McCarthy, D., Kuchnir, L., Kuczera, K., Lau, F. T. K., Mattos, C., Michnick, S., Ngo, T., Nguyen, D. T., Prodhom, B., Reiher, W. E., Roux, B., Schlenkrich, M., Smith, J. C., Stote, R., Straub, J., Watanabe, M., Wiórkiewicz-Kuczera, J., Yin, D., & Karplus, M. (1998). All-atom empirical potential for molecular modeling and dynamics studies of proteins. *The Journal of Physical Chemistry B, 102*, 3586–3616.
34. Best, R. B., Zhu, X., Shim, J., Lopes, P. E. M., Mittal, J., Feig, M., & MacKerell, A. D. (2012). Optimization of the additive CHARMM all-atom protein force field targeting improved sampling of the backbone ϕ, ψ and side-chain $\chi 1$ and $\chi 2$ dihedral angles. *Journal of Chemical Theory and Computation, 8*, 3257–3273.
35. Vanommeslaeghe, K., Hatcher, E., Acharya, C., Kundu, S., Zhong, S., Shim, J., Darian, E., Guvench, O., Lopes, P., Vorobyov, I., & Mackerell, A. D. (2010). CHARMM general force field: A force field for drug-like molecules compatible with the CHARMM all-atom additive biological force fields. *Journal of Computational Chemistry, 31*, 671–690.
36. Yu, W., He, X., Vanommeslaeghe, K., & MacKerell, A. D. (2012). Extension of the CHARMM general force field to sulfonyl-containing compounds and its utility in biomolecular simulations. *Journal of Computational Chemistry, 33*, 2451–2468.
37. Cornell, W. D., Cieplak, P., Bayly, C. I., Gould, I. R., Merz, K. M., Ferguson, D. M., Spellmeyer, D. C., Fox, T., Caldwell, J. W., & Kollman, P. A. (1995). A second generation force field for the simulation of proteins, nucleic acids, and organic molecules. *Journal of the American Chemical Society, 117*, 5179–5197.

38. Wang, J., Wolf, R. M., Caldwell, J. W., Kollman, P. A., & Case, D. A. (2004). Development and testing of a general amber force field. *Journal of Computational Chemistry, 25*, 1157–1174.
39. Friesner, R. A., Banks, J. L., Murphy, R. B., Halgren, T. A., Klicic, J. J., Mainz, D. T., Repasky, M. P., Knoll, E. H., Shelley, M., Perry, J. K., Shaw, D. E., Francis, P., & Shenkin, P. S. (2004). Glide: A new approach for rapid, accurate docking and scoring. 1. Method and assessment of docking accuracy. *Journal of Medicinal Chemistry, 47*, 1739–1749.
40. Eldridge, M. D., Murray, C. W., Auton, T. R., Paolini, G. V., & Mee, R. P. (1997). Empirical scoring functions: I. The development of a fast empirical scoring function to estimate the binding affinity of ligands in receptor complexes. *Journal of Computer-Aided Molecular Design, 11*, 425–445.
41. Wang, R., Lai, L., & Wang, S. (2002). Further development and validation of empirical scoring functions for structure-based binding affinity prediction. *Journal of Computer-Aided Molecular Design, 16*, 11–26.
42. Krammer, A., Kirchhoff, P. D., Jiang, X., Venkatachalam, C. M., & Waldman, M. (2005). LigScore: A novel scoring function for predicting binding affinities. *Journal of Molecular Graphics & Modelling, 23*, 395–407.
43. Ballester, P. J., & Mitchell, J. B. (2010). A machine learning approach to predicting protein-ligand binding affinity with applications to molecular docking. *Bioinformatics, 26*, 1169–1175.
44. Kinnings, S. L., Liu, N., Tonge, P. J., Jackson, R. M., Xie, L., & Bourne, P. E. (2011). A machine learning-based method to improve docking scoring functions and its application to drug repurposing. *Journal of Chemical Information and Modeling, 51*, 408–419.
45. Wójcikowski, M., Ballester, P. J., & Siedlecki, P. (2017). Performance of machine-learning scoring functions in structure-based virtual screening. *Scientific Reports, 7*, 46710.
46. Ain, Q., Aleksandrova, A., Roessler, F. D., & Ballester, P. J. (2015). Machine-learning scoring functions to improve structure-based binding affinity prediction and virtual screening. *Wiley Interdisciplinary Reviews Computational Molecular Science, 5*, 405–424.
47. Karplus, M., & McCammon, J. A. (2002). Molecular dynamics simulations of biomolecules. *Nature Structural Biology, 9*, 646–652.
48. Teilum, K., Olsen, J. G., & Kragelund, B. B. (2009). Functional aspects of protein flexibility. *Cellular and Molecular Life Sciences, 66*, 2231–2247.
49. Carlson, H. A. (2002). Protein flexibility is an important component of structure-based drug discovery. *Current Pharmaceutical Design, 8*, 1571–1578.
50. Lexa, K. W., & Carlson, H. A. (2011). Full protein flexibility is essential for proper hot-spot mapping. *Journal of the American Chemical Society, 133*, 200–202.
51. Sugita, Y., & Okamoto, Y. (1999). Replica-exchange molecular dynamics method for protein folding. *Chemical Physics Letters, 314*, 141–151.
52. Schlitter, J., Engels, M., & Krüger, P. (1994). Targeted molecular dynamics: A new approach for searching pathways of conformational transitions. *Journal of Molecular Graphics, 12*, 84–89.
53. Grinter, S. Z., & Zou, X. (2014). Challenges, applications, and recent advances of protein-ligand docking in structure-based drug design. *Molecules, 19*, 10150–10176.
54. Ewing, T. A., Makino, S., Skillman, A. G., & Kuntz, I. (2001). DOCK 4.0: Search strategies for automated molecular docking of flexible molecule databases. *Journal of Computer-Aided Molecular Design, 15*, 411–428.
55. Morris, G. M., Huey, R., Lindstrom, W., Sanner, M. F., Belew, R. K., Goodsell, D. S., & Olson, A. J. (2009). AutoDock4 and AutoDockTools4: Automated docking with selective receptor flexibility. *Journal of Computational Chemistry, 30*, 2785–2791.
56. Jorgensen, W. L., & Thomas, L. L. (2008). Perspective on free-energy perturbation calculations for chemical equilibria. *Journal of Chemical Theory and Computation, 4*, 869–876.
57. Raman, E. P., Vanommeslaeghe, K., & MacKerell, A. D. (2012). Site-specific fragment identification guided by single-step free energy perturbation calculations. *Journal of Chemical Theory and Computation, 8*, 3513–3525.

58. Guvench, O., & MacKerell, A. D., Jr. (2009). Computational fragment-based binding site identification by ligand competitive saturation. *PLoS Computational Biology, 5*, e1000435.
59. Raman, E. P., Yu, W., Guvench, O., & MacKerell, A. D. (2011). Reproducing crystal binding modes of ligand functional groups using site-identification by ligand competitive saturation (SILCS) simulations. *Journal of Chemical Information and Modeling, 51*, 877–896.
60. Raman, E. P., Yu, W., Lakkaraju, S. K., & MacKerell, A. D. (2013). Inclusion of multiple fragment types in the site identification by ligand competitive saturation (SILCS) approach. *Journal of Chemical Information and Modeling, 53*, 3384–3398.
61. Ustach, V. D., Lakkaraju, S. K., Jo, S., Yu, W., Jiang, W., & MacKerell, A. D. (2019). Optimization and evaluation of site-identification by ligand competitive saturation (SILCS) as a tool for target-based ligand optimization. *Journal of Chemical Information and Modeling, 59*, 3018–3035.
62. Yu, W., Lakkaraju, S., Raman, E. P., & MacKerell, A., Jr. (2014). Site-identification by ligand competitive saturation (SILCS) assisted pharmacophore modeling. *Journal of Computer-Aided Molecular Design, 28*, 491–507.
63. Yu, W., Lakkaraju, S. K., Raman, E. P., Fang, L., & MacKerell, A. D. (2015). Pharmacophore modeling using site-identification by ligand competitive saturation (SILCS) with multiple probe molecules. *Journal of Chemical Information and Modeling, 55*, 407–420.
64. Huang, N., Shoichet, B. K., & Irwin, J. J. (2006). Benchmarking sets for molecular docking. *Journal of Medicinal Chemistry, 49*, 6789–6801.
65. Durant, J. L., Leland, B. A., Henry, D. R., & Nourse, J. G. (2002). Reoptimization of MDL keys for use in drug discovery. *Journal of Chemical Information and Computer Sciences, 42*, 1273–1280.
66. Xue, L., Godden, J. W., Stahura, F. L., & Bajorath, J. (2003). Design and evaluation of a molecular fingerprint involving the transformation of property descriptor values into a binary classification scheme. *Journal of Chemical Information and Computer Sciences, 43*, 1151–1157.
67. Shim, J., & MacKerell, A. D. (2011). Computational ligand-based rational design: Role of conformational sampling and force fields in model development. *Medicinal Chemistry Communications, 2*, 356–370.
68. Gorre, M. E., Mohammed, M., Ellwood, K., Hsu, N., Paquette, R., Rao, P. N., & Sawyers, C. L. (2001). Clinical resistance to STI-571 cancer therapy caused by BCR-ABL gene mutation or amplification. *Science, 293*, 876–880.
69. Holohan, C., Van Schaeybroeck, S., Longley, D. B., & Johnston, P. G. (2013). Cancer drug resistance: An evolving paradigm. *Nature Reviews Cancer, 13*, 714–726.
70. Tanneeru, K., & Guruprasad, L. (2013). Ponatinib is a Pan-BCR-ABL kinase inhibitor: MD simulations and SIE study. *PLoS One, 8*, e78556.
71. Salesse, S., & Verfaillie, C. M. (2002). BCR/ABL: From molecular mechanisms of leukemia induction to treatment of chronic myelogenous leukemia. *Oncogene, 21*, 8547–8559.
72. Huang, W., Metcalf, C. A., Sundaramoorthi, R., Wang, Y., Zou, D., Thomas, R. M., Zhu, X., Cai, L., Wen, D., Liu, S., Romero, J., Qi, J., Chen, I., Banda, G., Lentini, S. P., Das, S., Xu, Q., Keats, J., Wang, F., Wardwell, S., Ning, Y., Snodgrass, J. T., Broudy, M. I., Russian, K., Zhou, T., Commodore, L., Narasimhan, N. I., Mohemmad, Q. K., Luliucci, J., Rivera, V. M., Dalgarno, D. C., Sawyer, T. K., Clackson, T., & Shakespeare, W. C. (2010). Discovery of 3-[2-(Imidazo[1,2-b]pyridazin-3-yl)ethynyl]-4-methyl-N-{4-[(4-methylpiperazin-1-yl)methyl]-3-(trifluoromethyl)phenyl}benzamide (AP24534), a potent, orally active pan-inhibitor of breakpoint cluster region-abelson (BCR-ABL) kinase including the T315I gatekeeper mutant. *Journal of Medicinal Chemistry, 53*, 4701–4719.
73. Hauser, K., Negron, C., Albanese, S. K., Ray, S., Steinbrecher, T., Abel, R., Chodera, J. D., & Wang, L. (2018). Predicting resistance of clinical Abl mutations to targeted kinase inhibitors using alchemical free-energy calculations. *Communications Biology, 1*, 70.
74. Norman, R. A., Toader, D., & Ferguson, A. D. (2012). Structural approaches to obtain kinase selectivity. *Trends in Pharmacological Sciences, 33*, 273–278.

75. Huang, D., Zhou, T., Lafleur, K., Nevado, C., & Caflisch, A. (2010). Kinase selectivity potential for inhibitors targeting the ATP binding site: A network analysis. *Bioinformatics, 26*, 198–204.
76. Wang, L., Berne, B. J., & Friesner, R. A. (2011). Ligand binding to protein-binding pockets with wet and dry regions. *Proceedings of the National Academy of Sciences of the United States of America, 108*, 1326–1330.
77. Robinson, D. D., Sherman, W., & Farid, R. (2010). Understanding kinase selectivity through energetic analysis of binding site waters. *ChemMedChem, 5*, 618–627.
78. Pearson, G., Robinson, F., Gibson, T., Xu, B., Karandikar, M., Berman, K., & Cobb, M. (2001). Mitogen-activated protein (MAP) kinase pathways: Regulation and physiological functions. *Endocrine Reviews, 22*, 153–183.
79. Lewis, T. S., Shapiro, P., & Ahn, N. G. (1998). Signal transduction through MAP kinase cascades. *Advances in Cancer Research, 74*, 49–139.
80. von Kriegsheim, A., Baiocchi, D., Birtwistle, M., Sumpton, D., Bienvenut, W., Morrice, N., Yamada, K., Lamond, A., Kalna, G., Orton, R., Gilbert, D., & Kolch, W. (2009). Cell fate decisions are specified by the dynamic ERK interactome. *Nature Cell Biology, 11*, 1458–1464.
81. Zhang, J., Zhou, B., Zheng, C., & Zhang, Z. (2003). A bipartite mechanism for ERK2 recognition by its cognate regulators and substrates. *The Journal of Biological Chemistry, 278*, 29901–29912.
82. Roberts, P. J., & Der, C. J. (2007). Targeting the Raf-MEK-ERK mitogen-activated protein kinase cascade for the treatment of cancer. *Oncogene, 26*, 3291–3310.
83. Bain, J., McLauchlan, H., Elliott, M., & Cohen, P. (2003). Thespecificities of protein kinase inhibitors: An update. *The Biochemical Journal, 371*, 199–204.
84. Tanoue, T., Adachi, M., Moriguchi, T., & Nishida, E. (2000). A conserved docking motif in MAP kinases common to substrates, activators and regulators. *Nature Cell Biology, 2*, 110–116.
85. Tanoue, T., Maeda, R., Adachi, M., & Nishida, E. (2001). Identification of a docking groove on ERK and p38 MAP kinases that regulates the specificity of docking interactions. *The EMBO Journal, 20*, 466–479.
86. Lee, T., Hoofnagle, A. N., Kabuyama, Y., Stroud, J., Min, X., Goldsmith, E. J., Chen, L., Resing, K. A., & Ahn, N. G. (2004). Docking motif interactions in MAP kinases revealed by hydrogen exchange mass spectrometry. *Molecular Cell, 14*, 43–55.
87. Zhang, F., Strand, A., Robbins, D., Cobb, M. H., & Goldsmith, E. J. (1994). Atomic structure of the MAP kinase ERK2 at 2.3 A resolution. *Nature, 367*, 704–711.
88. Ferrin, T. E., Huang, C. C., Jarvis, L. E., & Langridge, R. (1988). The MIDAS display system. *Journal of Molecular Graphics, 6*, 13–27.
89. Kuntz, I. D., Blaney, J. M., Oatley, S. J., Langridge, R., & Ferrin, T. E. (1982). A geometric approach to macromolecule-ligand interactions. *Journal of Molecular Biology, 161*, 269–288.
90. Pan, Y., Huang, N., Cho, S., & MacKerell, A. D. (2003). Consideration of molecular weight during compound selection in virtual target-based database screening. *Journal of Chemical Information and Computer Sciences, 43*, 267–272.
91. Jarvis, R. A., & Patrick, E. A. (1973). Clustering using a similarity measure based on shared nearest neighbors. *IEEE Transactions on Computers, C-22*, 1025–1034.
92. *Molecular operating environment (MOE)*. Chemical Computing Group Inc., 1010 Sherbrooke St. W, Suite 910, Montreal, Quebec, Canada H3A 2R7. Retrieved 2005, from https://www.chemcomp.com.
93. Godden, J. W., Xue, L., & Bajorath, J. (2000). Combinatorial preferences affect molecular similarity/diversity calculations using binary fingerprints and tanimoto coefficients. *Journal of Chemical Information and Computer Sciences, 40*, 163–166.
94. Lipinski, C. A., Lombardo, F., Dominy, B. W., & Feeney, P. J. (1997). Experimental and computational approaches to estimate solubility and permeability in drug discovery and development settings. *Advanced Drug Delivery Reviews, 23*, 3–26.

95. Canagarajah, B. J., Khokhlatchev, A., Cobb, M. H., & Goldsmith, E. J. (1997). Activation mechanism of the MAP kinase ERK2 by dual phosphorylation. *Cell, 90*, 859–869.
96. Foster, T. J., MacKerell, A. D., & Guvench, O. (2012). Balancing target flexibility and target denaturation in computational fragment-based inhibitor discovery. *Journal of Computational Chemistry, 33*, 1880–1891.
97. Zhong, S., & MacKerell, A. D. (2007). Binding response: A descriptor for selecting ligand binding site on protein surfaces. *Journal of Chemical Information and Modeling, 47*, 2303–2315.
98. Emrick, M. A., Lee, T., Starkey, P. J., Mumby, M. C., Resing, K. A., & Ahn, N. G. (2006). The gatekeeper residue controls autoactivation of ERK2 via a pathway of intramolecular connectivity. *Proceedings of the National Academy of Sciences of the United States of America, 103*, 18101–18106.
99. Barr, D., Oashi, T., Burkhard, K., Lucius, S., Samadani, R., Zhang, J., Shapiro, P., MacKerell, A. D., & van der Vaart, A. (2011). Importance of domain closure for the autoactivation of ERK2. *Biochemistry, 50*, 8038–8048.
100. Brooks, B. R., Brooks, C. L., Mackerell, A. D., Nilsson, L., Petrella, R. J., Roux, B., Won, Y., Archontis, G., Bartels, C., Boresch, S., Caflisch, A., Caves, L., Cui, Q., Dinner, A. R., Feig, M., Fischer, S., Gao, J., Hodoscek, M., Im, W., Kuczera, K., Lazaridis, T., Ma, J., Ovchinnikov, V., Paci, E., Pastor, R. W., Post, C. B., Pu, J. Z., Schaefer, M., Tidor, B., Venable, R. M., Woodcock, H. L., Wu, X., Yang, W., York, D. M., & Karplus, M. (2009). CHARMM: The biomolecular simulation program. *Journal of Computational Chemistry, 30*, 1545–1614.
101. van der Vaart, A., & Karplus, M. (2005). Simulation of conformational transitions by the restricted perturbation: Targeted molecular dynamics method. *The Journal of Chemical Physics, 122*, 114903.
102. Phillips, J. C., Braun, R., Wang, W., Gumbart, J., Tajkhorshid, E., Villa, E., Chipot, C., Skeel, R. D., Kalé, L., & Schulten, K. (2005). Scalable molecular dynamics with NAMD. *Journal of Computational Chemistry, 26*, 1781–1802.
103. Teeter, M. M., & Case, D. A. (1990). Harmonic and quasiharmonic descriptions of crambin. *The Journal of Physical Chemistry, 94*, 8091–8097.
104. Ichiye, T., & Karplus, M. (1991). Collective motions in proteins: A covariance analysis of atomic fluctuations in molecular dynamics and normal mode simulations. *Proteins: Structure, Function, and Genetics, 11*, 205–217.
105. Wagner, E. F., & Nebreda, A. R. (2009). Signal integration by JNK and p38 MAPK pathways in cancer development. *Nature Reviews Cancer, 9*, 537–549.
106. Feng, Y., & Li, Y. (2011). The role of p38 mitogen-activated protein kinase in the pathogenesis of inflammatory bowel disease. *Journal of Digestive Diseases, 12*, 327–332.
107. Tulapurkar, M. E., Almutairy, E. A., Shah, N. G., He, J., Puche, A. C., Shapiro, P., Singh, I. S., & Hasday, J. D. (2012). Febrile-range hyperthermia modifies endothelial and neutrophilic functions to promote extravasation. *American Journal of Respiratory Cell and Molecular Biology, 46*, 807–814.
108. O'Keefe, S. J., Mudgett, J. S., Cupo, S., Parsons, J. N., Chartrain, N. A., Fitzgerald, C., Chen, S. L., Lowitz, K., Rasa, C., Visco, D., et al. (2007). Chemical genetics define the roles of p38alpha and p38beta in acute and chronic inflammation. *The Journal of Biological Chemistry, 282*, 34663–34671.
109. Ferrari, G., Terushkin, V., Wolff, M. J., Zhang, X., Valacca, C., Poggio, P., Pintucci, G., & Mignatti, T. (2012). TGF-b1 induces endothelial cell apoptosis by shifting VEGF activation of p38(MAPK) from the prosurvival p38b to proapoptotic p38. *Molecular Cancer Research, 10*, 605–614.
110. Marber, M. S., Molkentin, J. D., & Force, T. (2010). Developing small molecules to inhibit kinases unkind to the heart: p38 MAPK as a case in point. *Drug Discovery Today Disease Mechanisms, 7*, e123–e127.

111. MacNee, W., Allan, R. J., Jones, I., De Salvo, M. C., & Tan, L. F. (2013). Efficacy and safety of the oral p38 inhibitor PH-797804 in chronic obstructive pulmonary disease: A randomised clinical trial. *Thorax, 68*, 738–745.
112. Shah, N. G., Tulapurkar, M. E., Ramarathnam, A., Brophy, A., Martinez, R., III, Hom, K., Hodges, T., Samadani, R., Singh, I. S., MacKerell, A. D., Shapiro, P., & Hasday, J. D. (2017). Novel noncatalytic substrate-selective p38a-specific MAPK inhibitors with endothelial-stabilizing and anti-inflammatory activity. *Journal of Immunology, 198*, 3296–3306.
113. Wang, Z., Harkins, P. C., Ulevitch, R. J., Han, J., Cobb, M. H., & Goldsmith, E. J. (1997). The structure of mitogen-activated protein kinase p38 at 2.1-A resolution. *Proceedings of the National Academy of Sciences of the United States of America, 94*, 2327–2332.
114. *Screening libraries from Maybridge, part of Thermo Fisher Scientific Inc.* https://www.maybridge.com.
115. Oashi, T., Ringer, A. L., Raman, E. P., & MacKerell, A. D. (2011). Automated selection of compounds with physicochemical properties to maximize bioavailability and druglikeness. *Journal of Chemical Information and Modeling, 51*, 148–158.
116. Barancík, M., Bohácová, V., Kvackajová, J., Hudecová, S., Krizanová, O., & Breier, A. (2001). SB203580, a specific inhibitor of p38-MAPK pathway, is a new reversal agent of P-glycoprotein-mediated multidrug resistance. *European Journal of Pharmaceutical Sciences, 14*, 29–36.
117. Raman, E. P., Lakkaraju, S. K., Denny, R. A., & MacKerell, A. D. (2017). Estimation of relative free energies of binding using pre-computed ensembles based on the single-step free energy perturbation and the site-identification by ligand competitive saturation approaches. *Journal of Computational Chemistry, 38*, 1238–1251.
118. Van Der Spoel, D., Lindahl, E., Hess, B., Groenhof, G., Mark, A. E., & Berendsen, H. J. C. (2005). GROMACS: Fast, flexible, and free. *Journal of Computational Chemistry, 26*, 1701–1718.
119. Lakkaraju, S. K., Raman, E. P., Yu, W., & MacKerell, A. D. (2014). Sampling of organic solutes in aqueous and heterogeneous environments using oscillating excess chemical potentials in grand canonical-like monte carlo-molecular dynamics simulations. *Journal of Chemical Theory and Computation, 10*, 2281–2290.
120. Lakkaraju, S. K., Yu, W., Raman, E. P., Hershfeld, A. V., Fang, L., Deshpande, D. A., & MacKerell, A. D. (2015). Mapping functional group free energy patterns at protein occluded sites: Nuclear receptors and G-protein coupled receptors. *Journal of Chemical Information and Modeling, 55*, 700–708.
121. Goldstein, D. M., Soth, M., Gabriel, T., Dewdney, N., Kuglstatter, A., Arzeno, H., Chen, J., Bingenheimer, W., Dalrymple, S. A., Dunn, J., Farrell, R., Frauchiger, S., La Fargue, J., Ghate, M., Graves, B., Hill, R. J., Li, F., Litman, R., Loe, B., McIntosh, J., McWeeney, D., Papp, E., Park, J., Reese, H. F., Roberts, R. T., Rotstein, D., San Pablo, B., Sarma, K., Stahl, M., Sung, M.-L., Suttman, R. T., Sjogren, E. B., Tan, Y., Trejo, A., Welch, M., Weller, P., Wong, B. R., & Zecic, H. (2011). Discovery of 6-(2,4-Difluorophenoxy)-2- [3-hydroxy-1-(2-hydroxyethyl)propylamino]-8-methyl-8H-pyrido- [2,3-d]pyrimidin-7-one (Pamapimod) and 6-(2,4-Difluorophenoxy)- 8-methyl-2-(tetrahydro-2H-pyran-4-ylamino)pyrido[2,3-d]pyrimidin- 7(8H)-one (R1487) as orally bioavailable and highly selective inhibitors of p38α mitogen-activated protein kinase. *Journal of Medicinal Chemistry, 54*, 2255–2265.
122. Wang, L., Wu, Y., Deng, Y., Kim, B., Pierce, L., Krilov, G., Lupyan, D., Robinson, S., Dahlgren, M. K., Greenwood, J., Romero, D. L., Masse, C., Knight, J. L., Steinbrecher, T., Beuming, T., Damm, W., Harder, E., Sherman, W., Brewer, M., Wester, R., Murcko, M., Frye, L., Farid, R., Lin, T., Mobley, D. L., Jorgensen, W. L., Berne, B. J., Friesner, R. A., & Abel, R. (2015). Accurate and reliable prediction of relative ligand binding potency in prospective drug discovery by way of a modern free-energy calculation protocol and force field. *Journal of the American Chemical Society, 137*, 2695–2703.
123. Del Moral, P., Doucet, A., & Jasra, A. (2006). Sequential Monte Carlo samplers. *Journal of the Royal Statistical Society Series B (Statistical Methodology), 68*, 411–436.

124. Broadbridge, R. J., & Sharma, R. P. (2000). The Src homology-2 domains (SH2 domains) of the protein tyrosine kinase p56lck: Structure, mechanism and drug design. *Current Drug Targets, 1*, 365–386.
125. Straus, D. B., & Weiss, A. (1992). Genetic evidence for the involvement of the lck tyrosine kinase in signal transduction through the T cell antigen receptor. *Cell, 70*, 585–593.
126. Pawson, T., & Gish, G. D. (1992). SH2 and SH3 domains: From structure to function. *Cell, 71*, 359–362.
127. Cousins-Wasti, R., Ingraham, R. H., Morelock, M. M., & Grygon, C. A. (1996). Determination of affinities for lck SH2 binding peptides using a sensitive fluorescence assay: Comparison between the pYEEIP and pYQPQP consensus sequences reveals context-dependent binding specificity. *Biochemistry, 35*, 16746–16752.
128. Marengere, L., Songyang, Z., Gish, G. D., Schaller, M. D., Parsons, J. T., Stern, M. J., Cantley, L. C., & Pawson, T. (1994). SH2 domain specificity and activity modified by a single residue. *Nature, 369*, 502–505.
129. Huang, N., Nagarsekar, A., Xia, G., Hayashi, J., & MacKerell, A. D. (2004). Identification of non-phosphate-containing small molecular weight inhibitors of the tyrosine kinase p56 Lck SH2 domain via in silico screening against the pY + 3 binding site. *Journal of Medicinal Chemistry, 47*, 3502–3511.
130. Macias, A. T., Mia, Y., Xia, G., Hayashi, J., & MacKerell, A. D. (2005). Lead validation and SAR development via chemical similarity searching; application to compounds targeting the pY+3 site of the SH2 domain of p56lck. *Journal of Chemical Information and Modeling, 45*, 1759–1766.

A Toolbox of Structural Biology and Enzyme Kinetics Reveals the Case for ERK Docking Site Inhibition

Rachel M. Sammons and Kevin N. Dalby

Abstract Extracellular signal–regulated kinase (ERK) is a mitogen-activated protein kinase (MAPK) that mediates cellular processes such as proliferation, differentiation, cell motility, and survival. Dysregulation of the ERK signaling pathway is believed to have a protumorigenic role in many cancers, and studies also implicate it in a variety of other proliferative diseases. Within the ERK signaling pathway, protein-protein interactions via enzyme-docking sites help generate signal specificity and direct ERK to subsequent binding partners or substrates. ERK possesses two known docking sites that are distinct from its catalytic site: the D- and F- recruitment sites (DRS and FRS). Over time, our group has characterized these sites through a combination of structural and kinetic studies, including computational and biochemical techniques, centering around a model ERK substrate EtsΔ138 (residues 1–138 of the transcription factor Ets-1). These studies are part of a growing effort to elucidate new insights into ERK signaling and to evaluate the role of each binding site in specific ERK interactions. Furthermore, the development of inhibitors that target these docking sites offers a way to impede both catalytic and noncatalytic functions of ERK, which may provide therapeutic benefit in disease states driven by ERK signaling. Here, we describe the features of the DRS and FRS of ERK, their roles in the phosphorylation of EtsΔ138, and the status, mechanisms, and implications of targeting these sites with inhibitors.

Keywords Kinase · ERK · Non-ATP competitive · BRAF · KRAS · Melanoma

R. M. Sammons
Targeted Therapeutic Drug Discovery and Development Program, The University of Texas at Austin, Austin, TX, USA

K. N. Dalby (✉)
Targeted Therapeutic Drug Discovery and Development Program, The University of Texas at Austin, Austin, TX, USA

Division of Chemical Biology and Medicinal Chemistry, College of Pharmacy, The University of Texas at Austin, Austin, TX, USA

Department of Oncology, Dell Medical School, The University of Texas at Austin, Austin, TX, USA
e-mail: dalby@austin.utexas.edu

P. Shapiro (ed.), *Next Generation Kinase Inhibitors*,
https://doi.org/10.1007/978-3-030-48283-1_6

ERK Overview

ERK1 and ERK2 constitute the endmost node of a three-tiered kinase phosphorylation cascade, transducing signals that are initiated by extracellular stimuli (e.g., cytokines and stresses) to culminate in the phosphorylation of at least 250 known substrates in various subcellular compartments [1]. This MAPK signaling pathway is stimulated by events such as ligands binding to receptor tyrosine kinases (RTKs) at the cell surface, causing RTK dimerization and activation via autophosphorylation. The active RTKs then recruit guanine nucleotide exchange factors and adaptor proteins, such as SOS and Grb, that facilitate the activation of Ras. Ras activation occurs upon its exchange of GDP for GTP. Active Ras leads to the phosphorylation and subsequent dimerization and activation of Raf isoforms, initiating the three-tiered MAPK phosphorylation cascade. Raf proteins (MAP 3Ks, or mitogen-activated protein kinase kinase kinases) phosphorylate and activate MEK1 and MEK2 (MAP 2Ks, or mitogen-activated protein kinase kinases), which are dual-specificity kinases that phosphorylate and activate ERK1 and ERK2. ERK pathway signaling upstream of Raf typically occurs at the plasma membrane [2] while the substrates of ERK are nuclear or extranuclear. Within the nucleus, ERK is responsible for the phosphorylation of transcription factors that govern the induction of genes involved in cell cycle progression, cell survival, differentiation, migration, and a variety of other vital cellular processes. Accordingly, abnormal ERK signaling is implicated in a wide array of pathologies, including cancers [3], neurological disorders and diseases [4], cardiovascular diseases [5, 6], insulin resistance [7], kidney diseases [8], and pulmonary diseases [9, 10]. As the critical arbiter of translating upstream pathway activity into tightly regulated downstream signaling outcomes, ERK is an attractive therapeutic target.

The two most-studied isoforms of ERK, ERK1 and ERK2, have a high sequence (85% [11]) and structural similarity. The structure and mechanism of ERK2 have been extensively characterized, so ERK2 is the focus of this discussion. However, it is notable that isoform-specific cellular functions of ERK1 and ERK2 are unclear, and the possible redundancy of their roles is a topic of significant discussion [12]. Studies suggest that ERK2 is often expressed at higher levels than ERK1 when observed phenotypes appear to be ERK2-dependent although the ratio of ERK1/ERK2 expression shows variation across different cell types and model systems [12].

Active ERK is a proline-directed serine/threonine protein kinase, catalyzing the phosphorylation of serine or threonine residues on substrates that contain the target sequence Ser/Thr-Pro (or preferentially, Pro-Xxx-Ser/Thr-Pro [13, 14]). In the phosphorylation reaction at the active site of ERK, the γ-phosphate of an ATP molecule is transferred to serine or threonine on the substrate by a single-step nucleophilic reaction with a dissociative transition state [15–17]. Figure 1 shows a model of this reaction mechanism, including critical active site residues of ERK2 that participate in electrostatic interactions. These and other vital residues, along with structural components of ERK2, are discussed in further detail below.

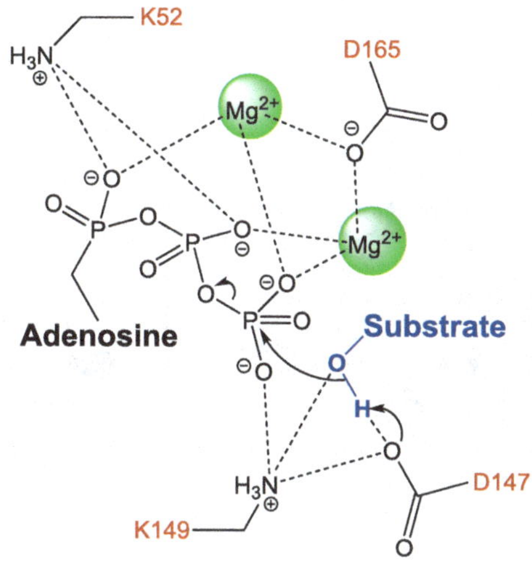

Fig. 1 ERK2 reaction mechanism [15, 17, 18, 125]. The scheme here shows an example of phosphoryl transfer from ATP to serine or threonine of a substrate protein by ERK2. Some of the key residues in the active site of ERK2 that are responsible for stabilizing phosphoryl transfer and coordination of magnesium ions are also depicted. Arrows symbolize the movement of electrons and bond formation/breakage. Dashed lines indicate electrostatic interactions

Like most protein kinases, the tertiary structure of ERK2 consists of a small N-terminal lobe (N-lobe) and a larger C-terminal lobe (C-lobe). The secondary structure of ERK2 is also highly conserved among kinases (Fig. 2a) and is reviewed in depth by R. Roskoski Jr. [18]. The N-lobe mainly consists of a five-stranded antiparallel β sheet (β1–β5) that aids in the binding and recognition of ATP [18]. The β1 and β2 strands are critical for interacting with the adenine base of ATP [18]. There is also a short glycine-rich loop between the β1 and β2 sheets that communicates with the β- and γ- phosphate groups of ATP to aid in cleavage of the γ-phosphate [18]. Additionally, Lys52 in the β3 sheet is known to facilitate ATP binding in addition to forming a salt bridge with Glu69 in the αC helix and the β- and γ- phosphates of ATP that is necessary for full kinase activity (Fig. 2b) [18, 19]. Lys52 stabilizes the reaction transition state and final products through these electrostatic interactions and is essential for proper orientation of ATP in the active site [15, 19].

In contrast, the C-lobe is mostly α-helical but contains four β-strands (β6-β9) where most of the catalytic residues are located [18]. The two most integral components of this lobe are the catalytic loop and the activation segment (also referred to as activation loop) (Fig. 2b). The activation segment starts with Asp165 (DFG motif) and ends with Glu195 (APE motif) [18]. It occurs after the catalytic loop in sequence and contains Thr183 and Tyr185, the two phosphorylation sites responsible for ERK2 activation. The activation loop is critical to substrate recognition and regulation of ERK2 signaling. The primary residues in the catalytic core are Lys52, Asp147, and Asp165 of the DFG motif, which together comprise a K/D/D motif, and His145, Arg146, and Asp147 (first Asp of the K/D/D motif), which form a

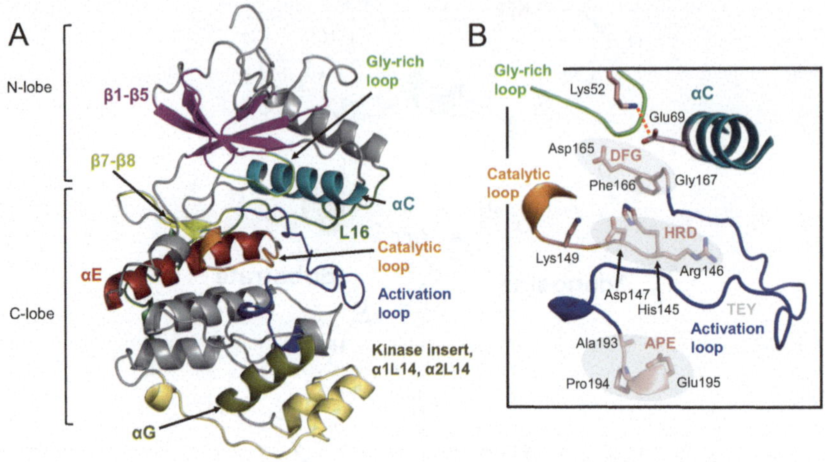

Fig. 2 ERK2 secondary structure and catalytic site [18, 23, 125]. (**a**) The structure of active ERK2 (PDB 2ERK [44]) is shown, including the glycine-rich loop (light green), the αC helix (teal), β-sheets β1-β5 (magenta), the catalytic loop (orange), the activation segment (blue), β-sheets β7 and β8 (yellow), the αE helix that forms part of the hydrophobic groove within the DRS (red), loop 16 (L16, dark green), the αG helix (gold), and the kinase insert domain with helices α1L14 and α2L14 (light orange). (**b**) A closer look at the key residues of the catalytic core, shown in pink. All other colored secondary structures correspond to the scheme in part (**a**). The activation loop begins with the DFG motif (Asp165/Phe166/Gly167) and ends with the APE motif (A193/Pro194/Glu195). It contains the TEY motif, Thr183/Glu184/Tyr285, where MEK1/2 phosphorylate threonine and tyrosine to activate ER2. The catalytic residues that are responsible for stabilizing transfer of the γ-phosphate of ATP to substrate serine/threonine residues, coordinating with Mg^{2+}, and electrostatic stabilization of the charged region of ATP/ADP are shown as well. These include the catalytic HRD motif (His145/Arg146/Asp147) and the K/D/D motif (Lys52, Asp147 of the HRD motif, and Asp165 of the DFG motif). The salt bridge between Lys52 of the K/D/D motif and Glu69 of the αC helix is also shown as a red dotted line

catalytic HRD motif. (Fig. 2b) [18]. Asp147 is located in the catalytic loop and is believed to be involved in the positioning of the substrate Ser/Thr sidechain hydroxyl group (–OH) for nucleophilic attack of the ATP γ-phosphate phosphorous atom [17, 18]. It is also believed that Asp147 acts as the catalytic base, accepting a proton from the substrate Ser/Thr sidechain –OH group to activate it for a nucleophilic reaction [15, 17]. Lys149 is involved in stabilization of the phosphoryl transfer reaction and transition state, working together with Lys52 and the Mg^{2+} ions coordinated in the ATP-binding site [18]. Lys149 strongly interacts with the γ-phosphate of ATP and helps appropriately position it in the active site [15]. Asp165 is part of the activation segment and binds the two Mg^{2+} ions that coordinate the phosphates of ATP [18, 20]. Interestingly, models have predicted that ERK2 activity and mechanism do not significantly change if one or two magnesium ions are present in the active site due to distribution of the extra negative charge [15]. However, other data show that the second magnesium ion appears to be essential for full physiological ERK2 activity [20]. Magnesium ions are believed to have a regulatory influence on cellular

ERK as ERK activity is thought to be susceptible to variations of free divalent magnesium concentrations in cells [21].

ERK2 is phosphorylated and activated by MEK1/2 on Thr183 and Tyr185 as mentioned above. Phosphorylation of Thr183 and Tyr185, part of a Thr-Xxx-Tyr motif in the activation segment (TEY for ERK2), is required for full activation of ERK2 and is marked by a 600,000-fold increase in catalytic efficiency [22]. Inactive, unphosphorylated ERK2 adopts a DFG-out conformation, such that the DFG motif sidechains are pointing away from the active site, and the active site is open. When Thr185/Tyr185 are phosphorylated, the activation segment undergoes a conformational change that extends the DFG motif toward the active site, and the active site closes to position the key catalytic residues discussed above [23]. Recently, analyses have suggested that accessible kinase conformations are more dynamic and nuanced than the classical DFG-in or DFG-out categories. The DFG-in conformation is required but not sufficient for full kinase activity, which must involve proper positioning of the αC helix, glycine-rich loop, and an extended activation loop to facilitate substrate binding. These requirements support the existence of a variety of inactive, intermediate kinase conformations that can share some (but not all) attributes with the fully active conformation [24].

In order for ERK2 substrates to undergo efficient phosphorylation at specific serine/threonine residues, they must possess a proline in the P + 1 position (where P is the target phospho-site). The substrate P + 1 proline adopts a trans, α-helical conformation and interacts with the phosphorylated Tyr185 of active ERK2, driving the target serine/threonine into the hydrophobic pocket of the active site within an appropriate distance of the ATP γ-phosphate [15]. Other amino acid substitutions in the P + 1 position are either too bulky or too flexible to optimally position the target P site [15].

However, there are many Ser/Thr-directed kinases like ERK2 that also recognize their substrates by short consensus sequences, and in total at least 356 kinases that phosphorylate their substrates on either threonine or serine residues [25]. It follows that the catalytic core and activation segment are not the only locations on ERK2 that are critical for facilitating binding interactions and catalysis. Additional distinct and structurally diverse protein-protein interaction sites (PPIs) on kinases are employed to promote recognition of specific substrates and binding partners. The two main PPI sites on ERK2 are known as the D-recruitment site and the F-recruitment site.

The D-Recruitment Site

The D-recruitment site (DRS) is distal to the active site on the surface of ERK2 (Fig. 3a). It is composed of a hydrophobic binding groove (Φ_{hyd}) flanked by two domains: the ED domain (Thr157/Thr158 of ERK2) and a charged region known as the common docking (CD) domain (Φ_{chg}), which contains the acidic residues Asp316 and Asp319. All MAPKs possess a DRS and a conserved Φ_{chg} region while

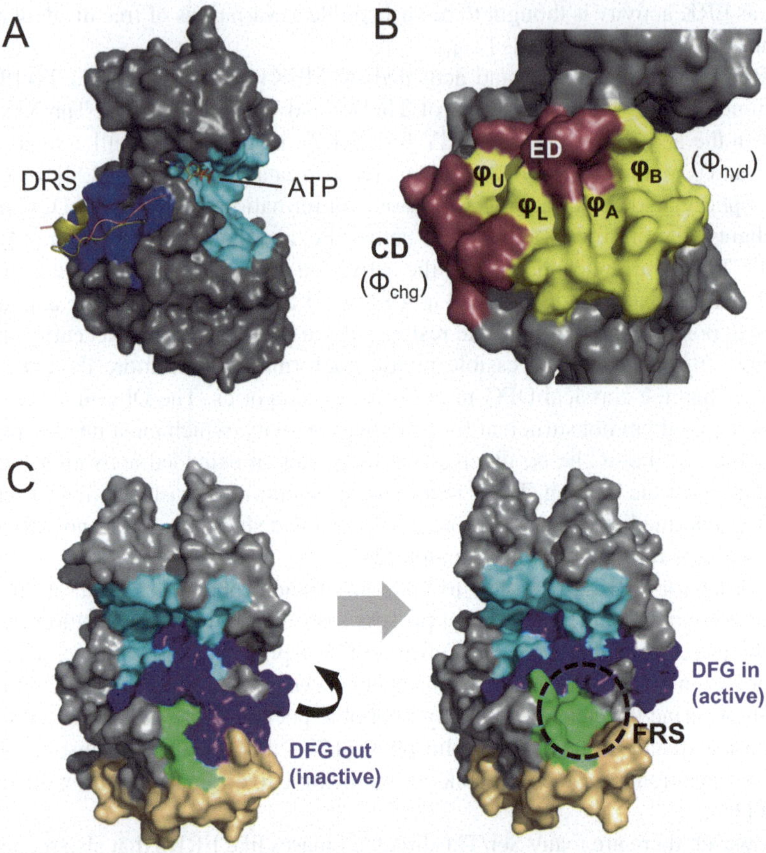

Fig. 3 The D-recruitment site and F-recruitment site of ERK2 [23, 52, 54]. (**a**) The D-recruitment site (dark blue) and the catalytic region (light blue) of active ERK2 (PDB 2ERK [44]) are shown. The stick structure of ATP is shown bound (aligned and superimposed in PyMol from 4GT3). Two example peptides, D-site peptides, are shown bound to the DRS from HePTP (yellow, PDB 2GPH [46]) and MEK2 (light orange, PDB 4H3Q [126]). (**b**) Detailed view of the DRS (PDB 2ERK [44]), showing the ED and CD domains in pink and the hydrophobic groove in yellow. The hydrophobic groove (Φ_{hyd}) is separated into four subpockets that interact with φ_U, φ_L, φ_A, and φ_B residues of different D-site consensus sequences [26, 27]. Φ_{chg} denotes the acidic CD domain. (**c**) The key residues of the FRS (green) are located between the active site (light blue, activation segment shown in purple) of ERK2 and the kinase insert domain (light orange). When ERK2 (PDB 1ERK [45], left panel) is inactive in the DFG-out conformation, the activation segment obscures the FRS. When ERK2 is doubly phosphorylated (PDB 2ERK [44], right panel), the activation segment undergoes a conformational change that exposes the hydrophobic FRS binding pocket

variability exists in Φ_{hyd} and the ED domain (ED in p38, SD in JNK, TT in ERK1/2, and EN in ERK5) that helps provide selective binding partner recognition. The hydrophobic groove of the ERK2 DRS is formed in part by the αE helix, shown earlier in Fig. 2a for reference. The DRS also contains a conserved cysteine residue (Cys159 of ERK2) that is solvent exposed and adjacent to the ED domain. The canonical motif that binds to the DRS of ERK2 is the D-site (also known as the D-motif/domain, δ-domain, kinase-interacting motif (KIM), D box, or DEJL motif/domain), which consists of the sequence $(Arg/Lys)_{2-3}–X_{2-6}–\varphi_A–X–\varphi_B$, or, more broadly, $\psi_{1-3}–X_{3-7}–\varphi_A–X–\varphi_B$, where ψ is a basic residue, φ_A and φ_B are hydrophobic residues, and X is any residue [26]. Many variations of D-site sequences exist as well, allowing ERK2-binding partners to occupy the DRS by different binding modes. For example, the DCC subtype of D-site, named for the transmembrane protein '*d*eleted in *c*olorectal *c*ancer,' docks with ERK2 according to the consensus sequence $(Arg/Lys)_{1-2}–X_{2-4}–\varphi_L–Pro–X–\varphi_A–X–\varphi_B$ [27]. The hematopoietic protein tyrosine phosphatase (HePTP) docks to ERK2 with a different subtype of D-site: $\varphi_U –X–X–(Arg/Lys)_{(2)} – X_{(5)}–\varphi_L–X–\varphi_A–X–\varphi_B$ [27]. In these sequences, φ_U, φ_L, φ_A, and φ_B are hydrophobic residues that bind in different pockets within the hydrophobic groove as shown in Fig. 3b.

The DRS of ERK2 interacts with many substrates, such as the transcription factors Ets-1 [28, 29] and Elk-1 [30, 31], caspase-9 [32], and the kinases RSK1 [33, 34] and MAPK-activated protein kinase MNK1 [35]. Phosphatases, like DUSP6 [35] and HePTP [36], and activators of ERK (MEK1/2 [37]) also engage the DRS along with scaffolding proteins such as PEA-15 [38, 39]. Many of these interactions influence the subcellular location of ERK. For example, DRS-mediated binding to the scaffolding protein PEA-15 or MEK1/2 can mediate the localization of ERK to the cytoplasm [40–43].

Many binding partners of ERK2 that utilize the DRS can bind both active and inactive ERK2 as the DRS does not undergo significant conformational changes upon dual phosphorylation of the activation segment. This structural conservation of the DRS is apparent by comparison of the crystal structures of active (PDB 2ERK [44]) and inactive (PDB 1ERK [45]) ERK2. In contrast, additional structures of ERK2 obtained from crystallography have revealed that binding events at the DRS can allosterically affect other structural features of ERK2. The crystal structure of a D-site peptide derived from HePTP (^{16}RLQERRGSNVALMLDV^{311}) in complex with inactive ERK2 showed that ERK2 undergoes conformational changes at the CD domain, loop 16, the activation loop, the glycine-rich loop, the N-terminus, and the MAPK insert that are distinct from both active and inactive ERK2 [46]. The CD domain is located at the N-terminus of loop 16 (Fig. 2a), which connects the N- and C-lobes and helps to stabilize the activation loop in active ERK2. Therefore, conformational changes in the CD domain and DRS upon docking can possibly transfer to the activation loop through loop 16. When ERK2 is bound to the HePTP peptide, its conformation represents an intermediate structure between fully active and inactive ERK2, more closely resembling active ERK2. In this conformation, Thr183/Tyr185 are solvent exposed and primed for modification. A crystal structure of ERK2 in complex with a peptide derived from MEK2 showed similar results [46]. These structures support that docking at the DRS can facilitate modifications of the

[1] Underlined amino acid codes denote basic (ψ) and hydrophobic (φ_A and φ_B) residues of the D-site sequence.

activation loop. A recent study found that two CD domain mutants (D319N and E320K) caused significantly different structural and functional changes in ERK2 depending on if the residues were solvent-exposed (D319N) or buried (E320K) [47]. This finding suggests that this compact region of negatively charged residues experiences high-energy electrostatic repulsion which may explain how changes at the DRS can thermodynamically drive alterations of other sites on ERK2 [47]. Changes in the MAPK insert and the activation loop of ERK2 upon DRS binding also suggest that the DRS can allosterically affect the F-recruitment site, discussed below.

The F-Recruitment Site

ERK1/2 and p38α are known to have an additional distinct docking site, called the F-recruitment site (FRS), which may be putatively found on ERK5 as well [48–50]. This docking site is not known to be canonically present in JNK2 or the other p38 isoforms although JNK1 has been shown to possess an "FRS-like" site that engages with activating kinases and phosphatases [51–53]. The FRS binds to proteins containing the F-site consensus sequence Phe-Xxx-Phe-Pro (FXFP), also known as the DEF motif (*D*ocking site for ERK, FXFP) [30]. The FRS is located adjacent to the active site and the MAPK insert. It consists of the critical hydrophobic residues Ile196, Met197, Leu198, Tyr231, Leu232, Leu235, and Tyr261 [52, 54]. When ERK is in its inactive conformation (DFG-out), the FRS is obscured by the activation segment, specifically by the residues Phe181 and Leu182 that are directly N-terminal to Thr183/Tyr185 [52]. The hydrophobic cavity of the FRS forms after the activation of the kinase when the activation segment adopts the DFG-in conformation (Fig. 3c) [52]. In this conformational change, Phe181 and Leu182 travel 23 Å away from the FRS [52], exposing the hydrophobic pocket.

The FRS of ERK is known to interact with several ERK substrates including c-Fos [33, 34], Elk-1 [31, 55], Ets-1 [29, 56, 57], PEA-15 [40], and nucleoporins [52], indicating it may play a role in the nuclear transport of ERK. The FRS also mediates binding to the kinase suppressor of Ras 1 (KSR1) [30, 58]. KSR1 is a scaffold protein that is known to localize ERK and other components of the ERK pathway at the cell membrane in order to facilitate the phosphorylation cascade [58]. The fact that activation of ERK exposes the FRS suggests that its function is likely associated with ERK interactions that occur postactivation while the D-site substrates are often nondiscriminatory against active and inactive ERK2. Proteins with F-sites can access the FRS by different binding modes in an analogous manner to D-site/DRS interactions. For example, the FRS mutation L198A/L235A disrupted Elk-1 binding but not GST-nup153c binding. Here, GST-nup153c is a GST-tagged and truncated construct of nucleoporin 153 that contains 18 Phe-Xxx-Phe sequences [52]. Therefore, these different binding modes at the FRS offer an additional level of protein recognition.

Docking Sites in Catalysis

Knowing that there are many variations in docking motif sequences, it follows that identifying substrates that use the DRS and FRS through atypical interactions can be difficult. Furthermore, substrates can utilize different combinations of docking sequences and sites on ERK2 and can access these sites using different binding modes. Therefore, the roles of the DRS and FRS in the mechanism of phosphorylation of a particular substrate can be complex. Here, we illustrate an example of how we have used a combination of structural studies and kinetics to determine how the ERK2 substrate Ets-1 interacts with docking sites during catalysis.

The Story of Ets-1

Steady-State Kinetics

In order to investigate the mechanism of ERK2, our group expressed and purified the N-terminal 138 residues of the transcription factor Ets-1 (EtsΔ138) as a model substrate [59]. ERK2 singly phosphorylates EtsΔ138 at Thr38. By measuring the initial rates of reaction for different concentrations of EtsΔ138 and $MgATP^{2-}$, we found that the bi-reactant kinetic model conformed to a random-ordered sequential binding mechanism for the formation of a ternary complex (Fig. 4a). In this model, both EtsΔ138 and $MgATP^{2-}$ have unrestrained access to the active site, and we did not make assumptions regarding the use of docking sites by EtsΔ138 [60]. The catalytic parameters for this simplified steady-state model are defined according to Eq. 1 below, in the absence of products [61]:

$$k_{obs} = \frac{k_{cat}[A][B]}{K_{iA}K_{mB} + K_{mB}[A] + K_{mA}[B] + [A][B]} \tag{1}$$

Here, k_{obs} is the observed reaction rate constant, k_{cat} is the catalytic constant (or turnover number), and [A] and [B] are the concentrations of the two substrates, A and B (EtsΔ138 and $MgATP^{2-}$). K_{mB} is the Michaelis constant for B when [A] is saturating and, similarly, K_{mA} is the Michaelis constant for A when [B] is saturating. K_{iA} is the dissociation constant of A in the absence of B. It followed from this analysis that $k_{cat} = 17\ s^{-1}$, $K_{i(Ets\text{-}1)} = 9.3\ \mu M$, $K_{i(ATP)} = 68\ \mu M$, $K_{m(Ets\text{-}1)} = 19\ \mu M$, and $K_{m(ATP)} = 140\ \mu M$ [59]. These data revealed that EtsΔ138 phosphorylation by ERK2 is highly efficient; therefore, EtsΔ138 is a good model substrate for investigating ERK2.

Empirical evidence from past studies and other research groups suggested that EtsΔ138 binding involves more than just the active site of ERK2 [30, 62]. Elk-1, another ERK2 substrate in the ETS family of transcription factors, had been found to dock to ERK2 via a D-site and to also possess an FXFP site [30]. Like Elk-1,

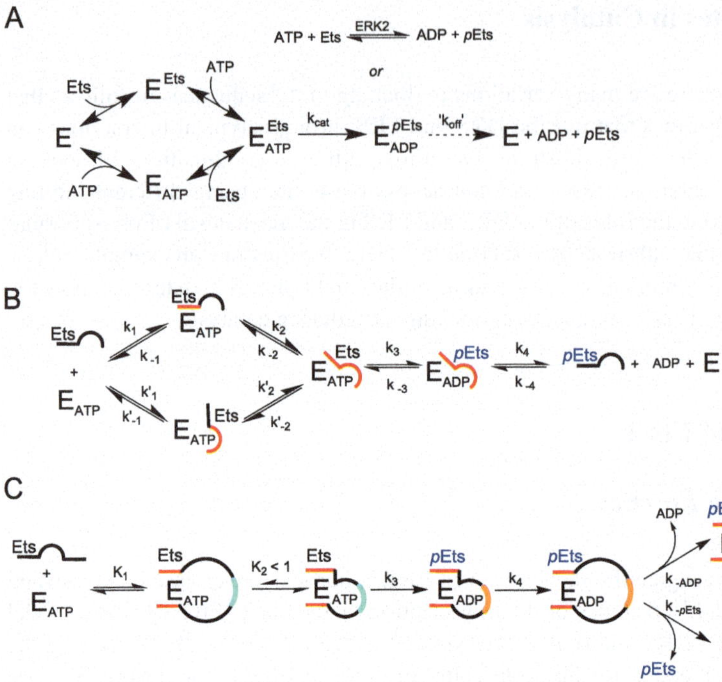

Fig. 4 Evolution of the Ets-1 phosphorylation mechanism. Schemes show ERK2 (E) reaction with EtsΔ138 (Ets) and ATP to yield phosphorylated EtsΔ138 (*p*Ets) and ADP. (**a**) Initial steady-state kinetics fit the model of a random-ordered sequential mechanism and the formation of a ternary complex. k_{cat} is the catalytic constant, and k_{off} is the apparent rate constant for product release. The shorthand for this mechanism is shown at the top of the panel [59]. (**b**) Further steady-state kinetics experiments suggested a docking site was involved in Ets phosphorylation [60]. The top path shows initial binding (red segment of Ets illustration) at the docking site of ERK2 (deemed to be the most likely pathway), and the bottom path shows initial binding at the active site. The values k_n and k_{-n}, where n indicates the reaction pathway step, indicate rate constants for forward and reverse reactions steps, respectively. (**c**) Presteady-state kinetics experiments resulted in a model with two partial rate limiting steps: rapid Ets phosphorylation (k_3) and product release (k_{-ADP} and k_{-pEts}) [63, 64]. Docking segments of Ets are illustrated in red while Thr38 is shown in cyan and phospho-Thr38 is shown in orange. The first step shows docking site engagement, and the second step shows active site binding. The third and fourth steps show phosphorylation of Ets, followed by disengagement from the active site binding. The remaining steps indicate random-ordered product release

Ets-1 contains a pointed (pnt) domain and encompasses several putative DEJL docking sequences, or D-sites, such as ^{15}KTEKVDLEL^{23} (see footnote 1) [60] and ^{110}KECFLELAPDF^{120} (see footnote 1) [28]. Particularly, Seidel & Graves (2002) identified Leu114, Leu116, and Phe120 as composing a potential docking interface [62].

We carried out full steady-state kinetic studies of the ERK2/EtsΔ138 reaction in the presence of the reaction products, phosphorylated EtsΔ138 (p-EtsΔ138) and $MgADP^{-}$, to investigate the possibility of a docking interaction [60]. P-EtsΔ138 was found to be a competitive inhibitor against EtsΔ138 and a mixed inhibitor with respect to $MgATP^{2-}$. Similarly, $MgADP^{-}$ was competitive with respect to $MgATP^{2-}$ and a mixed inhibitor against EtsΔ138. These observations supported the likelihood of a docking interaction and the consequential possibility of two ternary complexes, as shown in Fig. 4b, where binding initially occurs at either the active site or a docking site. However, the product inhibition observed for p-EtsΔ138 suggested that the phosphorylation consensus sequence of Ets-1 contributes little to the stability of the complex, so the transient docking interaction (upper pathway of Fig. 4b) was deemed the most likely productive enzyme/substrate encounter.

Presteady-State Kinetics

To further investigate the mechanism of EtsΔ138 phosphorylation by ERK2, we conducted a presteady-state kinetic analysis of the reaction using a rapid quench-flow apparatus [63]. The burst phase of the presteady-state reaction indicated two partially rate-limiting steps: rapid phosphorylation of EtsΔ138 and product release from ERK2. These steps have first-order rate constants of $109 \pm 9\ s^{-1}$ and $56 \pm 4\ s^{-1}$, respectively [63]. Phosphoryl transfer occurs once EtsΔ138 and $MgATP^{2-}$ are both bound to ERK2. Rapid quench-flow and stopped-flow experiments were also used to further assess product release, with $MgADP^{-}$ and p-EtsΔ138 forming and dissociating from abortive complexes with ERK2 [64]. Two abortive complexes can form during the reaction due to product inhibition: ERK2·EtsΔ138·ADP and ERK2·p-EtsΔ138·ATP. P-EtsΔ138 and ADP dissociate from ERK2 in random order and have little energetic interaction with one another (Fig. 4c). Rapid quench-flow data showed that ADP dissociates from ERK2 with a rate constant of $61 \pm 12\ s^{-1}$ while p- EtsΔ138 dissociates with a rate constant of $121 \pm 3.8\ s^{-1}$ (Fig. 4c) [64]. This observation validated ADP dissociation as a partial rate-limiting step, suggesting that Ets-1 has evolved to approach maximal catalytic efficiency. P-EtsΔ138 was found to bind to ERK2 20-fold more tightly than ADP with dissociation constants of approximately 7.3 and 165 μM, respectively [64]. The dissociation constants of p-EtsΔ138 and EtsΔ138 were very similar, further supporting the idea that the phosphorylation site sequence is not involved in complex stability. This notion indicated a mechanism of "proximity-induced catalysis" in which docking interactions outside of the active site facilitate substrate phosphorylation [65].

Mutational Studies

At this point, we knew little about Ets-1 docking to ERK2 or the relationship between potential docking events and the ERK2 active site. To examine the binding interactions of Ets-1 with ERK2, we began taking a combined kinetic and structural approach by implementing mutational studies. We first investigated a mutant of Phe120 (F120A) which is an EtsΔ138 residue implicated in a docking interface between ERK2 and Ets-1 [62]. We confirmed earlier data [62] that F120A reduced the specificity constant (k_{cat}/K_m) for the reaction by ~20 fold and found that F120A reduced the binding affinity of EtsΔ138 for ERK2 by ten-fold as compared to wild-type EtsΔ138 [57, 63, 65]. F120A is located in the globular pnt domain of EtsΔ138 and was found to not affect the catalytic rate constant (k_{cat}) (see Eq. 1) for the reaction when compared to wildtype EtsΔ138. Therefore, the mutation was predicted to primarily affect the stability of initial EtsΔ138 binding by interfering with a docking interaction. In further agreement with the proximity-induced catalysis model discussed above, mutations of the TP phosphorylation consensus motif (Pro39 to Asp, Arg, Val, Gly, Ala, Glu, and T38A/P39A) did not significantly alter the ability of EtsΔ138 to bind ERK2 [57, 65].

Ets-1 lacks canonical D-site and F-site sequences, but a peptide derived from the D-site of Elk-1 displaced EtsΔ138 from active and inactive ERK2 while a peptide based on the F-site of Elk-1 displaced EtsΔ138 from active ERK2 [57]. The pnt domain of Ets-1 (Ets Δ51–138) bound to ERK2 with similar affinity to the N-terminal domain of Ets-1 (EtsΔ1–52). This observation led to a model whereby ERK2 binds to two docking sequences on EtsΔ138 where the pnt domain was predicted to interact at the substrate binding groove and the N-terminal tail was predicted to bind the DRS. Knowing that the FRS pocket is inaccessible on inactive ERK2, and yet ERK2 binds EtsΔ138 with similar affinity regardless of its activation state, we ascertained that an allosteric effect of the F-site peptide could cause it to interfere with EtsΔ138 binding.

Cysteine footprinting was then used to identify the ERK2 DRS residues that interact with EtsΔ138 [28]. In this technique, ERK2 was first rendered "cysteine less" by mutation of cysteine residues to either Ala, Ser, or Leu, and then the DRS residues were systematically mutated to cysteines. We then measured the ability of EtsΔ138 to protect the DRS cysteine mutants from alkylation. EtsΔ138 protected Q117C, L113C, L119C, and H123C from alkylation, indicating that EtsΔ138 physically obscures these DRS residues and they may be critical for binding.

Structural Insights

To further support the kinetic data and mutational studies, we performed a series of computational modeling studies to explore Ets-1 binding to ERK2. This modeling was critical as no crystal structures of Ets-1 in complex with ERK2 exist to date. Initially, a molecular modeling simulation was performed to dock only the pnt domain of Ets (Δ29–138, PDB 2JV3) onto ERK2 [64]. These results predicted that the sterile alpha motif (SAM) within the pnt domain interacted with αG helix (Fig. 2a) of the MAPK insert/FRS region of ERK2, providing our first indication that the FRS is involved in Ets-1 binding [64]. We then modeled the N-terminus (EtsΔ1–40) and combined this data with the pnt domain model to generate the first full structural model of the EtsΔ138/ERK2 complex [29]. From this model, ^{10}TLTIIKT^{16} of EtsΔ138 was predicted to interact in the Φ_{hyd} region of the DRS with high flexibility. Therefore, the computational model suggested that both the DRS and the FRS contribute to positioning Thr38 near the ERK2 active site.

NMR studies were conducted to further develop and support the EtsΔ138/ERK2 binding model. In the first of these studies, backbone resonances were assigned to the residues of inactive ERK2, and perturbations of these resonances, or chemical shifts, were measured in the presence of EtsΔ138 [66, 67]. These chemical shift perturbations indicated the residues of ERK2 that are either directly engaged by EtsΔ138 or allosterically affected by EtsΔ138 binding. EtsΔ138 was found to interact with the DRS of inactive ERK2 at Φ_{hyd} (including residues Leu113, Leu155, and Tyr126) but not at Φ_{chg}, consistent with the computational modeling discussed above. EtsΔ138 also induced chemical shift perturbations in the FRS at the α2L14 helix, the αG helix (which contains the residues Tyr231 and Leu232 of the FRS), and the key FRS residue Tyr261. These data suggested that EtsΔ138 engages the FRS either directly or allosterically, but our computational model of the ERK2·EtsΔ138 complex and the competitive displacement of EtsΔ138 (and EtsΔ138 lacking N-terminal 1–24) by an F-site ligand supports the former. NMR data also showed that D-site ligands induced disruption of the β5 strand and linker between the N- and C- lobes, in line with the allosteric remodeling of the catalytic site that had been previously detected by crystal structures of ERK2 with D-site ligands [46]. Strict D-site ligands, however, did not cause chemical shift perturbations in the FRS. This observation suggested that EtsΔ138 and other ERK2-binding proteins with noncanonical docking site motifs may access different binding modes or cause different allosteric changes in ERK2.

In a follow-up study, Piserchio et al. evaluated the chemical shift perturbations of EtsΔ138 upon binding to ERK2 in order to validate the interactions that were suggested by ERK2 NMR data [56]. As expected, the N-terminal domain of EtsΔ138 is predominantly disordered before and after binding although a segment (Pro9-Ile14) that resembles the φ_A–X–φ_B motif of the canonical D-site sequence contacted the Φ_{hyd} region of the DRS. These residues were in line with predictions from our previous computational studies [29]. Other residues of the N-terminal portion of EtsΔ138 appear to engage the DRS transiently. In contrast, the C-terminal pnt domain of EtsΔ138 forms a rigid-body interaction with a region of the FRS, marked by Phe120 interaction with Tyr261 and Leu262 of ERK2 [66]. When comparing EtsΔ138 chemical shifts when bound to active versus inactive ERK2, Thr38 undergoes a significant perturbation along with the H0 helix of EtsΔ138 and areas around where F120 contacts the FRS. These chemical shift perturbations are reflective of the repositioning of Thr38 for catalysis. The proline of the P + 1 position (Pro39) was found to be critical for EtsΔ138 phosphorylation, in line with the mechanism of ERK2 discussed earlier in this review. The positioning of ^{38}TP^{39} by docking interactions was estimated to result in phosphorylation in up to 40% of molecular collisions [56]. Displacement of ^{38}TP^{39} using alanine spacers lowers k_{cat} values for ERK2, indicating the importance of optimal positioning of phosphorylation motifs that are provided by docking interactions.

Altogether, we have used a combination of mutational studies, kinetics, computational modeling, and NMR spectroscopy to evolve a detailed model of the mechanism of EtsΔ138 phosphorylation by ERK2. Though EtsΔ138 does not engage ERK2 through canonical D-site or F-site interactions, it utilizes both the DRS and FRS to increase productive encounters between its phosphorylation sequence and the catalytic site of ERK2.

Mechanisms of Docking Site Inhibition

Reversible Inhibition

Through the understanding of the role of the DRS and FRS in the mechanism of ERK2 that we have learned from studying Ets-1 phosphorylation, we can explore the effects of blocking these sites using peptide and small-molecule ligands. Kinase inhibitors that block substrate or other protein interactions are garnering attention, especially in the field of cancer drug discovery and development. This approach targets the molecular recognition requirement of the kinase mechanism discussed above, rather than the catalytic machinery of ERK itself, which allows for specific and selective manipulation of ERK signaling by avoiding ATP competition.

Here, we use an example of peptide ligands that engage the DRS and FRS of ERK2 as an illustration of the potential effects that docking site inhibitors can have on the mechanism of ERK2. We designed two peptides, Lig-D (FQRKTLQ-RRNLKGLNLNL (see footnote 1) derived from the D-site of yeast Ste7) and Lig-F (YAPRAPAKLAFQFPSR[2] from the F-site of mRNA export factor MEX67) that bind exclusively to the DRS and FRS of ERK2, respectively [29]. We then tested the ability of these peptides to inhibit EtsΔ138 phosphorylation by varying EtsΔ138 and ligand concentrations and measuring steady-state rates of reaction. Lig-D manifested as a nonlinear (hyperbolic) mixed-type inhibitor of EtsΔ138 phosphorylation. Mixed inhibition is described by Eq. 2 below [29]:

$$k_{\text{obs}} = \frac{k_{\text{cat}}^{\text{app}}[\text{S}]}{K_{\text{mS}}^{\text{app}}\left(\dfrac{1+\dfrac{[\text{I}]}{K_{\text{i}}^{\text{app}}}}{1+\dfrac{\beta[\text{I}]}{\alpha K_{\text{i}}^{\text{app}}}}\right)+[S]\left(\dfrac{1+\dfrac{[\text{I}]}{\alpha K_{\text{i}}^{\text{app}}}}{1+\dfrac{\beta[\text{I}]}{\alpha K_{\text{i}}^{\text{app}}}}\right)} \quad (2)$$

[2] Underlined residues correspond to the F-site sequence FXFP

Here, [S] is the concentration of substrate S, [I] is the concentration of inhibitor I, K_{mS}^{app} is the apparent Michaelis constant for substrate S (in this case, EtsΔ138), αK_i^{app} is the apparent *uncompetitive* inhibition constant for inhibitor I, and βk_{cat}^{app} is the apparent catalytic constant for the enzyme-inhibitor complex. This mechanism is shown in Fig. 5a where $\alpha = 8$ and $\beta = 1$ [29]. Lig-D is a partial inhibitor of EtsΔ138 phosphorylation and thus has limited influence on k_{cat} while increasing K_m, which accounts for the observed nonlinear behavior. This behavior can be attributed

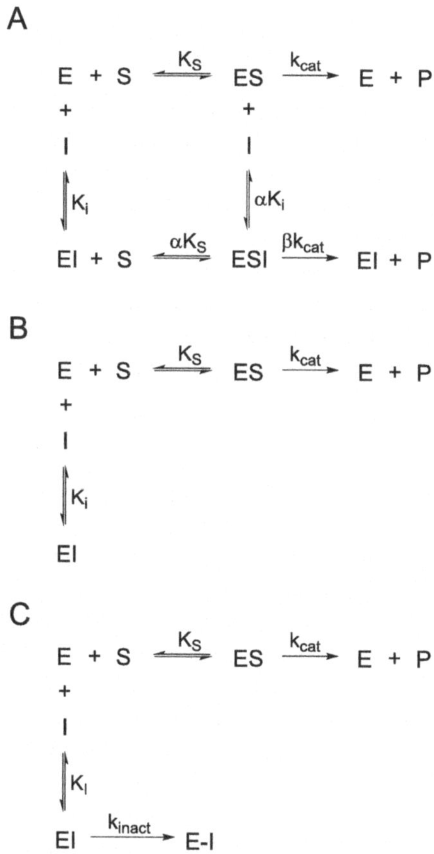

Fig. 5 Effects of docking site inhibitors on substrate phosphorylation [29, 81, 101]. In each case, enzyme (E) reacts with substrate (S) to yield product (P) or is inhibited by ligand (I). (**a**) Mechanism for mixed inhibition (hyperbolic). K_s is the dissociation constant for substrate S, αK_s is the apparent Michaelis constant for substrate S, αK_i is the apparent uncompetitive inhibition constant for inhibitor I, k_{cat} is the catalytic constant, and βk_{cat} is the apparent catalytic constant for the enzyme-inhibitor complex. In the case of Lig-D inhibition of EtsΔ138 phosphorylation, $\alpha = 8$ and $\beta = 1$ [29]. (**b**) Model for linear competitive inhibition as in the case of Lig-F inhibition of EtsΔ138 phosphorylation. K_s and k_{cat} are defined as in part (**a**). (**c**) Model for two-step covalent inhibition. K_I is the inhibition constant, or the concentration of inhibitor required to reach the half-maximal rate of enzyme inactivation, and k_{inact} is the maximal rate constant of enzyme inactivation

to the binding of the pnt domain to the FRS being largely unaffected by the Lig-D interaction.

On the other hand, Lig-F exhibited linear competitive inhibition of EtsΔ138 phosphorylation and an increase in K_m, as shown in Fig. 5b. This information indicated that Lig-F binding to the FRS was sufficient in this case to fully displace EtsΔ138. Linear competitive inhibition shown in Fig. 5b can be described by Eq. 3 below where K_i^{app} is the apparent *competitive* inhibition constant for inhibitor (I).

$$k_{obs} = \frac{k_{cat}^{app}[S]}{K_{mS}^{app}\left(1+[I]/K_i^{app}\right)} \tag{3}$$

Together, these examples show that a docking site inhibitor (1) may be fully competitive against ERK substrates, (2) may partially inhibit phosphorylation of substrates that bind to more than one region (mixed inhibition), or (3) may leave substrates that dock at other sites unaffected. However, this does not rule out the likelihood of allosteric communication between an inhibitor bound at the DRS or FRS and the active site. As discussed earlier, the occupation of the DRS can induce large conformational changes in the activation segment of ERK2 and can also affect the MAPK insert [23, 46]. This knowledge suggests that the binding of an inhibitor at the DRS could potentially affect substrate binding or other interactions that involve residues near the activation segment and the FRS. The FRS and active site are adjacent and are conformationally linked as indicated by the exposure of the FRS upon phosphorylation of the activation segment. Targeting the activation segment with inhibitors is expected to affect the FRS and vice versa. In 2012, Kummer et al. identified two *d*esigned *a*nkyrin *r*epeat *prote*ins (DARPins) that selectively bind and inhibit either active (doubly phosphorylated) or inactive ERK2 [68]. The DARPins bind mainly to the activation loop of ERK2 and adjacent regions, recognizing the conformational changes that occur upon phosphorylation of Thr183 and Tyr185. The regions where the DARPins make contact with ERK2 also encompass the key hydrophobic residues of the FRS, specifically Tyr231. This example not only illustrates the relationship between the FRS and the catalytic core of ERK2, but it also suggests that targeting the FRS with inhibitors provides an opportunity to selectively inhibit active ERK2.

In cases where ERK2 substrates can undergo multisite phosphorylation, docking site inhibitors can affect the observed rates of phosphorylation of different individual sites on a substrate that can regulate its activation or deactivation. Time-resolved NMR of Elk-1 phosphorylation showed that competition between docking motifs promoted different rates of phosphorylation of eight sites in the Elk-1 transcriptional activation domain, termed fast, intermediate, and slow sites based on their relative phosphorylation rates [69]. Phosphorylation of fast and intermediate sites on Elk-1 drove recruitment of the mediator coactivator complex and transcriptional activation while continued phosphorylation of slow sites promoted inactivation and limited Elk-1 transcriptional output [69]. Blocking DRS and FRS interactions by deleting the D-site or F-site on Elk-1 differentially affected the rates of phosphorylation at each phospho-site by ERK2. Thus, docking site inhibitors can potentially alter the accessibility of different phosphorylation sites either by blocking binding or by altering reaction rates.

Covalent Inhibition

Docking sites may be targeted by irreversible covalent inhibitors, provided they possess a solvent-exposed amino acid side chain that can function as a nucleophile. An example of such a residue is Cys179/Cys159, located adjacent to the ED domain in the DRS of ERK1/2. Development of covalent inhibitors for therapeutic purposes has long been met with concern for a variety of reasons, including toxicity, off-target reactivity, and haptenization [70, 71]. However, the benefits of covalent inhibition, including extended duration of action and high potency, can outweigh these risks with careful inhibitor design.

Irreversible covalent inhibitors can be interpreted as nonsubstrate-competitive regardless of their target location on functionally relevant enzyme surfaces since they can inherently overcome high substrate concentrations and affinities over time [71, 72]. Therefore, the duration of action of selective covalent inhibitors is theoretically limited by the half-life of their target protein in cells, which is more than 50 h for ERK1/2 [73]. This long turnover time suggests that covalent inhibitors can also potentially overcome issues with signaling pathway feedback mechanisms and acquired resistance in response to reversible targeted kinase inhibition [74–76]. Feedback activation of ERK through upregulation of the expression and activity of upstream pathway members can often occur in response to ERK inhibition. Reversible inhibitors can be displaced by shifts in equilibria of ERK activators and deactivators due to feedback signaling, or by increased expression of ERK substrates, while irreversible inhibitors are not vulnerable to such competitive displacement. The same principle illustrates how covalent ERK inhibitors can potentially overcome specific resistance mechanisms to inhibitors of upstream pathway components. In BRAF-V600E mutant melanoma, for example, resistance mechanisms to clinical ERK pathway inhibitors can culminate in increased signaling flux through the pathway, which overwhelms and outcompetes reversible inhibition to drive ERK reactivation [77, 78]. Irreversible covalent ERK inhibitors may also be capable of achieving complete inhibition of ERK, which may be necessary for inhibiting phenotypes associated with ERK activity [79].

Irreversible inhibitor design must involve a balance of reactivity and selectivity [70]. This balance requires an inhibitor that acts via a two-step model, involving initial reversible binding and a subsequent irreversible reaction step. Figure 5c illustrates this type of inhibitor mechanism, and the two-step covalent modification can be modeled using Eq. 4 [80, 81] below, assuming 1:1 enzyme/inhibitor stoichiometry.

$$k_{obs} = \frac{k_{inact}[I]}{K_I + [I]} \tag{4}$$

In this model, k_{obs} is described by the inhibitor concentration [I] and two parameters: the inhibition constant K_I, or the concentration of inhibitor required to reach the half-maximal rate of enzyme inactivation, and k_{inact}, or the maximal rate constant of enzyme inactivation. K_I is a descriptor of the inhibitor binding step although it is analogous to the Michaelis constant (K_m) in the basic Michaelis-Menten model and is, therefore, not the true binding affinity of the inhibitor. The rate constant k_{inact} is considered a metric of inhibitor reactivity and describes the second step of Fig. 5c where irreversible adduct formation occurs between the inhibitor and enzyme. Given sufficient time to react under ideal conditions, irreversible inhibitors will inactivate an enzyme with 1:1 stoichiometry, thus rendering them indistinguishable from one another at such endpoints. Therefore, it is necessary to characterize covalent inhibitors in terms of the kinetic parameters K_I and k_{inact} rather than conventional measures of inhibition like IC_{50} values.[3] Unlike IC_{50} values, these parameters are independent of reaction conditions.

Noncatalytic Effects

The implications of docking site inhibitors can reach far beyond direct effects on ERK catalysis. Numerous studies show that ERK has noncatalytic functions that are involved in regulatory interactions and signaling events. One key to these noncatalytic functions appears to be the conformation of the activation loop of ERK, which, as we have discussed here, can be altered by docking site interactions. In an early study in yeast, Bardwell et al. (1998) found that inactive Kss1 (ERK) can directly bind to the transcription factor Ste12 in yeast, leading to the inhibition of invasive filamentous growth [82]. They showed that activation of Kss1 by Ste7 (MEK) and the concomitant change in activation loop conformation alleviated this transcriptional repression without the requirement of Kss1 catalytic activity. They identified Tyr231 of Kss1 as a critical residue involved in Ste12 binding. Tyr231 in Kss1 corresponds to Tyr231 of the FRS of mammalian ERK2 and also forms a hydrogen bond with glutamate in the TEY motif of the activation segment of inactive Kss1.

In another study, Camps et al. found that direct binding of ERK2 to DUSP6 resulted in the activation of DUSP6, and this activation was allosteric and independent of ERK2 kinase activity [83]. They found that the *sevenmaker* mutant of ERK2, D319N, which is located in the DRS, prevented this allosteric activation of DUSP6.

[3] IC_{50} values are concentrations of an antagonist molecule that are required to observe a half-maximal inhibitory effect. These measurements are dependent on enzyme concentration, presence of competitive substrates, and duration of exposure to enzyme (if the inhibitors are time-dependent enzyme inactivators).

Hari et al. (2014) found that ATP-site inhibitors that trap the ERK2 activation loop in the inactive DFG-out conformation can prevent the noncatalytic activation of DUSP6 by ERK2 while inhibitors that trap ERK2 in the DFG-in conformation do not [84]. Together, these results show that the DRS and the activation loop, which can be influenced by interactions at both DRS and FRS residues, are critical for DUSP6 activation by ERK2.

The kinase-independent functions of ERK2 also include transcriptional repression of INFγ-responsive genes by direct binding to the promoter region sequence GAAAC [85]. This binding was found by mutational studies to involve positively charged residues within Lys257-Arg275 of ERK2, located within the MAPK insert domain and α2L14 ERK2 [85]. This binding sequence includes the FRS residue Tyr261 and is nearby other FRS residues as well. ERK1/2 can also competitively displace retinoblastoma protein (pRb) from lamin-A to promote cell cycle entry in a kinase-independent manner [86]. ERK can also activate PARP1 and topoisomerase αII regardless of kinase activity [87, 88]. However, ERK must be phosphorylated and in the active conformation in order to activate both PARP1 and topoisomerase αII.

As discussed earlier, docking sites on ERK are also involved in subcellular localization and scaffolding interactions that influence ERK activity but do not necessarily involve the catalytic apparatus of ERK. As mentioned earlier, MEK, PEA-15, KSR1, and nucleoporin binding all involve ERK docking sites and influence ERK transport/localization [38–43, 58]. Our studies indicate that ERK2 can bind PEA-15 and Ets-1 with affinities that do not significantly change with activation state, which is suggestive of noncatalytic ERK functions [38, 39, 57]. Therefore, it is essential to consider the effects of docking site inhibitors on ERK interactions that do not involve direct catalytic activity of ERK, whether these interactions directly involve the docking sites or are influenced by allosteric effects of the inhibitors.

Docking Site Inhibitor Development

Current DRS Inhibitors

Just as proteins can utilize different binding modes at the DRS, subgroups can also classify inhibitors of ERK that target the DRS based on their localized binding mode within the docking site. Current known DRS inhibitors engage mainly with residues at either the CD domain, the ED domain, and/or the hydrophobic docking groove.

Hydrophobic Groove and CD Domain Inhibitors

Hancock et al. (2005) discovered the first low-molecular-weight DRS-targeted ERK inhibitors through computer-aided drug design (CADD) and in silico screening using the hydrophobic cleft formed between the CD and ED domains on inactive ERK2 as an initial location for ligand placement [89]. Figure 6 shows two of the compounds resulting from this screening (compound **1.1** and **1.2**). Both of these compounds were confirmed to bind to ERK2 in vitro by fluorescence quenching assays with dissociation constants of approximately 5 μM. Treatment of HeLa cells with these compounds at 100 μM showed significant inhibition of the downstream ERK2 target RSK1 (**1.1**: ~50% inhibition, **1.2**: 20–25% inhibition), and compound **1.1** inhibited Elk-1 phosphorylation. Both RSK1 and Elk-1 are known to interact at the DRS as mentioned earlier. Compounds **1.1** and **1.2** also inhibited colony formation of several cancer cell lines by 50% at concentrations of approximately 15–25 μM. Computational docking of the compounds predicted that they both bind in the hydrophobic cleft of the DRS between the CD and ED domains and are within hydrogen-bonding distance of the CD domain aspartate residues.

The same research group performed an analogous in silico screening of active ERK2 to identify compounds that could potentially select for subtle conformational or flexibility differences in the DRS of the active versus the inactive enzyme [90]. Though the crystal structures of active (1ERK) and inactive (2ERK) ERK2 do not show significant structural differences in the DRS, they were able to identify new compounds that target active ERK2 but were not hits in their original screen of inactive ERK2. Figure 6 shows three of these compounds (compounds **1.3**, **1.4**, and **1.5**). These compounds were shown to directly bind to ERK2 in vitro with dissociation constants of 13–20 μM. Compound **1.3** exhibited the most potent overall inhibition of phosphorylation of downstream ERK targets and proliferation in cells. Interestingly, some of the hit compounds showed differential effects on Elk-1 and RSK1 phosphorylation in cells, consistent with the possibility for different binding modes of the two substrates and/or the compounds themselves.

In further studies stemming from these reports, compound **1.1** was further optimized by virtual screening of analogs (Boston et al.) [91] and synthetic chemistry to evaluate structure-activity relationship [92, 93]. The inhibitors identified by Boston et al. activated the intrinsic apoptosis pathway in cells, inhibiting proliferation and phosphorylation of caspase-9, RSK1, and Bad, which is downstream of RSK1 [91]. The compounds also showed the potential to preferentially target transformed cells over nontransformed cells. Furthermore, compound **1.1** was tested in a human lymphoma xenograft model and exhibited antitumor activity [94].

Other screenings have been performed to identify compounds that interact at the CD domain of the DRS. Kinoshita et al. used in silico methods to identify inhibitors **1.6** and **1.7** in Fig. 6, and this inhibition was confirmed by a biochemical assay that detected competitive displacement of a D-site peptide from the DRS [95]. Through computational docking, the authors predicted that these two compounds mainly interact with the "negative charge pool" (CD domain) of the DRS though they display no highly basic moieties.

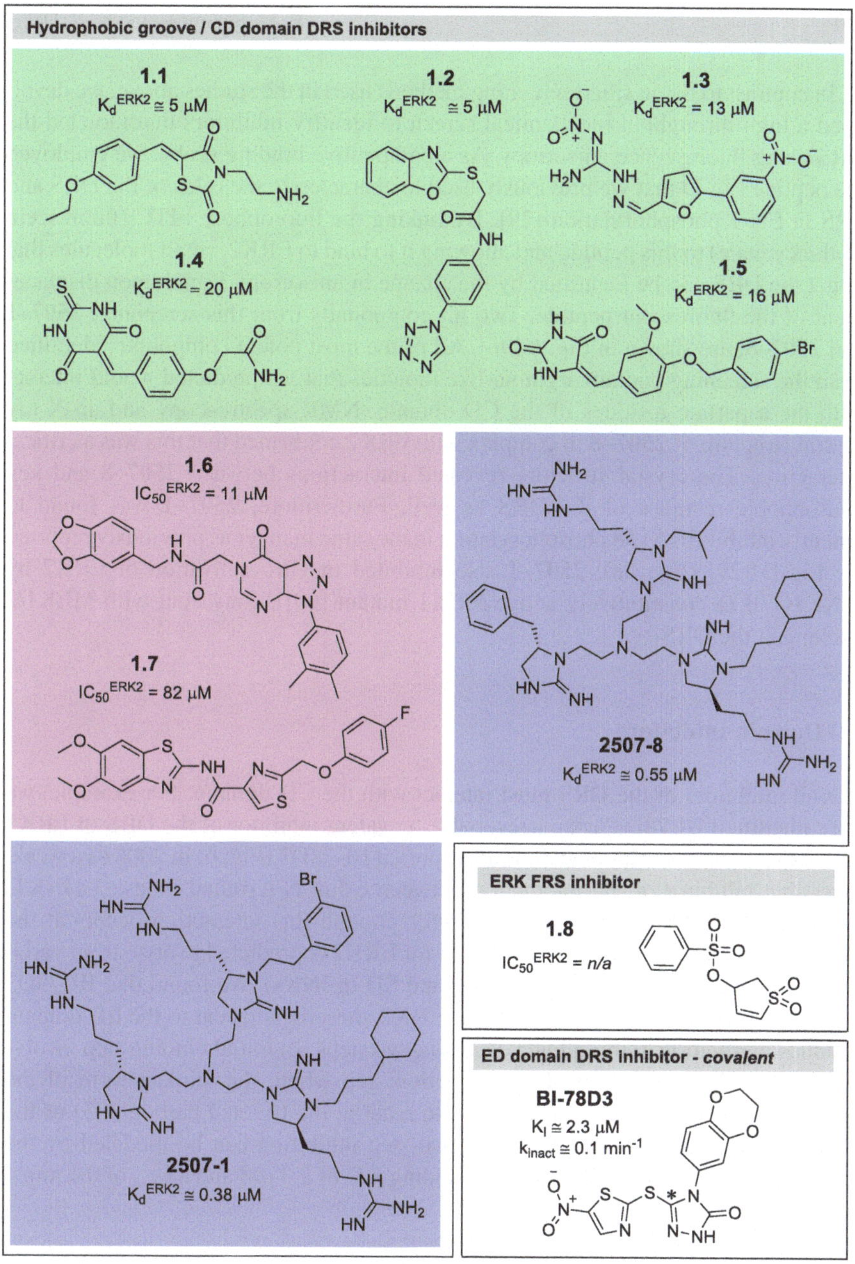

Fig. 6 Inhibitors that target the DRS and FRS of ERK. The compounds shown in this table are examples of docking site inhibitors. Compounds in green are reversible inhibitors that target the hydrophobic groove and CD domain of the DRS, identified using CADD and in silico screening [89, 90]. Compounds in pink are reversible CD domain inhibitors identified by in silico methods [95]. Compounds in blue are reversible hydrophobic groove/CD domain inhibitors identified by a high-throughput biochemical screen [96]. Also shown are a reversible FRS inhibitor [99] and a covalent inhibitor of the DRS ED domain [97]. Available IC_{50} or dissociation constant (K_d) values are shown for active and inactive ERK2, respectively. K_I and k_{inact} for the covalent inhibitor are given against active ERK2. *n/a* not available. *C5 carbon, site of nucleophilic addition on BI-78D3

In contrast to the in silico screening methods used in the studies above, we developed a high-throughput biochemical screen to identify inhibitors that targeted the DRS using fluorescence anisotropy. As a competitive binding probe, we employed the peptide Lig-D that we previously used to characterize the roles of the DRS and FRS in Ets-1 phosphorylation [29]. By linking the fluorophore FITC (fluorescein isothiocyanate) to this peptide and allowing it to bind to ERK2, small molecules that target the DRS can be identified by the change in anisotropy signal upon displacement of the fluorescent peptide. Two hit compounds from this screening, **2507–1** and **2507–8**, are shown in Fig. 6 [96]. All of the most potent compounds identified from the screening contain arginine-like moieties that we predicted would interact with the aspartate residues of the CD domain. NMR spectroscopy and an X-ray crystal structure of **2507–8** in complex with ERK2 confirmed that this was a critical interaction. The crystal structure revealed interactions between **2507–8** and key hydrophobic residues of the DRS as well. Furthermore, **2507–1** was found to potently inhibit EtsΔ138 phosphorylation in the same manner as previously reported for Lig-D [29] (Fig. 5a). **2507–1** also inhibited in vitro activation of ERK2 by MKK1G7B (a constitutively active MEK1 mutant [60]), consistent with MEK1/2 docking at the DRS.

ED Domain Inhibitors

Not all inhibitors of the DRS must interact with the CD domain. For example, we have identified BI-78D3 as an irreversible, covalent inhibitor of the DRS of ERK1 and ERK2 [97]. Stebbins et al. initially reported BI-78D3 (Fig. 6) in 2008 as a weak, reversible inhibitor of the interaction between c-Jun N-terminal kinase 1 (JNK1) and JNK-interacting protein 1 (JIP1) [98]. Though this interaction occurs at the DRS of JNK1, the selectivity of BI-78D3 for ERK2 is predicted to arise from variations of the ED domain (TT in ERK1/2 and SD in JNKs). We found that BI-78D3 forms a tetrahedral adduct at Cys159 of ERK2, directly adjacent to the ED domain residues. Formation of this adduct occurs in two steps: an initial binding step involving the ED domain, followed by a reaction step where the thiolate form of the Cys159 sidechain acts as a nucleophile to react at the trigonal carbon (C5) of the 1,2,4-triazol-3-one ring (Fig. 6). This two-step inhibition can be modeled by the scheme in Fig. 5c as described above, yielding a K_I of 2.3 μM and a k_{inact} of 0.1 min^{-1} (Fig. 6).

Current FRS Inhibitors

There have been fewer ventures into identifying FRS inhibitors compared to the number of studies that identify DRS inhibitors. Recently, a class of small molecules that targets the FRS of ERK2 was identified by Samadani et al. (2015) using virtual database screening [99]. The resulting thienyl benzenesulfonate scaffold molecule

(Fig. 6, compound **1.8**) was shown to interact with the FRS of ERK2 in a pocket exposed by Phe181 and Leu182. From the structure of compound **1.8** (Fig. 6), the two aromatic rings resemble the phenylalanine residues of the FXFP F-site motif buried in the hydrophobic pocket of the FRS. Compound **1.8** and its derivatives were found to inhibit Elk-1 phosphorylation by ERK and the expression of immediate early genes in the Fos family. A high-throughput biochemical assay to identify FRS inhibitors was recently reported by Miller et al. [100]. The method employed a proximity-based AlphaScreen (Perkin-Elmer) to detect the ability of small molecules to inhibit the phosphorylation of an F-site peptide. This screen was designed to employ high concentrations of ATP to select against ATP-competitive inhibitors. This screening method will likely be a useful tool for biochemical detection of FRS inhibitors. In addition to small molecules, numerous peptides containing the DEF consensus sequence have been generated in order to probe the FRS and its role in ERK catalysis and binding interactions [29, 55, 101].

The Future of Docking Site Inhibitors

The structural and kinetic studies that we have applied to characterize interactions at the DRS and FRS of ERK2 are critical for developing docking site inhibitors and have led to the discovery of 2507–1, 2507–8, and new mechanisms for BI-78D3. However, the DRS and FRS are not likely to be the only PPI sites on ERK. Recently, Herrero et al. identified a compound, DEL-22379, as targeting a putative dimerization interface on ERK2 [102]. The compound was an effective inhibitor of proliferation in ERK pathway-driven tumor cells, even in models of MEK and B-Raf inhibitor resistance. This study indicated that this region on ERK2 is biologically relevant albeit the dimerization of ERK2 and its potential roles are debated [57, 103–106].

Variations in docking locations have been identified for other MAPKs as well, suggesting this same possibility for ERK1/2. Francis et al. used a combination of NMR and small angle X-ray scattering to show that HePTP engages p38α residues beyond the established DRS [107]. Additionally, Glatz et al. (2013) found that ERK5 interacts with MKK5 outside of the DRS region as well [108]. These additional interactions that occur external to established docking sites likely contribute to specificity of binding and signaling. These cases illustrate that the continued identification and evaluation of molecules that bind outside of the kinase active site are critical for the discovery of new PPI sites and potential advances in drug development.

Without explicit structural data, protein-protein interactions can be challenging to characterize, making inhibitors of such interactions a useful tool. In 2010, Comess et al. developed a biochemical screening method for detection of p38α and JNK1 inhibitors that bind at any exposed surface of the proteins without bias [53]. This involved exposure of the proteins to small molecules and subsequent removal of any weakly bound compounds by ultrafiltration. Mass spectrometry was then used to identify the remaining high-affinity compounds, and NMR and/or X-ray crystallography were used to determine the binding sites of active compounds. The screen identified both ATP-competitive and non-ATP competitive inhibitors. Of interest, a non-ATP competitive inhibitor of JNK1 activation was found to bind in the region of JNK1 bordered by the activation loop and the kinase insert region, which is analogous to the FRS of ERK2 [51]. This study shows that small molecule inhibitors can reveal protein docking interactions on MAPKs, and these interaction sites need not be previously identified or fully understood.

Docking sites on MAPKs are more superficial and solvent exposed than the ATP-binding pocket, which limits the potency of docking site inhibitors. Typically, selective small-molecule inhibitors of ERK (and kinases in general) that are ATP competitive have nanomolar potencies, which is necessary for overcoming ATP binding in cells. In contrast, known small-molecule docking site inhibitors of ERK typically have micromolar potencies. Although substrate proteins like those that dock at the DRS and FRS are typically present in lower concentrations (relative to their K_m values) than ATP in cells and may interact with ERK transiently; as in the case of Ets-1, it is essential to improve the potencies of DRS and other docking site inhibitors for drug design purposes [109, 110]. Two ways to overcome this issue are (1) development of covalent docking site inhibitors like BI-78D3, and (2) multifunctional and multivalent docking site inhibitors.

Development of covalent inhibitors may follow a structure-guided approach in order to functionalize reversible docking site inhibitors with reactive moieties that can target nearby cysteines [111] or other circumstantial nucleophilic residues. Structure-guided design has been employed to build inhibitors that irreversibly target Cys164 in the active site of ERK2 [112]. New targets for small reactive molecules can also be identified by selectivity profiling against the kinome. Browne et al. (2019) have recently developed a chemoproteomic strategy to profile the reactivity of covalent inhibitors with cysteine thiols across the proteome [113]. This approach, termed CITe-ID (*C*ovalent *I*nhibitor *T*arget Sit*e* *Id*entification), can identify cysteine residues for potential drug targeting as well as off-target effects of existing covalent inhibitors.

However, off-target effects of inhibitors are not always undesirable. Multifunctional inhibitors that target more than one MAPK can be beneficial in targeting disease states in which more than one signaling pathway contributes to pathology. For example, in cancers, crosstalk between ERK, JNK, and PI3K/Akt signaling pathways can occur [114–118], making single-agent inhibitors of multiple MAPKs or combinations of multiple inhibitors attractive therapeutic options [119–121]. Such treatments could be a vehicle to preemptively block the development of resistance that is often observed for targeted single-kinase inhibition in cancers wherein the activation of alternative signaling pathways can perpetuate tumor growth. Inhibitors can also be engineered to target more than one binding site on the same kinase. Furthermore, improved potency and selectivity of ERK docking site inhibitors can be achieved by building multivalent inhibitors, where docking site inhibitors are chemically linked to ATP-competitive inhibitors [122].

Docking site inhibitors can also be designed to have more than one mechanism of action. For example, PROTACs (*pro*teolysis-*ta*rgeting *c*himeric molecules) are multifunctional inhibitors that bind to a target protein and recruit E3 ubiquitin ligase to induce polyubiquitination and proteasomal degradation of the target [123, 124]. Functionalizing ERK docking site inhibitors as PROTACs could overcome observed potency issues by globally decreasing ERK levels, thereby improving effective inhibition of ERK signaling.

Summary

ERK docking site inhibitors add diversity to the available approaches of targeting ERK signaling for potential therapeutic purposes. They also serve as biochemical tools to probe protein-protein interactions that occur at docking sites, involving both catalytic and noncatalytic functions of ERK. Our detailed investigations into Ets-1 phosphorylation by ERK2 show that docking site interactions are crucial for the catalytic efficiency of ERK2, yet illustrate that docking site roles and the definitions of docking interactions are not always clear upon initial analyses. This knowledge demonstrates the importance of using combinations of kinetic and structural methodologies to answer unsolved questions about kinase interactions.

References

1. Eblen, S. T. (2018). Extracellular-regulated kinases: Signaling from Ras to ERK substrates to control biological outcomes. *Advances in Cancer Research, 138*, 99–142.
2. Roskoski, R., Jr. (2019). Targeting ERK1/2 protein-serine/threonine kinases in human cancers. *Pharmacological Research, 142*, 151–168.
3. Santarpia, L., Lippman, S. M., & El-Naggar, A. K. (2012). Targeting the MAPK-RAS-RAF signaling pathway in cancer therapy. *Expert Opinion on Therapeutic Targets, 16*(1), 103–119.
4. Chico, L. K., Van Eldik, L. J., & Watterson, D. M. (2009). Targeting protein kinases in central nervous system disorders. *Nature Reviews Drug Discovery, 8*(11), 892–909.
5. Muslin, A. J. (2008). MAPK signalling in cardiovascular health and disease: Molecular mechanisms and therapeutic targets. *Clinical Science (London, England), 115*(7), 203–218.
6. Gallo, S., et al. (2019). ERK: A key player in the pathophysiology of cardiac hypertrophy. *International Journal of Molecular Sciences, 20*(9), 2164.
7. Tanti, J. F., & Jager, J. (2009). Cellular mechanisms of insulin resistance: Role of stress-regulated serine kinases and insulin receptor substrates (IRS) serine phosphorylation. *Current Opinion in Pharmacology, 9*(6), 753–762.
8. Omori, S., et al. (2006). Extracellular signal-regulated kinase inhibition slows disease progression in mice with polycystic kidney disease. *J Am Soc Nephrol, 17*(6), 1604–1614.
9. Pelaia, G., et al. (2005). Mitogen-activated protein kinases and asthma. *Journal of Cellular Physiology, 202*(3), 642–653.
10. Mercer, B. A., et al. (2004). Extracellular regulated kinase/mitogen activated protein kinase is up-regulated in pulmonary emphysema and mediates matrix metalloproteinase-1 induction by cigarette smoke. *The Journal of Biological Chemistry, 279*(17), 17690–17696.

11. Boulton, T. G., & Cobb, M. H. (1991). Identification of multiple extracellular signal-regulated kinases (ERKs) with antipeptide antibodies. *Cell Regulation, 2*(5), 357–371.
12. Busca, R., Pouyssegur, J., & Lenormand, P. (2016). ERK1 and ERK2 map kinases: Specific roles or functional redundancy? *Frontiers in Cell and Development Biology, 4*, 53.
13. Davis, R. J. (1993). The mitogen-activated protein kinase signal transduction pathway. *The Journal of Biological Chemistry, 268*(20), 14553–14556.
14. Gonzalez, F. A., Raden, D. L., & Davis, R. J. (1991). Identification of substrate recognition determinants for human ERK1 and ERK2 protein kinases. *The Journal of Biological Chemistry, 266*(33), 22159–22163.
15. Turjanski, A. G., Hummer, G., & Gutkind, J. S. (2009). How mitogen-activated protein kinases recognize and phosphorylate their targets: A QM/MM study. *Journal of the American Chemical Society, 131*(17), 6141–6148.
16. Admiraal, S. J., & Herschlag, D. (1995). Mapping the transition state for ATP hydrolysis: Implications for enzymatic catalysis. *Chemistry & Biology, 2*(11), 729–739.
17. Adams, J. A. (2001). Kinetic and catalytic mechanisms of protein kinases. *Chemical Reviews, 101*(8), 2271–2290.
18. Roskoski, R., Jr. (2012). ERK1/2 MAP kinases: Structure, function, and regulation. *Pharmacological Research, 66*(2), 105–143.
19. Robinson, M. J., et al. (1996). Mutation of position 52 in ERK2 creates a nonproductive binding mode for adenosine 5′-triphosphate. *Biochemistry, 35*(18), 5641–5646.
20. Waas, W. F., & Dalby, K. N. (2003). Physiological concentrations of divalent magnesium ion activate the serine/threonine specific protein kinase ERK2. *Biochemistry, 42*(10), 2960–2970.
21. Waas, W. F., et al. (2004). A kinetic approach towards understanding substrate interactions and the catalytic mechanism of the serine/threonine protein kinase ERK2: Identifying a potential regulatory role for divalent magnesium. *Biochimica et Biophysica Acta, 1697*(1-2), 81–87.
22. Prowse, C. N., & Lew, J. (2001). Mechanism of activation of ERK2 by dual phosphorylation. *The Journal of Biological Chemistry, 276*(1), 99–103.
23. Hoofnagle, A. N., et al. (2001). Changes in protein conformational mobility upon activation of extracellular regulated protein kinase-2 as detected by hydrogen exchange. *Proceedings of the National Academy of Sciences of the United States of America, 98*(3), 956–961.
24. Modi, V., & Dunbrack, R. L., Jr. (2019). Defining a new nomenclature for the structures of active and inactive kinases. *Proceedings of the National Academy of Sciences of the United States of America, 116*(14), 6818–6827.
25. Wilson, L. J., et al. (2018). New perspectives, opportunities, and challenges in exploring the human protein kinome. *Cancer Research, 78*(1), 15–29.
26. Garai, A., et al. (2012). Specificity of linear motifs that bind to a common mitogen-activated protein kinase docking groove. *Science Signaling, 5*(245), ra74.
27. Zeke, A., et al. (2015). Systematic discovery of linear binding motifs targeting an ancient protein interaction surface on MAP kinases. *Molecular Systems Biology, 11*(11), 837.
28. Abramczyk, O., et al. (2007). Expanding the repertoire of an ERK2 recruitment site: Cysteine footprinting identifies the D-recruitment site as a mediator of Ets-1 binding. *Biochemistry, 46*(32), 9174–9186.
29. Lee, S., et al. (2011). A model of a MAPK*substrate complex in an active conformation: A computational and experimental approach. *PLoS One, 6*(4), e18594.
30. Jacobs, D., et al. (1999). Multiple docking sites on substrate proteins form a modular system that mediates recognition by ERK MAP kinase. *Genes & Development, 13*(2), 163–175.
31. Fantz, D. A., et al. (2001). Docking sites on substrate proteins direct extracellular signal-regulated kinase to phosphorylate specific residues. *The Journal of Biological Chemistry, 276*(29), 27256–27265.
32. Martin, M. C., et al. (2008). The docking interaction of caspase-9 with ERK2 provides a mechanism for the selective inhibitory phosphorylation of caspase-9 at threonine 125. *The Journal of Biological Chemistry, 283*(7), 3854–3865.

33. Burkhard, K. A., Chen, F., & Shapiro, P. (2011). Quantitative analysis of ERK2 interactions with substrate proteins: Roles for kinase docking domains and activity in determining binding affinity. *The Journal of Biological Chemistry, 286*(4), 2477–2485.
34. Dimitri, C. A., et al. (2005). Spatially separate docking sites on ERK2 regulate distinct signaling events in vivo. *Current Biology, 15*(14), 1319–1324.
35. Tanoue, T., et al. (2000). A conserved docking motif in MAP kinases common to substrates, activators and regulators. *Nature Cell Biology, 2*(2), 110–116.
36. Piserchio, A., et al. (2012). Docking interactions of hematopoietic tyrosine phosphatase with MAP kinases ERK2 and p38alpha. *Biochemistry, 51*(41), 8047–8049.
37. Bardwell, A. J., et al. (2001). A conserved docking site in MEKs mediates high-affinity binding to MAP kinases and cooperates with a scaffold protein to enhance signal transmission. *The Journal of Biological Chemistry, 276*(13), 10374–10386.
38. Callaway, K., et al. (2007). The anti-apoptotic protein PEA-15 is a tight binding inhibitor of ERK1 and ERK2, which blocks docking interactions at the D-recruitment site. *Biochemistry, 46*(32), 9187–9198.
39. Callaway, K., Rainey, M. A., & Dalby, K. N. (2005). Quantifying ERK2-protein interactions by fluorescence anisotropy: PEA-15 inhibits ERK2 by blocking the binding of DEJL domains. *Biochimica et Biophysica Acta, 1754*(1-2), 316–323.
40. Mace, P. D., et al. (2013). Structure of ERK2 bound to PEA-15 reveals a mechanism for rapid release of activated MAPK. *Nature Communications, 4*, 1681.
41. Formstecher, E., et al. (2001). PEA-15 mediates cytoplasmic sequestration of ERK MAP kinase. *Developmental Cell, 1*(2), 239–250.
42. Adachi, M., Fukuda, M., & Nishida, E. (2000). Nuclear export of MAP kinase (ERK) involves a MAP kinase kinase (MEK)-dependent active transport mechanism. *The Journal of Cell Biology, 148*(5), 849–856.
43. Zheng, C. F., & Guan, K. L. (1994). Cytoplasmic localization of the mitogen-activated protein kinase activator MEK. *The Journal of Biological Chemistry, 269*(31), 19947–19952.
44. Canagarajah, B. J., et al. (1997). Activation mechanism of the MAP kinase ERK2 by dual phosphorylation. *Cell, 90*(5), 859–869.
45. Zhang, F., et al. (1994). Atomic structure of the MAP kinase ERK2 at 2.3 A resolution. *Nature, 367*(6465), 704–711.
46. Zhou, T., et al. (2006). Docking interactions induce exposure of activation loop in the MAP kinase ERK2. *Structure, 14*(6), 1011–1019.
47. Taylor, C. A. T., et al. (2019). Functional divergence caused by mutations in an energetic hotspot in ERK2. *Proceedings of the National Academy of Sciences of the United States of America, 116*(31), 15514–15523.
48. Galanis, A., Yang, S. H., & Sharrocks, A. D. (2001). Selective targeting of MAPKs to the ETS domain transcription factor SAP-1. *The Journal of Biological Chemistry, 276*(2), 965–973.
49. Tzarum, N., et al. (2013). DEF pocket in p38alpha facilitates substrate selectivity and mediates autophosphorylation. *The Journal of Biological Chemistry, 288*(27), 19537–19547.
50. Elkins, J. M., et al. (2013). X-ray crystal structure of ERK5 (MAPK7) in complex with a specific inhibitor. *Journal of Medicinal Chemistry, 56*(11), 4413–4421.
51. Liu, X., et al. (2016). A conserved motif in JNK/p38-specific MAPK phosphatases as a determinant for JNK1 recognition and inactivation. *Nature Communications, 7*, 10879.
52. Lee, T., et al. (2004). Docking motif interactions in MAP kinases revealed by hydrogen exchange mass spectrometry. *Molecular Cell, 14*(1), 43–55.
53. Comess, K. M., et al. (2011). Discovery and characterization of non-ATP site inhibitors of the mitogen activated protein (MAP) kinases. *ACS Chemical Biology, 6*(3), 234–244.
54. Sheridan, D. L., et al. (2008). Substrate discrimination among mitogen-activated protein kinases through distinct docking sequence motifs. *The Journal of Biological Chemistry, 283*(28), 19511–19520.
55. Piserchio, A., et al. (2015). Structural and dynamic features of F-recruitment site driven substrate phosphorylation by ERK2. *Scientific Reports, 5*, 11127.

56. Piserchio, A., et al. (2017). Local destabilization, rigid body, and fuzzy docking facilitate the phosphorylation of the transcription factor Ets-1 by the mitogen-activated protein kinase ERK2. *Proceedings of the National Academy of Sciences of the United States of America, 114*(31), E6287–E6296.
57. Callaway, K. A., et al. (2006). Properties and regulation of a transiently assembled ERK2. Ets-1 signaling complex. *Biochemistry, 45*(46), 13719–13733.
58. McKay, M. M., Ritt, D. A., & Morrison, D. K. (2009). Signaling dynamics of the KSR1 scaffold complex. *Proceedings of the National Academy of Sciences of the United States of America, 106*(27), 11022–11027.
59. Waas, W. F., & Dalby, K. N. (2001). Purification of a model substrate for transcription factor phosphorylation by ERK2. *Protein Expression and Purification, 23*(1), 191–197.
60. Waas, W. F., & Dalby, K. N. (2002). Transient protein-protein interactions and a random-ordered kinetic mechanism for the phosphorylation of a transcription factor by extracellular-regulated protein kinase 2. *The Journal of Biological Chemistry, 277*(15), 12532–12540.
61. Cornish-Bowden, A. (2012). Fundamentals of enzyme kinetics (4th ed., Vol. xviii, 498p). Weinheim: Wiley-VCH.
62. Seidel, J. J., & Graves, B. J. (2002). An ERK2 docking site in the pointed domain distinguishes a subset of ETS transcription factors. *Genes & Development, 16*(1), 127–137.
63. Waas, W. F., et al. (2003). Two rate-limiting steps in the kinetic mechanism of the serine/threonine specific protein kinase ERK2: A case of fast phosphorylation followed by fast product release. *Biochemistry, 42*(42), 12273–12286.
64. Callaway, K., et al. (2010). Phosphorylation of the transcription factor Ets-1 by ERK2: Rapid dissociation of ADP and phospho-Ets-1. *Biochemistry, 49*(17), 3619–3630.
65. Rainey, M. A., et al. (2005). Proximity-induced catalysis by the protein kinase ERK2. *Journal of the American Chemical Society, 127*(30), 10494–10495.
66. Piserchio, A., et al. (2011). Solution NMR insights into docking interactions involving inactive ERK2. *Biochemistry, 50*(18), 3660–3672.
67. Piserchio, A., Dalby, K. N., & Ghose, R. (2012). Assignment of backbone resonances in a eukaryotic protein kinase—ERK2 as a representative example. *Methods in Molecular Biology, 831*, 359–368.
68. Kummer, L., et al. (2012). Structural and functional analysis of phosphorylation-specific binders of the kinase ERK from designed ankyrin repeat protein libraries. *Proceedings of the National Academy of Sciences of the United States of America, 109*(34), E2248–E2257.
69. Mylona, A., et al. (2016). Opposing effects of Elk-1 multisite phosphorylation shape its response to ERK activation. *Science, 354*(6309), 233–237.
70. Johnson, D. S., Weerapana, E., & Cravatt, B. F. (2010). Strategies for discovering and derisking covalent, irreversible enzyme inhibitors. *Future Medicinal Chemistry, 2*(6), 949–964.
71. Barf, T., & Kaptein, A. (2012). Irreversible protein kinase inhibitors: Balancing the benefits and risks. *Journal of Medicinal Chemistry, 55*(14), 6243–6262.
72. Garuti, L., Roberti, M., & Bottegoni, G. (2011). Irreversible protein kinase inhibitors. *Current Medicinal Chemistry, 18*(20), 2981–2994.
73. Schwanhausser, B., et al. (2011). Global quantification of mammalian gene expression control. *Nature, 473*(7347), 337–342.
74. Singh, J., et al. (2011). The resurgence of covalent drugs. *Nature Reviews Drug Discovery, 10*(4), 307–317.
75. Kwak, E. L., et al. (2005). Irreversible inhibitors of the EGF receptor may circumvent acquired resistance to gefitinib. *Proceedings of the National Academy of Sciences of the United States of America, 102*(21), 7665–7670.
76. Kobayashi, S., et al. (2005). An alternative inhibitor overcomes resistance caused by a mutation of the epidermal growth factor receptor. *Cancer Research, 65*(16), 7096–7101.
77. Lake, D., Correa, S. A., & Muller, J. (2016). Negative feedback regulation of the ERK1/2 MAPK pathway. *Cellular and Molecular Life Sciences, 73*(23), 4397–4413.

78. Johnson, G. L., et al. (2014). Molecular pathways: Adaptive kinome reprogramming in response to targeted inhibition of the BRAF-MEK-ERK pathway in cancer. *Clinical Cancer Research, 20*(10), 2516–2522.
79. Albeck, J. G., Mills, G. B., & Brugge, J. S. (2013). Frequency-modulated pulses of ERK activity transmit quantitative proliferation signals. *Molecular Cell, 49*(2), 249–261.
80. Copeland, R. A. (2000). Enzymes: A practical introduction to structure, mechanism, and data analysis (2nd ed., Vol. xvi, 397p). New York: J. Wiley.
81. Kitz, R., & Wilson, I. B. (1962). Esters of methanesulfonic acid as irreversible inhibitors of acetylcholinesterase. *The Journal of Biological Chemistry, 237*, 3245–3249.
82. Bardwell, L., et al. (1998). Repression of yeast Ste12 transcription factor by direct binding of unphosphorylated Kss1 MAPK and its regulation by the Ste7 MEK. *Genes & Development, 12*(18), 2887–2898.
83. Camps, M., et al. (1998). Catalytic activation of the phosphatase MKP-3 by ERK2 mitogen-activated protein kinase. *Science, 280*(5367), 1262–1265.
84. Hari, S. B., Merritt, E. A., & Maly, D. J. (2014). Conformation-selective ATP-competitive inhibitors control regulatory interactions and noncatalytic functions of mitogen-activated protein kinases. *Chemistry & Biology, 21*(5), 628–635.
85. Hu, S., et al. (2009). Profiling the human protein-DNA interactome reveals ERK2 as a transcriptional repressor of interferon signaling. *Cell, 139*(3), 610–622.
86. Rodriguez, J., et al. (2010). ERK1/2 MAP kinases promote cell cycle entry by rapid, kinase-independent disruption of retinoblastoma-lamin A complexes. *The Journal of Cell Biology, 191*(5), 967–979.
87. Cohen-Armon, M., et al. (2007). DNA-independent PARP-1 activation by phosphorylated ERK2 increases Elk1 activity: A link to histone acetylation. *Molecular Cell, 25*(2), 297–308.
88. Shapiro, P. S., et al. (1999). Extracellular signal-regulated kinase activates topoisomerase IIalpha through a mechanism independent of phosphorylation. *Molecular and Cellular Biology, 19*(5), 3551–3560.
89. Hancock, C. N., et al. (2005). Identification of novel extracellular signal-regulated kinase docking domain inhibitors. *Journal of Medicinal Chemistry, 48*(14), 4586–4595.
90. Chen, F., et al. (2006). Characterization of ATP-independent ERK inhibitors identified through in silico analysis of the active ERK2 structure. *Bioorganic & Medicinal Chemistry Letters, 16*(24), 6281–6287.
91. Boston, S. R., et al. (2011). Characterization of ERK docking domain inhibitors that induce apoptosis by targeting Rsk-1 and caspase-9. *BMC Cancer, 11*, 7.
92. Li, Q., et al. (2009). Structure-activity relationship (SAR) studies of 3-(2-amino-ethyl)-5-(4-ethoxy-benzylidene)-thiazolidine-2,4-dione: Development of potential substrate-specific ERK1/2 inhibitors. *Bioorganic & Medicinal Chemistry Letters, 19*(21), 6042–6046.
93. Jung, K. Y., et al. (2013). Structural modifications of (Z)-3-(2-aminoethyl)-5-(4-ethoxybenzylidene)thiazolidine-2,4-dione that improve selectivity for inhibiting the proliferation of melanoma cells containing active ERK signaling. *Organic & Biomolecular Chemistry, 11*(22), 3706–3732.
94. Dai, B., et al. (2009). Extracellular signal-regulated kinase positively regulates the oncogenic activity of MCT-1 in diffuse large B-cell lymphoma. *Cancer Research, 69*(19), 7835–7843.
95. Kinoshita, T., et al. (2016). Identification of allosteric ERK2 inhibitors through in silico biased screening and competitive binding assay. *Bioorganic & Medicinal Chemistry Letters, 26*(3), 955–958.
96. Sammons, R. M., et al. (2019). A novel class of common docking domain inhibitors that prevent ERK2 activation and substrate phosphorylation. *ACS Chemical Biology, 14*(6), 1183–1194.
97. Kaoud, T. S., et al. (2019). Modulating multi-functional ERK complexes by covalent targeting of a recruitment site in vivo. *Nature Communications, 10*(1), 5232.

98. Stebbins, J. L., et al. (2008). Identification of a new JNK inhibitor targeting the JNK-JIP interaction site. *Proceedings of the National Academy of Sciences of the United States of America, 105*(43), 16809–16813.
99. Samadani, R., et al. (2015). Small-molecule inhibitors of ERK-mediated immediate early gene expression and proliferation of melanoma cells expressing mutated BRaf. *The Biochemical Journal, 467*(3), 425–438.
100. Miller, C. J., Muftuoglu, Y., & Turk, B. E. (2017). A high throughput assay to identify substrate-selective inhibitors of the ERK protein kinases. *Biochemical Pharmacology, 142*, 39–45.
101. Lee, S., et al. (2011). Examining docking interactions on ERK2 with modular peptide substrates. *Biochemistry, 50*(44), 9500–9510.
102. Herrero, A., et al. (2015). Small molecule inhibition of ERK dimerization prevents tumorigenesis by RAS-ERK pathway oncogenes. *Cancer Cell, 28*(2), 170–182.
103. Lidke, D. S., et al. (2010). ERK nuclear translocation is dimerization-independent but controlled by the rate of phosphorylation. *The Journal of Biological Chemistry, 285*(5), 3092–3102.
104. Kaoud, T. S., et al. (2011). Activated ERK2 is a monomer in vitro with or without divalent cations and when complexed to the cytoplasmic scaffold PEA-15. *Biochemistry, 50*(21), 4568–4578.
105. Burack, W. R., & Shaw, A. S. (2005). Live cell imaging of ERK and MEK: Simple binding equilibrium explains the regulated nucleocytoplasmic distribution of ERK. *The Journal of Biological Chemistry, 280*(5), 3832–3837.
106. Casar, B., Pinto, A., & Crespo, P. (2008). Essential role of ERK dimers in the activation of cytoplasmic but not nuclear substrates by ERK-scaffold complexes. *Molecular Cell, 31*(5), 708–721.
107. Francis, D. M., et al. (2011). Structural basis of p38alpha regulation by hematopoietic tyrosine phosphatase. *Nature Chemical Biology, 7*(12), 916–924.
108. Glatz, G., et al. (2013). Structural mechanism for the specific assembly and activation of the extracellular signal regulated kinase 5 (ERK5) module. *The Journal of Biological Chemistry, 288*(12), 8596–8609.
109. Breen, M. E., & Soellner, M. B. (2015). Small molecule substrate phosphorylation site inhibitors of protein kinases: Approaches and challenges. *ACS Chemical Biology, 10*(1), 175–189.
110. Knight, Z. A., & Shokat, K. M. (2005). Features of selective kinase inhibitors. *Chemistry & Biology, 12*(6), 621–637.
111. Liu, Q., et al. (2013). Developing irreversible inhibitors of the protein kinase cysteinome. *Chemistry & Biology, 20*(2), 146–159.
112. Ward, R. A., et al. (2015). Structure-guided design of highly selective and potent covalent inhibitors of ERK1/2. *Journal of Medicinal Chemistry, 58*(11), 4790–4801.
113. Browne, C. M., et al. (2019). A Chemoproteomic strategy for direct and proteome-wide covalent inhibitor target-site identification. *Journal of the American Chemical Society, 141*(1), 191–203.
114. Adler, V., et al. (2005). Functional interactions of Raf and MEK with Jun-N-terminal kinase (JNK) result in a positive feedback loop on the oncogenic Ras signaling pathway. *Biochemistry, 44*(32), 10784–10795.
115. Ritt, D. A., et al. (2016). Inhibition of Ras/Raf/MEK/ERK pathway signaling by a stress-induced phospho-regulatory circuit. *Molecular Cell, 64*(5), 875–887.
116. Jokinen, E., & Koivunen, J. P. (2015). MEK and PI3K inhibition in solid tumors: Rationale and evidence to date. *Therapeutic Advances in Medical Oncology, 7*(3), 170–180.
117. Fallahi-Sichani, M., et al. (2015). Systematic analysis of BRAF(V600E) melanomas reveals a role for JNK/c-Jun pathway in adaptive resistance to drug-induced apoptosis. *Molecular Systems Biology, 11*(3), 797.
118. Miura, H., et al. (2018). Cell-to-cell heterogeneity in p38-mediated cross-inhibition of JNK causes stochastic cell death. *Cell Reports, 24*(10), 2658–2668.

119. Gossage, L., & Eisen, T. (2010). Targeting multiple kinase pathways: A change in paradigm. *Clinical Cancer Research, 16*(7), 1973–1978.
120. Knight, Z. A., Lin, H., & Shokat, K. M. (2010). Targeting the cancer kinome through polypharmacology. *Nature Reviews Cancer, 10*(2), 130–137.
121. Rao, S., et al. (2019). A multitargeted probe-based strategy to identify signaling vulnerabilities in cancers. *The Journal of Biological Chemistry, 294*(21), 8664–8673.
122. Lechtenberg, B. C., et al. (2017). Structure-guided strategy for the development of potent bivalent ERK inhibitors. *ACS Medicinal Chemistry Letters, 8*(7), 726–731.
123. Gu, S., et al. (2018). PROTACs: An emerging targeting technique for protein degradation in drug discovery. *BioEssays, 40*(4), e1700247.
124. An, S., & Fu, L. (2018). Small-molecule PROTACs: An emerging and promising approach for the development of targeted therapy drugs. *eBioMedicine, 36*, 553–562.
125. Kornev, A. P., et al. (2006). Surface comparison of active and inactive protein kinases identifies a conserved activation mechanism. *Proceedings of the National Academy of Sciences of the United States of America, 103*(47), 17783–17788.
126. Gogl, G., Toro, I., & Remenyi, A. (2013). Protein-peptide complex crystallization: A case study on the ERK2 mitogen-activated protein kinase. *Acta Crystallographica Section D Biological Crystallography, 69*(Pt 3), 486–489.

Novel Stabilized Peptide Inhibitors of Protein Kinases

Leah G. Helton, Ameya J. Limaye, George N. Bendzunas, and Eileen J. Kennedy

Abstract Protein kinases are critical components of diverse signaling pathways. While all kinases share a conserved kinase domain, there is considerable diversity among kinases within the additional flanking domains and sequences that may regulate processes such as catalytic function, substrate phosphorylation, or serve as regulatory domains. These other domains are often evolutionarily divergent across the kinase superfamily and provide unique handles for selective targeting of a kinase of interest. As an alternative to small-molecule inhibitors for kinases, this chapter focuses on the development of constrained peptide scaffolds that target allosteric regulatory mechanisms or spatiotemporal kinase regulation. Constrained peptides can have many advantages over nonmodified peptides including increased proteolytic stability and improved permeation into cells. In contrast to small molecules, peptides also provide elongated surfaces that can bind shallow, hydrophobic regions on proteins and can be strategically applied to inhibit protein-protein interactions. Several examples of constrained peptide inhibitors are discussed in this section and their limitations and opportunities within this inhibitor class.

Keywords Constrained peptide · Stapled peptide · EGFR · PKA · AKAP disruptor · PKI · cAMP

Leah G. Helton, Ameya J. Limaye, and George N. Bendzunas contributed equally.

L. G. Helton · A. J. Limaye · G. N. Bendzunas · E. J. Kennedy (✉)
Department of Pharmaceutical and Biomedical Sciences, University of Georgia, College of Pharmacy, Augusta, GA, USA
e-mail: ekennedy@uga.edu

P. Shapiro (ed.), *Next Generation Kinase Inhibitors*,
https://doi.org/10.1007/978-3-030-48283-1_7

Introduction

Protein kinases play an essential role in cellular signal transduction. The specificity of signaling pathways demonstrates that kinases have evolved divergent substrate recognition capabilities all the while, in most cases at least, conserving the activity of their catalytic domain. The ability of these proteins to receive diverse regulatory inputs and convey information to specific appropriate substrates using the common core function of phosphorylation is the result of an intricate balancing act. The requirement to balance conservation of activity and plasticity defines an axis which determines catalytic activity, substrate specificity, and regulatory interactions.

As a strategy for selective kinase inhibition, allosteric disruption of protein kinases may offer a more selective form of regulation by targeting unique regions or surfaces that are imperative for overall kinase function. Protein-protein interaction (PPI) surfaces, whether intramolecular or intermolecular, often require relatively large, shallow, and hydrophobic surfaces that are particularly well suited for peptide targeting. However, native peptides are inherently susceptible to various processes including proteolytic cleavage, lack of solubility, and loss of the secondary structural fold that may be required for PPIs [1]. In order to circumvent the issues seen with native peptides, constrained peptides were developed to "lock" the peptide in a favorable conformation and embed the backbone, which makes the peptide resistant to proteolytic cleavage (Fig. 1) [2]. In addition, various chemical modifications can be made in order to improve the hydrophilicity, specificity, and biological relevance of the compound [3].

One synthetic strategy for constraining peptides is hydrocarbon stapling [4]. In this approach, nonnatural olefinic amino acids are incorporated into a peptide sequence of interest during solid-phase synthesis, and the olefinic side chains are subsequently joined together to form an all-hydrocarbon staple using ring-closing metathesis chemistry. In the case of peptide helices, the secondary structural fold of the helix can be synthetically reinforced by incorporation of a staple by positioning the olefinic amino acids around one or two helical turns (Fig. 1). Hydrocarbon-stapled peptides possess the potential to have multiple favorable properties includ-

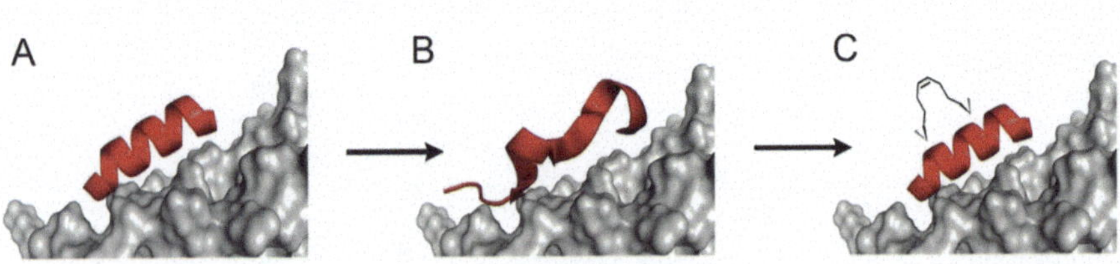

Fig. 1 Targeting protein-protein interactions (PPIs) with constrained peptides. (**a**) PPI interfaces often involve secondary structural elements such as alpha-helices or beta-sheets that mediate and stabilize the protein complex. (**b**) Peptide mimics of a PPI interface that are modified may be subject to loss of its secondary structural fold and, therefore, have a reduced affinity for its target interface. (**c**) Chemical modifications can be introduced into the peptide sequence to reinforce the secondary structure and, thereby, improve the biological inhibitory activity of the peptide as a strategy for PPI disruption

ing reinforced helical conformation, resistance to proteolytic degradation, and enhanced cell permeability through an active transport mechanism [1, 5]. Stapled peptides have been designed to engage a wide variety of targets to disrupt a PPI of interest. In this chapter, multiple examples of constrained peptides, including hydrocarbon-stapled peptides, will be discussed that specifically disrupt allosteric or spatiotemporal regulation of diverse kinases.

Targeting Receptor Tyrosine Kinase Dimerization with Stapled Peptides

Oligomerization and stable and transient interactions are common mechanisms of kinase regulation and play a crucial role in a diverse set of signaling pathways. In the case of receptor tyrosine kinases (RTKs), the activation mechanism is usually dependent on dimerization of either the extracellular receptor or intracellular kinase domain [6, 7]. Although numerous small-molecule inhibitors have targeted RTKs, mostly through ATP-competitive inhibition, drug resistance remains a major problem partly due to the complex mechanism of RTK activation [8, 9]. However, due to the extensive interfaces involved in RTK dimerization, these surfaces can be exploited for allosteric kinase inhibition.

Targeting the Extracellular Region of EGFR with Constrained Peptides

One example of a kinase that is regulated via dimerization is the epidermal growth factor receptor (EGFR/HER1/ErbB1). EGFR is a transmembrane receptor composed of an ectodomain, a transmembrane region, a juxtamembrane region, and an intracellular tyrosine kinase domain. Upon binding of an extracellular growth factor, EGFR may homodimerize or heterodimerize with other Erb family receptors to elicit its role in cell proliferation and differentiation (Fig. 2) [10, 11]. EGFR, and fellow ErbB family proteins HER2, HER3, and HER4, are commonly mutated in a variety of cancers, and, therefore, a significant amount of research has focused on developing therapeutics to inhibit these receptors and the downstream signaling pathways [12–14]. While the majority of EGFR inhibitors target either the growth factor binding site or the active site of EGFR, one can additionally take advantage of the wide variety of protein surfaces involved in ErbB dimerization for targeted inhibition.

Dimerization of EGFR plays a crucial role in regulating EGFR activation, and there are multiple mechanisms by which allosteric inhibition of dimerization could be targeted: inhibition of ectodomain oligomerization, inhibition of dimerization arm interactions, inhibition of coiled coil juxtamembrane formation, and inhibition

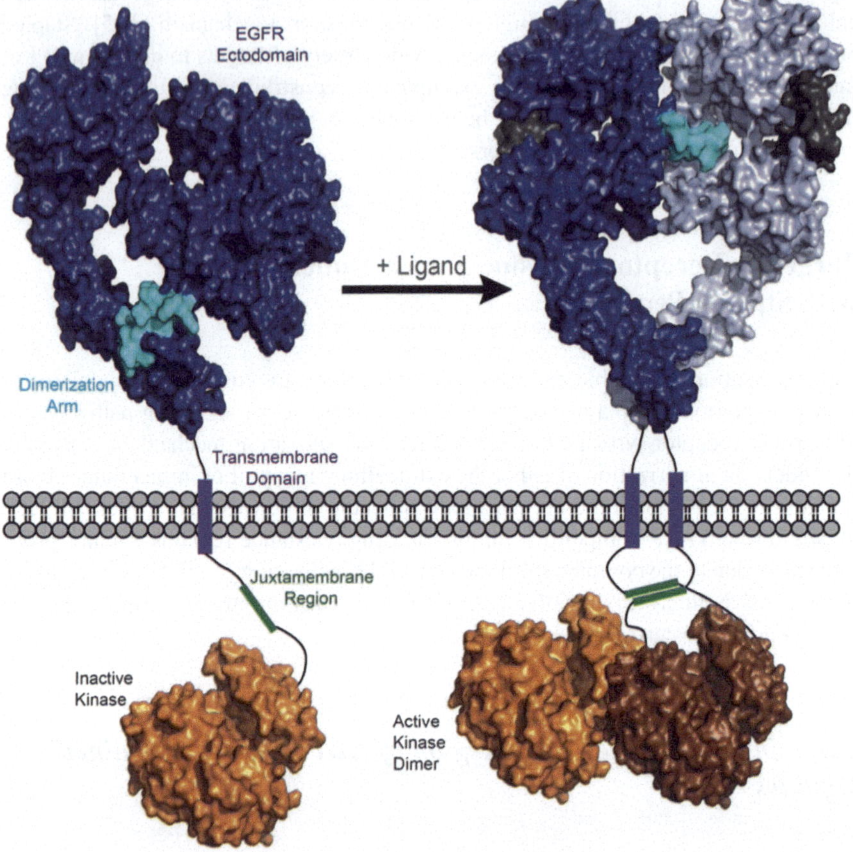

Fig. 2 Schematic of EGFR dimerization and activation. The EGFR ectodomain is composed of four domains that undergo a distinct conformational change upon ligand binding, thereby allowing the dimerization arms (cyan) to interact with and stabilize the receptor dimer. The intracellular kinase domains also undergo a conformational change to form an asymmetric dimer that is stabilized by the coiled coil arrangement of the juxtamembrane dimer. (PDB IDs: 2GS6, 3NJP, and 1NQL)

of asymmetric kinase dimerization (Fig. 3). Allosteric inhibition of EGFR kinase activity via receptor oligomerization had not been successfully targeted with small-molecule inhibitors [15], thereby leaving a gap in drug development that peptide therapeutics may be well-suited to fill.

Homodimerization of EGFR is mediated by a "dimerization arm" that undergoes a substantial conformational change upon binding to an extracellular ligand [16, 17]. The conformational change promotes dimerization and subsequent activation of the intracellular kinase domain. One strategy of targeting EGFR dimerization focuses on disrupting the "dimerization arm" beta loop structure that is essential for stabilizing the EGFR homo or heterodimer (Fig. 2). Various mimics of the dimeriza-

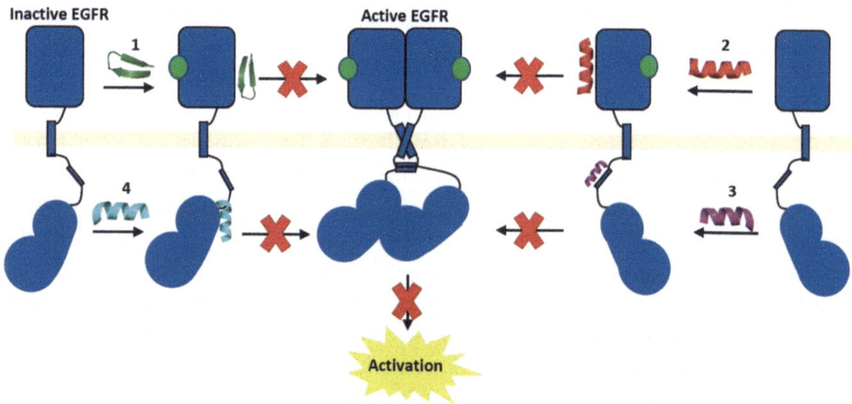

Fig. 3 Allosteric disruption of RTK dimerization and activation. (**1**) Beta-loop peptide macrocycle mimics of the dimerization arm structure, (**2**) disruption of ectodomain interactions essential for homo- or heterodimerization as strategies to block ectodomain dimerization. (**3**) All-hydrocarbon-stapled peptides targeting the coiled coil juxtamembrane region prevent formation and stabilization of the kinase dimer. (**4**) Direct targeting of the asymmetric kinase dimer interface as an approach for allosteric kinase inhibition

tion arm have been developed that contain additional synthetic constraints to structurally reinforce the beta-turn conformer including the introduction of a cross-strand disulfide bridge, a selenylsulfide bridge, or a triazolyl bridge [18–21]. These peptide-based dimerization arm mimics were shown to have inhibitory effects on EGFR dimerization and activation. A major shortcoming of these particular chemistries is that, although the chemical constraint introduced into the peptide sequence helped reinforce the structural shape of the peptide to effectively bind its target, none of these modifications were found to enhance cell permeation of the dimerization arm mimics. While this physical property is not detrimental for extracellular targets such as the ectodomain of RTKs, other chemistries may need to be employed for targeting intracellular targets.

Targeting the Intracellular Region of EGFR with Stapled Peptides

An example of peptides targeting intracellular targets is the development of constrained alpha-helical peptides targeting the intracellular juxtamembrane region of EGFR. The juxtamembrane region forms a coiled coil dimer in order to assemble and stabilize the asymmetric kinase domain dimer [22]. Peptides were designed to mimic and inhibit the coiled coil interactions to allosterically disrupt EGFR activation [23]. The alpha-helical conformer was structurally reinforced through introduction of all-hydrocarbon staples that were shown to enhance cell permeation. The lead peptide in this study effectively disrupted EGFR dimerization and inhibited cell proliferation when treating cells with a micromolar range dosing [23].

Another intracellular target of EGFR is the asymmetric kinase dimer interface that is a requisite for dimerization-mediated kinase activation [24]. In this case, the N-lobe of one kinase domain interacts directly with the C-lobe of the other kinase domain, and this interaction is primarily mediated by several alpha-helices. As a strategy to allosterically inhibit EGFR activation, hydrocarbon-stapled peptides were developed to mimic the H-helix derived from the C-lobe of the kinase domain, thereby occluding kinase dimer formation and activation [25]. Sequences were optimized using in silico strategies to improve the efficacy of the compounds to approximate IC50 values of 5–10 μM. These cell-permeable peptide inhibitors were found to inhibit EGFR activation and downstream AKT activation. In addition, the lead compound from this study also caused a fortuitous reduction in EGFR protein expression levels in cells through an unknown mechanism [25].

Overall, EGFR has served as an archetype model of RTKs for targeted allosteric inhibition using peptide inhibitors due to the fact that EGFR has been extensively characterized both structurally and biochemically, and numerous PPIs have been identified as critical components of its activation mechanism. While a basis for proof-of-concept work has been completed, further development and optimization of these allosteric inhibitors may lead to a therapeutic with clinical success. Since they target discrete surfaces distal to the ATP-binding site, they may additionally fill a niche by serving as a second-line therapy after drug resistance mutations arise in patients. While EGFR highlights the diverse strategies that can be applied for therapeutic intervention using constrained peptides, these mechanisms can be translated to a variety of receptor tyrosine kinases and intracellular protein kinases that are critically regulated by PPIs.

RTKs as Peptide Inhibitor Targets

RTKs are commonly mutated or overexpressed in a multitude of cancers and diseases, and the current FDA-approved therapeutics are predominantly small-molecule inhibitors and a rapidly expanding class of antibody-based therapeutics [26]. The conserved ATP-binding pocket of tyrosine kinases makes specificity a challenging goal for small-molecule inhibitors, and off-target effects are of significant clinical concern [27]. Monoclonal antibodies are emerging as an alternative targeting mechanism since they are designed to complement a relatively large surface area of the protein, thereby enhancing target selectivity. A major drawback of antibody therapies is their inability to access the intracellular space, thereby reducing them to RTK targets in the case of the kinase superfamily. In addition, resistance has been found to be largely inevitable with both small-molecule and antibody-based therapeutics, thereby prompting the need for alternative therapeutics with unique targeting sites. By disrupting specific PPIs with evolutionarily divergent surfaces that are involved in RTK regulation, peptide therapeutics may serve to bridge the gap between small molecules and antibodies by providing a relatively large binding surface area that can target shallow pockets or patches while also having the potential to permeate cells. The increased potential by constrained peptides to target unique PPIs opens the door to entirely unique strategies for regulating signaling pathways within the cell.

Disruption of Spatiotemporal Regulation of Kinases with Stapled Peptides

Another indirect strategy for kinase inhibition involves disruption of spatial and temporal regulation for a given kinase. Where a kinase resides in the cell at any given time will greatly influence its cellular activity by limiting access to potential interactors within its localized environment including substrates and other interacting proteins. Thus, formation of highly organized molecular complexes is critical in determining the precise timing and location of signal transduction events that occur in response to secondary messengers [28]. One family of scaffold proteins known to exert such spatiotemporal control over cellular enzymes is A kinase anchoring proteins (AKAPs).

A Kinase Anchoring Proteins (AKAPs)

AKAPs share the common feature of docking protein kinase A (PKA) and serve as platforms to coordinate phosphorylation-dephosphorylation events by scaffolding protein kinases and phosphatases along with their appropriate substrates [29]. AKAPs also form multiprotein assemblies that are localized to specific subcellular locations, thereby orienting the scaffolded signaling enzymes to their distinct substrates. In consequence, AKAP-mediated microsignaling complexes are important spatiotemporal regulators of PKA-mediated signaling [28, 29].

Initial clues for the compartmentalization of protein kinases came from early experiments with cyclic adenosine monophosphate (cAMP) signaling during the late 1970s. cAMP was previously identified as an activator of protein kinase A (PKA) [30]. PKA is a hetero-tetrameric holoenzyme complex that is composed of two regulatory (R) subunits that bind and inhibit two catalytic (C) subunits. Following extracellular stimuli such as activation of G-protein coupled receptors (GPCRs), activated adenylate cyclase (AC) synthesizes cAMP that then binds to R subunits of PKA, releasing catalytically active C subunits [31]. Although it was previously hypothesized that cAMP was diffused throughout the cell, it was later shown in cardiac tissue that while both prostaglandin E_1 and epinephrine could increase intracellular cAMP levels, only epinephrine stimulation led to an increase in glycogen phosphorylase activity and contraction [32, 33], thereby demonstrating that specific subcellular sites for cAMP accumulation existed to result in PKA activation [29, 30].

Parallel research also revealed two distinct forms of PKA: cytoplasmic type I PKA and particulate type II PKA, hinting at a differential regulation of PKA activation through distinct intracellular compartments [34]. Subsequently, microtubule-associated protein, MAP 2, was the first example shown to anchor PKA to microtubules through interactions with the regulatory domain of PKA [29]. Further experimentation using PKA RII probes to perform protein-protein blotting allowed for the discovery of several more PKA anchoring proteins that were ultimately classified under the family of A kinase anchoring proteins (AKAPs) [29, 30]. At present, over 30 mammalian AKAPs have been reported and experimentally verified [35].

Anchoring of PKA only denotes one aspect of AKAP family's scaffolding functions. AKAPs form multivalent protein assemblies with other signaling enzymes to integrate multiple second messenger signaling cascades along with their feedback loops and localize these signaling events to specific intracellular sites [29, 36]. Some notable examples of cellular proteins scaffolded by AKAPs to distinct subcellular locations are adenylate cyclase (AC), protein kinase C (PKC), protein phosphatase 1, 2A and 2B (PP1, PP2A, PP2B), calcineurin (CaN), phosphodiesterase 4D3 and 3A (PDE4D3, PDE3A), L-type calcium ion channels, actin cytoskeleton, and tubulin [37–39]. Vastly different cellular responses can be elicited from AKAP complexes based upon which other proteins are present in an AKAP complex at any given time.

Functional Aspects of AKAP Complexes

An important function of AKAP-mediated protein scaffolding and complex formation is achieving signaling specificity. Balancing substrate phosphorylation and dephosphorylation provides an elegant manner for modulation of a cellular response. Indeed, AKAPs have been shown to localize with GPCRs and scaffold various proteins including AC, PDE, and PKA. In a typical PKA signaling event, hormone binding to the GPCR is followed by the activation of GαS subunit, stimulation of AC activity, and subsequent cAMP synthesis [40]. In turn, cAMP binds and activates PKA that catalyzes phosphorylation of downstream substrates while unbound cAMP is hydrolyzed to adenosine monophosphate (AMP) by PDE. This confines synthesis, function, and degradation of cAMP to a localized scaffold and greatly improves signaling efficiency [37, 41].

An example of this is AKAP5/79/150. One of the best-studied AKAPs, it was shown to orchestrate Ca^{2+}-dependent signaling events in postsynaptic neurons by scaffolding PKC, protein phosphatase 2B (PP2B), and calmodulin (CaM) while tethered to the glutamate receptor ion channels (AMPA receptor). Increased neuronal Ca^{2+} levels were found to increase Ca^{2+}/CaM binding to AKAP79 while disengaging inhibited PKC from the scaffold. Increased Ca^{2+}/CaM interaction with AKAP79 was also critical for the activation of complexed PP2B. Formation of such a complex provides for the generation of localized pools of second messenger responsive enzymes at localized points within the cell [42, 43].

While RI-selective AKAP complexes are considered to be primarily localized to the cytoplasm, RII-selective AKAPs are predominantly membrane-associated through diverse mechanisms. Some AKAPs may be modified to promote membrane interactions though the addition of myristoyl or palmitoyl moieties, including AKAP12 and AKAP18 [44]. AKAP12 (Gravin) is known to scaffold PKC and PKA to the cellular cytoskeleton; however, its subcellular distribution is dynamically regulated as it is determined by activation of PKC and CaM binding [44–46]. AKAP350 predominantly localizes at the centrosome and scaffolds a mecca of signaling enzymes such as PKA, PKN (Protein Kinase N1), PP1, and PP2A [44, 47]. Research has also found AKAP350 in the Golgi area at different stages of the cell cycle, implicating its scaffolding functions in directing PKA to specific compartmentalized substrates during cell division [47, 48]. Apart from these specific examples, AKAP complexes play a critical role in regulating precisely timed signaling events that impact a wide range of cellular functions including cytoskeletal dynamics, cell cycle progression, channel regulation, and apoptosis along with physiological functions such as memory formation, sperm motility, T-cell activation, and cardiac function [38, 44, 48, 49]. As such, they are critical regulators of specific PKA signaling events and may serve as an effective, indirect strategy for targeted disruption of altered AKAP-mediated PKA signaling in disease states.

Targeting AKAP Complexes

Given the extent of scaffolding and spatiotemporal control exerted by AKAPs on cellular functions, AKAP complexes have long been considered viable targets for disease intervention [38, 39, 44]. The majority of this work has focused on targeting PKA RI and RII domains and their anchoring by AKAPs, primarily due to the availability of high-resolution crystal structures, well-defined binding motifs, and conserved PKA-binding domain across multiple AKAPs [44].

Targeting PKA RII Anchoring by AKAPs

Early work was focused on identifying the binding sites on the RII domain of PKA that were required for its interactions with AKAPs. These studies identified the first 30 amino acid residues of PKA RII to be essential for AKAP interaction (docking/dimerization (D/D) domain), and RII dimerization was considered a prerequisite for anchoring by forming a binding groove at the D/D dimer interface [50–52]. Deletion studies performed on the reciprocal binding surfaces of multiple AKAPs revealed common helical regions essential for their anchoring interaction with PKA RII [30]. This led to the current understanding whereby AKAPs at least partly interact with PKA regulatory subunits via an amphipathic helical binding sequence [29, 30].

Ht-31, derived from the helical binding sequence of the RII-selective AKAP, AKAP-Lbc, was one of the first peptide disruptors aimed at AKAP-RII PKA interaction [53]. A stearated version of this peptide was subsequently developed to improve its cell permeability [54]. Several other peptide disruptors were also modelled after other AKAPs including TAT-AKAD and AKAP-IS [44]. Although these peptides have served as useful tools in understanding the functional aspects of AKAP-PKA scaffolding and PKA regulation, they have notable drawbacks such as poor cell permeability, loss of secondary structure in solution, and potential for proteolysis [55].

As a strategy to overcome some of these shortcomings, AKAP disruptors were later developed that incorporated an all-hydrocarbon staple to reinforce the secondary structure of the alpha-helical peptide [56]. Multiple peptides were designed based on the anchoring helix derived from several AKAPs. While most AKAP anchoring helices are relatively hydrophobic, three sequences were chosen for library design that were intrinsically more hydrophilic since the hydrocarbon staple notably increases hydrophobicity of the overall compound: RI-anchoring disruptor (RIAD), AKAP220, and small-membrane AKAP (smAKAP). From this library screen, a stapled peptide analog of the binding helix derived from AKAP220, STAD-2, was found to permeate cells, have up to 40-fold selectivity for PKA RII over PKA RI with a K_D value in the low nanomolar range, and could inhibit AKAP-PKA RII scaffolded interactions and signaling in cells [56, 57] and, thereby, serves as a cell-permeable tool for perturbing spatial and temporal regulation of PKA (Fig. 4).

Targeting PKA RI Anchoring by AKAPs

While the PKA RII isoform has been shown to bind AKAPs in the low nanomolar range, PKA RI is generally considered to have weaker interactions with AKAPs in the high nanomolar to low micromolar range [58]. Notably, some PKA RI-selective AKAPs bind in the low nanomolar affinity with the RI isoform [58–60]. Due to its

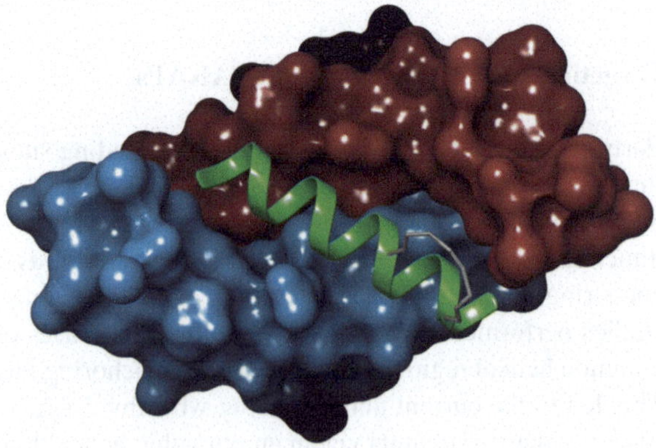

Fig. 4 Stapled AKAP inhibitor bound to PKA RII. Schematic representation of STAD-2 peptide (in green) bound to the docking/dimerization domains of PKA RII (in blue and red). STAD-2 mimics and occludes the helical binding interaction of AKAPs with PKA RII

site-specific localization, PKA RII is also markedly distinct from PKA RI, which is mostly cytosolic while PKA RII is associated with cytoskeletal elements and intracellular cellular organelles [61]. In addition, structural analysis of the D/D domains on RI and RII revealed certain critical differences between their engagement with AKAP-docking helices. The D/D domain of PKA RI forms a shallow, hydrophobic patch that interacts with two helical turns of an AKAP helix. On the contrary, the D/D domain of PKA RII forms a markedly deeper cleft that engages with the AKAP helix over four helical turns [62, 63].

Due in part to the lack of a clear consensus sequence for RI-specific AKAP binding, a limited number of RI-specific peptide disruptors have been developed [64]. The first RI-selective AKAP inhibitor peptide was identified from a peptide array library derived from the dual-selective AKAP, D-AKAP2 [65]. This peptide, PV-38, was found to have selectivity for the RI-isoform with a KD value of 5 nM while binding the RII-isoform in the high nanomolar range and, when transfected in cells, could disrupt PKA RI-AKAP interactions [65]. Subsequently, another RI-selective peptide disruptor, termed RI-anchoring disruptor (RIAD), was designed using a bioinformatics approach [66]. Although RIAD was shown to over 1000-fold selectivity for PKA RI over the PKA RII isoform, it also did not readily permeate cells. Subsequently, a cell-permeable hydrocarbon-stapled analog of RIAD, termed RI-STAD-2, was developed [67]. This peptide disruptor was shown to be RI-selective with single nanomolar affinity toward PKA RI and could disrupt interactions between PKA RI and AKAPs within cells.

Targeting AKAP Complexes Beyond PKA Interactions

Although AKAPs were initially characterized as having the commonality of docking PKA, AKAPs are now understood to scaffold a variety of diverse proteins. Their ability to scaffold and localize multiple signaling enzymes, organelles, and receptors while orchestrating tightly controlled signaling events warrants deeper investigation. Currently, the only available tools to dissect these complexes include various peptides described above that uncouple PKA anchoring to the AKAP complexes. A major shortcoming of this approach is that most cells typically express between 10 and 15 AKAPs at any given time [39], and, thus, an individual AKAP of interest cannot be selectively targeted using this approach.

As an alternative approach, one could envision targeting the PPI mediated by a protein that only binds a small subset of AKAPs. One example of this is PKC. PKC, a major cellular kinase known for controlling a plethora of signaling cascades and diverse cellular processes, has been shown to directly interact with only a handful of AKAPs including AKAP12, APAP79, AKAP1, AKAP7, AKAP9, AKAP13, and Ezrin [39]. Its interaction with discrete signaling complexes results in various cellular effects such as altered actin cytoskeleton dynamics and suppression of cell migration and invasiveness when bound to AKAP12 [46, 68] and altered neuronal plasticity when bound to AKAP79 [42, 43]. Targeting AKAP-mediated PKC scaffolding may provide invaluable information on the various roles of PKC signaling via AKAP complexes, the role of localized pools of calcium on PKC activity, and how different PKC isoforms may be differentially compartmentalized and regulated. As more biochemical and structural information of PPI interfaces involving AKAPs becomes available, further peptide-based disruptors can be developed to selectively target an AKAP of interest. Overall, selective disruption of AKAP complex formation by inhibiting the docking of one or more kinases provides a route for altering and evaluating the effects and significance of the individual components of an AKAP signaling complex on localized signaling. Further, such probes can additionally provide a route to improve our understanding of the potential allosteric effects of AKAPs on their partner kinases.

Pseudosubstrate Inhibition of Kinases with Stabilized Peptides

Another strategy for allosteric kinase inhibition is through targeting sites within the kinase domain that are distal to the ATP-binding pocket that ultimately affect catalysis. The ability of kinases to receive diverse regulatory inputs and convey signals to various substrates via a phosphorylation mechanism is the result of an intricate balancing act. Kinases have to harmonize multiple facets including catalytic activity, substrate specificity, and regulatory interactions, and this is achieved through both plasticity and conservation. The specificity of signaling pathways demonstrates that kinases have evolved divergent substrate recognition capabilities while maintaining conservation of the active site. Additionally, some kinases, including PKA, PKC, and PKG, have a pseudosubstrate binding domain within the C-lobe of the kinase domain, which acts as an additional regulatory mechanism [69, 70].

Kinase Pseudosubstrate Interactions

In the case of PKA, substrates and pseudosubstrates interact with the kinase in overlapping regions within an extended groove located across the face of the C-lobe between the D and G helices [71] (Fig. 5a). This region contains the majority of contact points responsible for determining substrate specificity between protein kinases. While every kinase has substrate recognition motifs that engage the substrate-binding groove, many kinases can actually recognize a family of related sequences with a range of affinities. This spectrum of substrate affinity may be important in the dynamics of signal transduction by influencing the order of substrate phosphorylation events within the cell [72]. Further, the binding of pseudosubstrates within the substrate-binding region can result in partial steric occlusion of the substrate-binding groove, thereby inhibiting kinase activity through an allosteric mechanism [73].

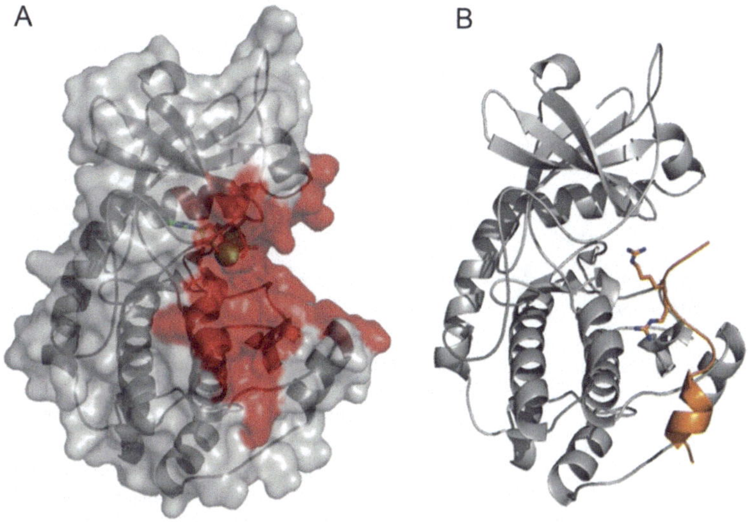

Fig. 5 The interface between PKA and a PKI-derived peptide. (**a**) The substrate binding groove on PKA (red) extends across the region between the C-lobe and N-lobe between the D and G helices. (**b**) PKI (5–24, shown in orange) serves as a pseudosubstrate by partly occupying the substrate binding groove to prevent catalytic activity. The side chains of arginine residues 18 and 19 are shown and are required for high-affinity binding (PDB 1ATP)

The pseudosubstrate region may be encoded within the full-length kinase such as on the regulatory domain of PKC [74] or on the C-terminal tail of myosin light chain kinase [75]. Alternatively, the pseudosubstrate region may be located on a separate protein. Examples include the R-subunits of PKA and the endogenous cAMP-dependent protein kinase inhibitor (PKI) [76]. As a strategy for allosteric inhibition of PKA, PKI was extensively explored.

Protein Kinase Inhibitor (PKI) as a Pseudosubstrate

PKI was discovered in the early 1970s as a non-ATP-competitive, heat-stable inhibitor of PKA [76]. This small, 11 kDa protein has two known functional regions: a nuclear export sequence (NES) to transport PKA out of the nucleus and a high-affinity pseudosubstrate region that inhibits the catalytic function of PKA (Fig. 6a) [77]. It is both a selective and potent inhibitor of PKA kinase activity with a K_i of 2 nM [78]. Through analysis of multiple truncations of PKI, it was discovered that only a short stretch of residues of PKI was required for inhibition (residues 5–24) and a peptide mimicking this region was found to have both potency and selectivity comparable to that of the full-length protein (Fig. 6b) [79–81]. This peptide representing PKI (5–24) has been termed IP20. Within this peptide there exists a sequence that resembles the consensus substrate sequence that is phosphorylated by PKA. The

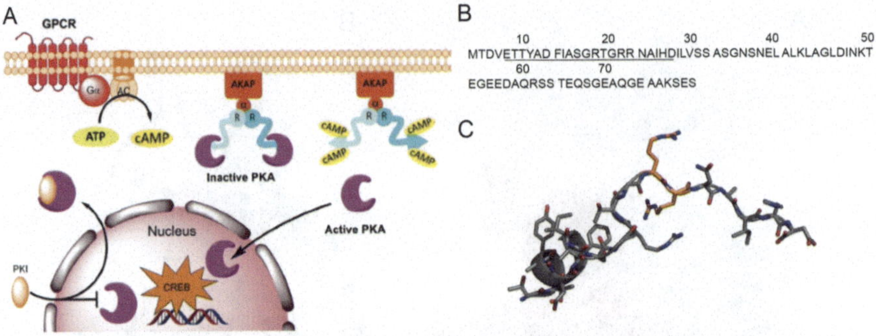

Fig. 6 PKI as a pseudosubstrate inhibitor of PKA. (**a**) PKI directly interacts with PKA and serves as both a pseudosubstrate inhibitor and a nuclear export transporter for PKA. (**b**) PKI is a small, 11 kDa protein. The sequence of PKI is shown, and the residues that comprise the IP20 peptide are underlined. (**c**) The IP20 peptide adopts a partially helical structure upon binding to PKA; this helical portion provided a location for the incorporation of an all-hydrocarbon staple. The C-terminus of the peptide must adopt a highly specific orientation for the arginine residues to interact properly (PDB 1ATP)

peptide contains the pseudosubstrate sequence Arg–Arg–X–S*–Y, where X represents a small residue, S* represents the phosphoacceptor residue that is replaced by a nonphosphorylatable residue as the pseudosubstrate, and Y represents a large hydrophobic residue [69]. The two arginine residues (residues R18 and R19 in PKI) are critical for the high-affinity binding of the peptide where glycine substitutions at these positions decrease the inhibitory potential of the peptide up to 500-fold [81] (Fig. 6c). Although this consensus sequence results in optimal binding, there is considerable variability among PKA substrates with only one third containing this sequence in its entirety [72]. This optimal consensus sequence results not only in high-affinity binding interactions with PKA but also high selectivity. IP20 was tested against multiple, diverse kinases including phosphorylase kinase, skeletal muscle myosin light chain kinase, PKC, casein kinase II, and cGMP-dependent protein kinase (PKG) and demonstrates no inhibition of these kinases in in vitro assays even when the peptide was tested at millimolar concentrations [79].

Stapled PKI Mimics as Pseudosubstrates for PKA

Although IP20 has been used for many years as an investigational tool, it has several drawbacks that are commonly seen in naturally occurring peptides including a lack of cell penetration and susceptibility to proteolytic cleavage. Cell permeation of IP20 can be enhanced via modifications such as myristoylation [69]; however, the hydrophobic nature of the myristoyl moiety may contribute to mislocalization by promoting membrane interactions/embedding and, thus, may limit its ability to interact with PKA at various subcellular locations. Additionally, attempts to improve the proteolytic stability of the IP20 peptide have been made though incorporation of D-stereoisomeric form of arginine in position 18 and protection of the C-terminal aspartate side chain with a cyclohexyl ester group [82]. Although this did increase the half-life of the peptide, it did not address cell permeability, and, consequently, this peptide still required microinjection dosing. The issues of cell permeation and stability were subsequently addressed via the addition of an all-hydrocarbon staple. Using this technique, a pseudosubstrate inhibitor of PKA was created that shared many of the favorable properties of IP20 but which could additionally accumulate within the cytosol [83].

Initial attempts to create a hydrocarbon-stapled version of IP20 introduced the staple into a helical portion located on the N-terminus (Fig. 6c). Unfortunately, this resulted in an approximately seven-fold loss in affinity for PKA-C as compared to the nonmodified parent peptide [83]. This reduction in affinity may reflect a ramification of nucleated helicity induced by the staple into less-structured regions of the peptide that have been shown to be required for high biological potency [84]. However, Scott et al. had previously established that extending the peptide by four residues toward the N-terminus resulted in a 24-residue peptide with a binding affinity that was comparable to IP20 [81]. These four additional residues provided space for the staple to be shifted closer to the N-terminus and, upon evaluation, it was discovered that these stapled IP24 analogs bound with comparable affinities to their nonstapled counterparts with K_D values in the 500–600 picomolar range [83]. To date, this stapled peptide has the highest reported target affinity among all published hydrocarbon-stapled peptides, largely owing to the naturally high-affinity interaction between PKA and the pseudosubstrate sequence of PKI. Further characterization to determine the inhibitory potential found that in vitro K_i values ranged from 25 to 35 nM. Additionally, the stapled version of the peptide was found to readily permeate cells, localize within the cytoplasm, and inhibit PKA substrate phosphorylation in a dose-dependent manner [83].

Targeting Other Kinases with Pseudosubstrates

Considering the success of the approach to develop a hydrocarbon-stapled pseudosubstrate inhibitor of PKA, it lays the foundation for designing other constrained pseudosubstrate inhibitor peptides as a strategy for high target selectivity. Table 1 shows pseudosubstrate sequences that have been identified for a number of protein kinases. Peptides based on these autoinhibitory pseudosubstrate sequences have been developed for many of the kinases listed; however, they suffer the same short comings of the original IP20 peptides, namely an inability to permeate cells.

One of the first crystal structures of an autoinhibited protein kinase was the myosin light chain kinase (MLCK) family member twitchin [75]. The autoinhibitory sequence is located within a 60 residue C-terminal tail [85], similar to Ca^{2+}/calmodulin-dependent protein kinases (CaMKII) and MLCK members [73]. In the autoinhibited state of these kinases, the C-terminal tail extends over the sur-

Table 1 Examples of pseudosubstrate sequences identified for diverse kinases

Protein kinase		Sequence	Refs.
PKA			
RI	(88–107)	VVKGRRRRGAISAEVYTEED	[89]
PKI	(5–24)	TTYADFIASGRTGRRNAIHD	[80]
PKC			
α	(15–31)	DVANRFARKGALRQKNV	[90]
β I and II	(15–31)	ESTVRFARKGALRQKNV	[91]
γ	(14–30)	GPRPLFCRKGALRQKVV	[92]
ε	(149–165)	ERMRPRKRQGAVRRRVH	[93]
δ	(137–153)	AMFPTMNRRGAIKQAKI	[94]
ζ	(109–125)	EKAESIYRRGARRWRKL	[94]
PKG			
α	(54–67)	GPRTTRAQGISAEP	[95]
β	(70–83)	GEPRTKRQAISAEP	[96]
Cam-II PK			
α	(280–307)	CMHRQETVDCLKKFNARRKLKGAILTTM	[97]
β	(281–308)	MMHRQETVECLKKFNARRKLKGAILTTM	[98]
γ	(281–308)	MMHRQETVECLKKFNARRKLKGAILTTM	[99]
δ	(281–308)	MMHRQETVDCLKKFNARRKLKGAILTTM	[100]
Myosin light chain kinase			
Smooth muscle	(787–810)	SKDRMKKYMARRKWQKTGHAVRAI	[101]
Skeletal muscle	(570–593)	RLLKKYLMKRRWKKNFIAVSAA	[102]
Twitchin	(5421–5443)	SRYTKIRDSIKTKYDAWPEPLPP	[75]

face of the cleft between the two lobes of the kinase domain and makes extensive contacts with both the substrate-binding site and the ATP-binding pocket. Calmodulin binding to a portion of this pseudosubstrate region results in a conformational change that removes the autoinhibitory sequence from the binding site [86]. A 22-residue peptide based on the pseudosubstrate region was shown to inhibit MLCK activity with a K_i of 46 nM [87]. However, since this MLCK pseudosubstrate peptide sequence overlaps with the calmodulin-binding region, it acted as both a calmodulin and MLCK antagonist. This overlap resulted in undesired inhibition of CaMKII. Further screening of peptide libraries with related sequences resulted in the identification of "Peptide 18" that had an IC_{50} of 50 nM for MLCK and only inhibits CaMKII at a 4000-fold greater concentration [88].

As with MLCK, CaMKII possesses an auto inhibitory sequence in its C-terminus tail that wraps around and interacts with its substrate-binding region and ATP-binding pocket [103]. This region also binds calmodulin, thereby allowing for the regulation of kinase activity. Peptide inhibitors of CaMKII derived from the sequence between positions 281 and 319 were evaluated, and it was found that peptide 290–309 possessed an IC_{50} of 52 nM for CaMKII inhibition [104]. The N-terminal of the CaMKII 290–309 peptide also contains an autophosphorylation site and has been used to create the autocamtide series of peptide substrates for

CaMKII research [105]. By substituting the Thr phosphoacceptor residue for an Ala, they found that this resulted in highly selective CaMKII pseudosubstrate inhibitor peptides AIP [106] and AC3-I [107]. The presence of an alpha-helical portion of the autoinhibitory sequence adjacent to the pseudosubstrate region identified in the structure obtained by Rellos et al. suggests that this may be a potential candidate for design of a hydrocarbon-stapled analog [103].

PKC consists of a family of closely related kinases that contain an N-terminus autoinhibitory pseudosubstrate sequence. The pseudosubstrate sequence of PKC was first described in 1987, and a synthetic peptide based on residues 19–36 of this sequence was found to inhibit PKC with a K_i of 150 nM [74]. Due to the similarity of the pseudosubstrate sequence of the α, β, and γ isoforms, this peptide inhibits these three isoforms with comparable potency. Emphasizing the importance of individual amino acids in determining binding and inhibition properties, the Arg at position 22 was found to be crucial for activity of this peptide [108]. Attempts have been made to improve the cell permeability and proteolytic stability of this peptide through myristoylation [69] and retro-inverso synthesis, respectively [109]. Further, the difference in the substrate consensus sequence of PKC ζ was exploited in efforts to create an isoform-specific inhibitory peptide for PKC [110]. The ζ inhibitory peptide (ZIP) was used extensively to investigate the role of PKC ζ in synaptic plasticity; however, recent work shows that ZIP promiscuously binds all PKC isoforms and interferes with PKC targeting and localization [111].

Like PKC, the autoinhibitory sequence of PKG is located in the N-terminus of the same polypeptide containing the catalytic domain; however PKG's mechanism of activation is more akin to that of PKA than PKC. The regulatory domain of PKG shares 28% homology with PKA while the catalytic domain of PKG shares 41% identity with that of PKA [112]. This is hardly surprising since both PKA and PKG depend on the binding of cyclic nucleotides to their regulatory regions for activation. PKGIβ is the only member of the six isoforms that contains the prototypical PKG substrate recognition sequence in its autoinhibitory domain; other PKGs have only a single basic residue at the P^{-2} or P^{-3} location [113]. This less–than-ideal pseudosubstrate sequence may reflect a reduced requirement for high-specificity binding due to fact that the autoinhibitory sequence is located on the same polypeptide chain as the catalytic domain.

The remarkable affinity of the PKA pseudosubstrate inhibitors as compared to other kinases regulated by pseudosubstrates may be due to the fact that the regulatory domains of PKA are located on separate proteins and, therefore, require higher affinity than the autoinhibitory sequences located within the same polypeptide chain as the kinase domain. Future research into adapting pseudosubstrate inhibitory domains into effective inhibitory peptides will likely require introduction of point mutations to increase the affinity of the sequence for the substrate recognition domain.

Conclusions

Overall, constrained peptides offer many advantages over nonmodified sequences, namely the potential for improved cell permeation and proteolytic stability. However, many challenges still exist. Although hydrocarbon stapling has been shown to generally improve the extent of cell permeation, peptides may still be localized within intracellular vesicles and, therefore, cannot reach their target of interest [5]. As of now, there are no clear design rules to strategically design a highly cell-permeable hydrocarbon-stapled peptide that has little to no intracellular vesicle accumulation. Further, an overall negative net charge can be detrimental to permeation and, thus, this strategy may not be amenable for all sequences of interest [114]. In addition, while the introduction of a synthetic constraint on a helical peptide often results in an analog with enhanced potency for its target due to reinforcement of the peptide conformer in solution, it can also be detrimental to binding. As shown with the stapled PKI pseudosubstrate peptide [83], our initial design of this compound resulted in a notable loss of affinity when introducing the peptide staple, likely by inducing helicity in a portion of the sequence that needed to be nonhelical. The positioning of the staple is extremely critical since it nucleates helicity around the staple position [115]. Another limitation of hydrocarbon peptide stapling is the added effect of enhanced hydrophobicity to the overall physical properties of the peptide. Since many of these designed peptides are ultimately earmarked to be assayed in cell-based assays, it is critical to ensure solubility in an aqueous buffer at a given pH. This step may require further optimization of the peptide sequence itself of addition of water-solubilizing moieties such as short PEG linkers to promote hydrophilicity of the compound. Thus, for a sequence of interest, a relatively small library of analogs may often be required for testing where various factors are modified such as staple position, overall net charge, hydrophilicity, and its ability to accumulate in the cellular cytosol.

As a whole, kinases are a rich field for targeting using constrained peptides. While the kinase domain itself is conserved among the kinase superfamily, kinases are highly divergent in their modes of regulation, activation, and intracellular location. These aspects of kinase control often require shallow binding surfaces on the kinase itself, and these surfaces are often unique for small kinase subsets. By taking advantage of these unique regulatory surfaces on kinases, one can strategically exploit their divergent regulatory mechanisms using peptide-based disruptors that can competitively target these shallow binding surfaces. As more and more kinase structures become available, coupled with an increased understanding of kinase regulation and dynamics, a variety of creative approaches can be taken to target these regulatory surfaces on a kinase of interest with high selectivity by disrupting its required processes for activation.

References

1. Verdine, G. L., & Hilinski, G. J. (2012). Stapled peptides for intracellular drug targets. *Methods in Enzymology, 503*, 3–33. https://doi.org/10.1016/B978-0-12-396962-0.00001-X. PubMed PMID: 22230563.
2. Cromm, P. M., Spiegel, J., & Grossmann, T. N. (2015). Hydrocarbon stapled peptides as modulators of biological function. *ACS Chemical Biology, 10*(6), 1362–1375. https://doi.org/10.1021/cb501020r. Epub 2015/03/24. PubMed PMID: 25798993.
3. Wu, Y., Kaur, A., Fowler, E., Wiedmann, M. M., Young, R., Galloway, W., Olsen, L., Sore, H. F., Chattopadhyay, A., Kwan, T. T., Xu, W., Walsh, S. J., de Andrade, P., Janecek, M., Arumugam, S., Itzhaki, L. S., Lau, Y. H., & Spring, D. R. (2019). Toolbox of diverse linkers for navigating the cellular efficacy landscape of stapled peptides. *ACS Chemical Biology, 14*(3), 526–533. https://doi.org/10.1021/acschembio.9b00063. Epub 2019/02/01. PubMed PMID: 30702850.
4. Blackwell, H. E., Sadowsky, J. D., Howard, R. J., Sampson, J. N., Chao, J. A., Steinmetz, W. E., O'Leary, D. J., & Grubbs, R. H. (2001). Ring-closing metathesis of olefinic peptides: Design, synthesis, and structural characterization of macrocyclic helical peptides. *The Journal of Organic Chemistry, 66*(16), 5291–5302. https://doi.org/10.1021/jo015533k. Epub 2001/08/04. PubMed PMID: 11485448.
5. Walensky, L. D., & Bird, G. H. (2014). Hydrocarbon-stapled peptides: Principles, practice, and progress. *Journal of Medicinal Chemistry, 57*(15), 6275–6288. https://doi.org/10.1021/jm4011675. Epub 2014/03/08. PubMed PMID: 24601557; PMCID: PMC4136684.
6. Lemmon, M. A., & Schlessinger, J. (2010). Cell signaling by receptor tyrosine kinases. *Cell, 141*(7), 1117–1134. https://doi.org/10.1016/j.cell.2010.06.011. Epub 2010/07/07. PubMed PMID: 20602996; PMCID: PMC2914105.
7. Mendrola, J. M., Shi, F., Park, J. H., & Lemmon, M. A. (2013). Receptor tyrosine kinases with intracellular pseudokinase domains. *Biochemical Society Transactions, 41*(4), 1029–1036. https://doi.org/10.1042/BST20130104. Epub 2013/07/19. PubMed PMID: 23863174; PMCID: PMC3777422.
8. Roskoski, R., Jr. (2019). Properties of FDA-approved small molecule protein kinase inhibitors. *Pharmacological Research, 144*, 19–50. https://doi.org/10.1016/j.phrs.2019.03.006. Epub 2019/03/17. PubMed PMID: 30877063.
9. Ferguson, F. M., & Gray, N. S. (2018). Kinase inhibitors: The road ahead. *Nature Reviews Drug Discovery, 17*(5), 353–377. https://doi.org/10.1038/nrd.2018.21. Epub 2018/03/17. PubMed PMID: 29545548.
10. Lemmon, M. A. (2009). Ligand-induced ErbB receptor dimerization. *Experimental Cell Research, 315*(4), 638–648. https://doi.org/10.1016/j.yexcr.2008.10.024. Epub 2008/11/29. PubMed PMID: 19038249; PMCID: PMC2667204.
11. Endres, N. F., Barros, T., Cantor, A. J., & Kuriyan, J. (2014). Emerging concepts in the regulation of the EGF receptor and other receptor tyrosine kinases. *Trends in Biochemical Sciences, 39*(10), 437–446. https://doi.org/10.1016/j.tibs.2014.08.001. Epub 2014/09/23. PubMed PMID: 25242369.
12. Singh, D., Attri, B. K., Gill, R. K., & Bariwal, J. (2016). Review on EGFR inhibitors: Critical updates. *Mini Reviews in Medicinal Chemistry, 16*(14), 1134–1166. Epub 2016/03/22. PubMed PMID: 26996617.
13. Roskoski, R., Jr. (2014). The ErbB/HER family of protein-tyrosine kinases and cancer. *Pharmacological Research, 79*, 34–74. https://doi.org/10.1016/j.phrs.2013.11.002. Epub 2013/11/26. PubMed PMID: 24269963.
14. Nagano, T., Tachihara, M., & Nishimura, Y. (2018). Mechanism of resistance to epidermal growth factor receptor-tyrosine kinase inhibitors and a potential treatment strategy. *Cells, 7*(11), 212. https://doi.org/10.3390/cells7110212. Epub 2018/11/18. PubMed PMID: 30445769; PMCID: PMC6262543.

15. Tebbutt, N., Pedersen, M. W., & Johns, T. G. (2013). Targeting the ERBB family in cancer: Couples therapy. *Nature Reviews Cancer, 13*(9), 663–673. https://doi.org/10.1038/nrc3559. Epub 2013/08/21. PubMed PMID: 23949426.
16. Dawson, J. P., Berger, M. B., Lin, C. C., Schlessinger, J., Lemmon, M. A., & Ferguson, K. M. (2005). Epidermal growth factor receptor dimerization and activation require ligand-induced conformational changes in the dimer interface. *Molecular and Cellular Biology, 25*(17), 7734–7742. https://doi.org/10.1128/MCB.25.17.7734-7742.2005. Epub 2005/08/19. PubMed PMID: 16107719; PMCID: PMC1190273.
17. Ogiso, H., Ishitani, R., Nureki, O., Fukai, S., Yamanaka, M., Kim, J. H., Saito, K., Sakamoto, A., Inoue, M., Shirouzu, M., & Yokoyama, S. (2002). Crystal structure of the complex of human epidermal growth factor and receptor extracellular domains. *Cell, 110*(6), 775–787. Epub 2002/09/26. PubMed PMID: 12297050.
18. Mizuguchi, T., Ohara, N., Iida, M., Ninomiya, R., Wada, S., Kiso, Y., Saito, K., & Akaji, K. (2012). Evaluation of dimerization-inhibitory activities of cyclic peptides containing a beta-hairpin loop sequence of the EGF receptor. *Bioorganic & Medicinal Chemistry, 20*(19), 5730–5737. https://doi.org/10.1016/j.bmc.2012.08.013. Epub 2012/09/11. PubMed PMID: 22959765.
19. Mizuguchi, T., Uchimura, H., Kakizawa, T., Kimura, T., Yokoyama, S., Kiso, Y., & Saito, K. (2009). Inhibitory effect of a dimerization-arm-mimetic peptide on EGF receptor activation. *Bioorganic & Medicinal Chemistry Letters, 19*(12), 3279–3282. https://doi.org/10.1016/j.bmcl.2009.04.080. Epub 2009/05/08. PubMed PMID: 19419869.
20. Hanold, L. E., Oruganty, K., Ton, N. T., Beedle, A. M., Kannan, N., & Kennedy, E. J. (2015). Inhibiting EGFR dimerization using triazolyl-bridged dimerization arm mimics. *PLoS One, 10*(3), e0118796. https://doi.org/10.1371/journal.pone.0118796. Epub 2015/03/20. PubMed PMID: 25790232; PMCID: PMC4366150.
21. Hanold, L. E., Watkins, C. P., Ton, N. T., Liaw, P., Beedle, A. M., & Kennedy, E. J. (2015). Design of a selenylsulfide-bridged EGFR dimerization arm mimic. *Bioorganic & Medicinal Chemistry, 23*(12), 2761–2766. https://doi.org/10.1016/j.bmc.2015.03.040. Epub 2015/04/05. PubMed PMID: 25840798; PMCID: PMC4451384.
22. Jura, N., Endres, N. F., Engel, K., Deindl, S., Das, R., Lamers, M. H., Wemmer, D. E., Zhang, X., & Kuriyan, J. (2009). Mechanism for activation of the EGF receptor catalytic domain by the juxtamembrane segment. *Cell, 137*(7), 1293–1307. https://doi.org/10.1016/j.cell.2009.04.025. Epub 2009/07/01. PubMed PMID: 19563760; PMCID: PMC2814540.
23. Sinclair, J. K., & Schepartz, A. (2014). Influence of macrocyclization on allosteric, juxtamembrane-derived, stapled peptide inhibitors of the epidermal growth factor receptor (EGFR). *Organic Letters, 16*(18), 4916–4919. https://doi.org/10.1021/ol502426b. Epub 2014/09/11. PubMed PMID: 25207804; PMCID: PMC4168776.
24. Zhang, X., Gureasko, J., Shen, K., Cole, P. A., & Kuriyan, J. (2006). An allosteric mechanism for activation of the kinase domain of epidermal growth factor receptor. *Cell, 125*(6), 1137–1149. https://doi.org/10.1016/j.cell.2006.05.013. Epub 2006/06/17. PubMed PMID: 16777603.
25. Fulton, M. D., Hanold, L. E., Ruan, Z., Patel, S., Beedle, A. M., Kannan, N., & Kennedy, E. J. (2018). Conformationally constrained peptides target the allosteric kinase dimer interface and inhibit EGFR activation. *Bioorganic & Medicinal Chemistry, 26*(6), 1167–1173. https://doi.org/10.1016/j.bmc.2017.08.051. Epub 2017/09/16. PubMed PMID: 28911855; PMCID: PMC5837902.
26. Yamaoka, T., Kusumoto, S., Ando, K., Ohba, M., & Ohmori, T. (2018). Receptor tyrosine kinase-targeted cancer therapy. *International Journal of Molecular Sciences, 19*(11), 3491. https://doi.org/10.3390/ijms19113491. Epub 2018/11/09. PubMed PMID: 30404198; PMCID: PMC6274851.
27. Zhang, J., Yang, P. L., & Gray, N. S. (2009). Targeting cancer with small molecule kinase inhibitors. *Nature Reviews Cancer, 9*(1), 28–39. https://doi.org/10.1038/nrc2559. Epub 2008/12/24. PubMed PMID: 19104514.

28. Langeberg, L. K., & Scott, J. D. (2005). A-kinase-anchoring proteins. *Journal of Cell Science, 118*(Pt 15), 3217–3220. https://doi.org/10.1242/jcs.02416. Epub 2005/08/05. PubMed PMID: 16079273.
29. Wong, W., & Scott, J. D. (2004). AKAP signalling complexes: Focal points in space and time. *Nature Reviews Molecular Cell Biology, 5*(12), 959–970. https://doi.org/10.1038/nrm1527. Epub 2004/12/02. PubMed PMID: 15573134.
30. Scott, J. D., Dessauer, C. W., & Tasken, K. (2013). Creating order from chaos: Cellular regulation by kinase anchoring. *Annual Review of Pharmacology and Toxicology, 53*, 187–210. https://doi.org/10.1146/annurev-pharmtox-011112-140204. Epub 2012/10/10. PubMed PMID: 23043438; PMCID: PMC3540170.
31. Taylor, S. S., Kim, C., Cheng, C. Y., Brown, S. H., Wu, J., & Kannan, N. (2008). Signaling through cAMP and cAMP-dependent protein kinase: Diverse strategies for drug design. *Biochimica et Biophysica Acta, 1784*(1), 16–26. https://doi.org/10.1016/j.bbapap.2007.10.002. Epub 2007/11/13. PubMed PMID: 17996741; PMCID: PMC2561045.
32. Hayes, J. S., Brunton, L. L., Brown, J. H., Reese, J. B., & Mayer, S. E. (1979). Hormonally specific expression of cardiac protein kinase activity. *Proceedings of the National Academy of Sciences of the United States of America, 76*(4), 1570–1574. https://doi.org/10.1073/pnas.76.4.1570. Epub 1979/04/01. PubMed PMID: 221898; PMCID: PMC383431.
33. Brunton, L. L., Hayes, J. S., & Mayer, S. E. (1979). Hormonally specific phosphorylation of cardiac troponin I and activation of glycogen phosphorylase. *Nature, 280*(5717), 78–80. Epub 1979/07/05. PubMed PMID: 15305586.
34. Corbin, J. D., Sugden, P. H., Lincoln, T. M., & Keely, S. L. (1977). Compartmentalization of adenosine 3′:5′-monophosphate and adenosine 3′:5′-monophosphate-dependent protein kinase in heart tissue. *The Journal of Biological Chemistry, 252*(11), 3854–3861. Epub 1977/06/10. PubMed PMID: 16921.
35. Burgers, P. P., Bruystens, J., Burnley, R. J., Nikolaev, V. O., Keshwani, M., Wu, J., Janssen, B. J., Taylor, S. S., Heck, A. J., & Scholten, A. (2016). Structure of smAKAP and its regulation by PKA-mediated phosphorylation. *The FEBS Journal, 283*(11), 2132–2148. https://doi.org/10.1111/febs.13726. Epub 2016/03/31. PubMed PMID: 27028580; PMCID: PMC4980077.
36. Greenwald, E. C., & Saucerman, J. J. (2011). Bigger, better, faster: Principles and models of AKAP anchoring protein signaling. *Journal of Cardiovascular Pharmacology, 58*(5), 462–469. https://doi.org/10.1097/FJC.0b013e31822001e3. Epub 2011/05/13. PubMed PMID: 21562426; PMCID: PMC3173587.
37. Kapiloff, M. S., Rigatti, M., & Dodge-Kafka, K. L. (2014). Architectural and functional roles of A kinase-anchoring proteins in cAMP microdomains. *The Journal of General Physiology, 143*(1), 9–15. https://doi.org/10.1085/jgp.201311020. Epub 2014/01/01. PubMed PMID: 24378903; PMCID: PMC3874566.
38. Carnegie, G. K., Means, C. K., & Scott, J. D. (2009). A-kinase anchoring proteins: From protein complexes to physiology and disease. *IUBMB Life, 61*(4), 394–406. https://doi.org/10.1002/iub.168. Epub 2009/03/26. PubMed PMID: 19319965; PMCID: PMC2682206.
39. Esseltine, J. L., & Scott, J. D. (2013). AKAP signaling complexes: Pointing towards the next generation of therapeutic targets? *Trends in Pharmacological Sciences, 34*(12), 648–655. https://doi.org/10.1016/j.tips.2013.10.005. Epub 2013/11/19. PubMed PMID: 24239028; PMCID: PMC3879114.
40. Torres-Quesada, O., Mayrhofer, J. E., & Stefan, E. (2017). The many faces of compartmentalized PKA signalosomes. *Cellular Signalling, 37*, 1–11. https://doi.org/10.1016/j.cellsig.2017.05.012. Epub 2017/05/23. PubMed PMID: 28528970.
41. Malbon, C. C., Tao, J., & Wang, H. Y. (2004). AKAPs (A-kinase anchoring proteins) and molecules that compose their G-protein-coupled receptor signalling complexes. *The Biochemical Journal, 379*(Pt 1), 1–9. https://doi.org/10.1042/BJ20031648. Epub 2004/01/13. PubMed PMID: 14715081; PMCID: PMC1224059.

42. Gold, M. G., Stengel, F., Nygren, P. J., Weisbrod, C. R., Bruce, J. E., Robinson, C. V., Barford, D., & Scott, J. D. (2011). Architecture and dynamics of an A-kinase anchoring protein 79 (AKAP79) signaling complex. *Proceedings of the National Academy of Sciences of the United States of America, 108*(16), 6426–6431. https://doi.org/10.1073/pnas.1014400108. Epub 2011/04/06. PubMed PMID: 21464287; PMCID: PMC3081024.
43. Faux, M. C., & Scott, J. D. (1997). Regulation of the AKAP79-protein kinase C interaction by Ca^{2+}/Calmodulin. *The Journal of Biological Chemistry, 272*(27), 17038–17044. https://doi.org/10.1074/jbc.272.27.17038. Epub 1997/07/04. PubMed PMID: 9202019.
44. Troger, J., Moutty, M. C., Skroblin, P., & Klussmann, E. (2012). A-kinase anchoring proteins as potential drug targets. *British Journal of Pharmacology, 166*(2), 420–433. https://doi.org/10.1111/j.1476-5381.2011.01796.x. Epub 2011/11/30. PubMed PMID: 22122509; PMCID: PMC3417477.
45. Tao, J., Shumay, E., McLaughlin, S., Wang, H. Y., & Malbon, C. C. (2006). Regulation of AKAP-membrane interactions by calcium. *The Journal of Biological Chemistry, 281*(33), 23932–23944. https://doi.org/10.1074/jbc.M601813200. Epub 2006/06/10. PubMed PMID: 16762919.
46. Guo, L. W., Gao, L., Rothschild, J., Su, B., & Gelman, I. H. (2011). Control of protein kinase C activity, phorbol ester-induced cytoskeletal remodeling, and cell survival signals by the scaffolding protein SSeCKS/GRAVIN/AKAP12. *The Journal of Biological Chemistry, 286*(44), 38356–38366. https://doi.org/10.1074/jbc.M111.258830. Epub 2011/09/10. PubMed PMID: 21903576; PMCID: PMC3207390.
47. Takahashi, M., Shibata, H., Shimakawa, M., Miyamoto, M., Mukai, H., & Ono, Y. (1999). Characterization of a novel giant scaffolding protein, CG-NAP, that anchors multiple signaling enzymes to centrosome and the golgi apparatus. *The Journal of Biological Chemistry, 274*(24), 17267–17274. https://doi.org/10.1074/jbc.274.24.17267. Epub 1999/06/08. PubMed PMID: 10358086.
48. Diviani, D., & Scott, J. D. (2001). AKAP signaling complexes at the cytoskeleton. *Journal of Cell Science, 114*(8), 1431–1437.
49. Ercu, M., & Klussmann, E. (2018). Roles of A-kinase anchoring proteins and phosphodiesterases in the cardiovascular system. *Journal of Cardiovascular Development and Disease, 5*(1), 14. https://doi.org/10.3390/jcdd5010014. Epub 2018/02/21. PubMed PMID: 29461511; PMCID: PMC5872362.
50. Hausken, Z. E., Dell'Acqua, M. L., Coghlan, V. M., & Scott, J. D. (1996). Mutational analysis of the A-kinase anchoring protein (AKAP)-binding site on RII. Classification of side chain determinants for anchoring and isoform selective association with AKAPs. *The Journal of Biological Chemistry, 271*(46), 29016–29022. https://doi.org/10.1074/jbc.271.46.29016. Epub 1996/11/15. PubMed PMID: 8910553.
51. Scott, J. D., Stofko, R. E., McDonald, J. R., Comer, J. D., Vitalis, E. A., & Mangili, J. A. (1990). Type II regulatory subunit dimerization determines the subcellular localization of the cAMP-dependent protein kinase. *The Journal of Biological Chemistry, 265*(35), 21561–21566. Epub 1990/12/15. PubMed PMID: 2147685.
52. Luo, Z., Shafit-Zagardo, B., & Erlichman, J. (1990). Identification of the MAP 2- and P75-binding domain in the regulatory subunit (RII beta) of type II cAMP-dependent protein kinase. Cloning and expression of the cDNA for bovine brain RII beta. *The Journal of Biological Chemistry, 265*(35), 21804–21810. Epub 1990/12/15. PubMed PMID: 2254332.
53. Carr, D. W., Stofko-Hahn, R. E., Fraser, I. D., Bishop, S. M., Acott, T. S., Brennan, R. G., & Scott, J. D. (1991). Interaction of the regulatory subunit (RII) of cAMP-dependent protein kinase with RII-anchoring proteins occurs through an amphipathic helix binding motif. *The Journal of Biological Chemistry, 266*(22), 14188–14192. Epub 1991/08/05. PubMed PMID: 1860836.
54. Vijayaraghavan, S., Goueli, S. A., Davey, M. P., & Carr, D. W. (1997). Protein kinase A-anchoring inhibitor peptides arrest mammalian sperm motility. *The Journal of Biological*

Chemistry, 272(8), 4747–4752. https://doi.org/10.1074/jbc.272.8.4747. Epub 1997/02/21. PubMed PMID: 9030527.

55. Calejo, A. I., & Tasken, K. (2015). Targeting protein-protein interactions in complexes organized by A kinase anchoring proteins. *Frontiers in Pharmacology, 6*, 192. https://doi.org/10.3389/fphar.2015.00192. Epub 2015/10/07. PubMed PMID: 26441649; PMCID: PMC4562273.
56. Wang, Y., Ho, T. G., Bertinetti, D., Neddermann, M., Franz, E., Mo, G. C., Schendowich, L. P., Sukhu, A., Spelts, R. C., Zhang, J., Herberg, F. W., & Kennedy, E. J. (2014). Isoform-selective disruption of AKAP-localized PKA using hydrocarbon stapled peptides. *ACS Chemical Biology, 9*(3), 635–642. https://doi.org/10.1021/cb400900r. Epub 2014/01/16. PubMed PMID: 24422448; PMCID: PMC3985448.
57. Mo, G. C., Ross, B., Hertel, F., Manna, P., Yang, X., Greenwald, E., Booth, C., Plummer, A. M., Tenner, B., Chen, Z., Wang, Y., Kennedy, E. J., Cole, P. A., Fleming, K. G., Palmer, A., Jimenez, R., Xiao, J., Dedecker, P., & Zhang, J. (2017). Genetically encoded biosensors for visualizing live-cell biochemical activity at super-resolution. *Nature Methods, 14*(4), 427–434. https://doi.org/10.1038/nmeth.4221. Epub 2017/03/14. PubMed PMID: 28288122; PMCID: PMC5388356.
58. Means, C. K., Lygren, B., Langeberg, L. K., Jain, A., Dixon, R. E., Vega, A. L., Gold, M. G., Petrosyan, S., Taylor, S. S., Murphy, A. N., Ha, T., Santana, L. F., Tasken, K., & Scott, J. D. (2011). An entirely specific type I A-kinase anchoring protein that can sequester two molecules of protein kinase A at mitochondria. *Proceedings of the National Academy of Sciences of the United States of America, 108*(48), E1227–E1235. https://doi.org/10.1073/pnas.1107182108. Epub 2011/11/16. PubMed PMID: 22084075; PMCID: PMC3228425.
59. Pidoux, G., Witczak, O., Jarnaess, E., Myrvold, L., Urlaub, H., Stokka, A. J., Kuntziger, T., & Tasken, K. (2011). Optic atrophy 1 is an A-kinase anchoring protein on lipid droplets that mediates adrenergic control of lipolysis. *The EMBO Journal, 30*(21), 4371–4386. https://doi.org/10.1038/emboj.2011.365. Epub 2011/10/11. PubMed PMID: 21983901; PMCID: PMC3230380.
60. Ruppelt, A., Mosenden, R., Gronholm, M., Aandahl, E. M., Tobin, D., Carlson, C. R., Abrahamsen, H., Herberg, F. W., Carpen, O., & Tasken, K. (2007). Inhibition of T cell activation by cyclic adenosine 5′-monophosphate requires lipid raft targeting of protein kinase A type I by the A-kinase anchoring protein ezrin. *Journal of Immunology, 179*(8), 5159–5168. Epub 2007/10/04. PubMed PMID: 17911601.
61. Herberg, F. W., Maleszka, A., Eide, T., Vossebein, L., & Tasken, K. (2000). Analysis of A-kinase anchoring protein (AKAP) interaction with protein kinase A (PKA) regulatory subunits: PKA isoform specificity in AKAP binding. *Journal of Molecular Biology, 298*(2), 329–339. https://doi.org/10.1006/jmbi.2000.3662. Epub 2000/04/15. PubMed PMID: 10764601.
62. Sarma, G. N., Kinderman, F. S., Kim, C., von Daake, S., Chen, L., Wang, B. C., & Taylor, S. S. (2010). Structure of D-AKAP2:PKA RI complex: Insights into AKAP specificity and selectivity. *Structure, 18*(2), 155–166. https://doi.org/10.1016/j.str.2009.12.012. Epub 2010/02/18. PubMed PMID: 20159461; PMCID: PMC3090270.
63. Kinderman, F. S., Kim, C., von Daake, S., Ma, Y., Pham, B. Q., Spraggon, G., Xuong, N. H., Jennings, P. A., & Taylor, S. S. (2006). A dynamic mechanism for AKAP binding to RII isoforms of cAMP-dependent protein kinase. *Molecular Cell, 24*(3), 397–408. https://doi.org/10.1016/j.molcel.2006.09.015. Epub 2006/11/04. PubMed PMID: 17081990; PMCID: PMC1855097.
64. Kennedy, E. J., & Scott, J. D. (2015). Selective disruption of the AKAP signaling complexes. *Methods in Molecular Biology, 1294*, 137–150. https://doi.org/10.1007/978-1-4939-2537-7_11. Epub 2015/03/19. PubMed PMID: 25783883; PMCID: PMC4722817.
65. Burns-Hamuro, L. L., Ma, Y., Kammerer, S., Reineke, U., Self, C., Cook, C., Olson, G. L., Cantor, C. R., Braun, A., & Taylor, S. S. (2003). Designing isoform-specific peptide disruptors of protein kinase A localization. *Proceedings of the National Academy of Sciences of*

the United States of America, 100(7), 4072–4077. https://doi.org/10.1073/pnas.2628038100. Epub 2003/03/21.PubMed PMID: 12646696; PMCID: PMC153050.
66. Carlson, C. R., Lygren, B., Berge, T., Hoshi, N., Wong, W., Tasken, K., & Scott, J. D. (2006). Delineation of type I protein kinase A-selective signaling events using an RI anchoring disruptor. *The Journal of Biological Chemistry, 281*(30), 21535–21545. https://doi.org/10.1074/jbc.M603223200. Epub 2006/05/27. PubMed PMID: 16728392.
67. Wang, Y., Ho, T. G., Franz, E., Hermann, J. S., Smith, F. D., Hehnly, H., Esseltine, J. L., Hanold, L. E., Murph, M. M., Bertinetti, D., Scott, J. D., & Herberg, F. W. (2015). Kennedy EJ. PKA-type I selective constrained peptide disruptors of AKAP complexes. *ACS Chemical Biology, 10*(6), 1502–1510. https://doi.org/10.1021/acschembio.5b00009. Epub 2015/03/15. PubMed PMID: 25765284; PMCID: PMC4475429.
68. Su, B., Bu, Y., Engelberg, D., & Gelman, I. H. (2010). SSeCKS/Gravin/AKAP12 inhibits cancer cell invasiveness and chemotaxis by suppressing a protein kinase C-Raf/MEK/ERK pathway. *The Journal of Biological Chemistry, 285*(7), 4578–4586. https://doi.org/10.1074/jbc.M109.073494. Epub 2009/12/19. PubMed PMID: 20018890; PMCID: PMC2836062.
69. Eichholtz, T., de Bont, D. B., de Widt, J., Liskamp, R. M., & Ploegh, H. L. (1993). A myristoylated pseudosubstrate peptide, a novel protein kinase C inhibitor. *The Journal of Biological Chemistry, 268*(3), 1982–1986. Epub 1993/01/25. PubMed PMID: 8420972.
70. Mitchell, R. D., Glass, D. B., Wong, C. W., Angelos, K. L., & Walsh, D. A. (1995). Heat-stable inhibitor protein derived peptide substrate analogs: Phosphorylation by cAMP-dependent and cGMP-dependent protein kinases. *Biochemistry, 34*(2), 528–534. https://doi.org/10.1021/bi00002a018. Epub 1995/01/17. PubMed PMID: 7819246.
71. Knighton, D. R., Zheng, J. H., Ten Eyck, L. F., Ashford, V. A., Xuong, N. H., Taylor, S. S., & Sowadski, J. M. (1991). Crystal structure of the catalytic subunit of cyclic adenosine monophosphate-dependent protein kinase. *Science, 253*(5018), 407–414. Epub 1991/07/26. PubMed PMID: 1862342.
72. Kemp, B. E., Parker, M. W., Hu, S., Tiganis, T., & House, C. (1994). Substrate and pseudosubstrate interactions with protein kinases: Determinants of specificity. *Trends in Biochemical Sciences, 19*(11), 440–444. Epub 1994/11/01. PubMed PMID: 7855883.
73. Kemp, B. E., Pearson, R. B., & House, C. M. (1991). Pseudosubstrate-based peptide inhibitors. *Methods in Enzymology, 201*, 287–304. Epub 1991/01/01. PubMed PMID: 1943770.
74. House, C., & Kemp, B. E. (1987). Protein kinase C contains a pseudosubstrate prototope in its regulatory domain. *Science, 238*(4834), 1726–1728. Epub 1987/12/18. PubMed PMID: 3686012.
75. Hu, S. H., Parker, M. W., Lei, J. Y., Wilce, M. C., Benian, G. M., & Kemp, B. E. (1994). Insights into autoregulation from the crystal structure of twitchin kinase. *Nature, 369*(6481), 581–584. https://doi.org/10.1038/369581a0. Epub 1994/06/16. PubMed PMID: 8202162.
76. Walsh, D. A., Ashby, C. D., Gonzalez, C., Calkins, D., Fischer, E. H., & Krebs, E. G. (1971). Purification and characterization of a protein inhibitor of adenosine 3′,5′-monophosphate-dependent protein kinases. *The Journal of Biological Chemistry, 246*(7), 1977–1985. Epub 1971/04/10. PubMed PMID: 4324557.
77. Hauer, J. A., Barthe, P., Taylor, S. S., Parello, J., & Padilla, A. (1999). Two well-defined motifs in the cAMP-dependent protein kinase inhibitor (PKIalpha) correlate with inhibitory and nuclear export function. *Protein Science, 8*(3), 545–553. https://doi.org/10.1110/ps.8.3.545. Epub 1999/03/26. PubMed PMID: 10091657; PMCID: PMC2144290.
78. Demaille, J. G., Peters, K. A., & Fischer, E. H. (1977). Isolation and properties of the rabbit skeletal muscle protein inhibitor of adenosine 3′,5′-monophosphate dependent protein kinases. *Biochemistry, 16*(14), 3080–3086. Epub 1977/07/12. PubMed PMID: 196623.
79. Scott, J. D., Fischer, E. H., Demaille, J. G., & Krebs, E. G. (1985). Identification of an inhibitory region of the heat-stable protein inhibitor of the cAMP-dependent protein kinase. *Proceedings of the National Academy of Sciences of the United States of America, 82*(13), 4379–4383. https://doi.org/10.1073/pnas.82.13.4379. Epub 1985/07/01. PubMed PMID: 2989819; PMCID: PMC390417.

80. Scott, J. D., Fischer, E. H., Takio, K., Demaille, J. G., & Krebs, E. G. (1985). Amino acid sequence of the heat-stable inhibitor of the cAMP-dependent protein kinase from rabbit skeletal muscle. *Proceedings of the National Academy of Sciences of the United States of America, 82*(17), 5732–5736. https://doi.org/10.1073/pnas.82.17.5732. Epub 1985/09/01. PubMed PMID: 3898070; PMCID: PMC390626.
81. Scott, J. D., Glaccum, M. B., Fischer, E. H., & Krebs, E. G. (1986). Primary-structure requirements for inhibition by the heat-stable inhibitor of the cAMP-dependent protein kinase. *Proceedings of the National Academy of Sciences of the United States of America, 83*(6), 1613–1616. https://doi.org/10.1073/pnas.83.6.1613. Epub 1986/03/01. PubMed PMID: 3456605; PMCID: PMC323133.
82. Fernandez, A., Mery, J., Vandromme, M., Basset, M., Cavadore, J. C., & Lamb, N. J. (1991). Effective intracellular inhibition of the cAMP-dependent protein kinase by microinjection of a modified form of the specific inhibitor peptide PKi in living fibroblasts. *Experimental Cell Research, 195*(2), 468–477. Epub 1991/08/01. PubMed PMID: 2070829.
83. Manschwetus, J. T., Bendzunas, G. N., Limaye, A. J., Knape, M. J., Herberg, F. W., & Kennedy, E. J. (2019). A stapled peptide mimic of the pseudosubstrate inhibitor PKI inhibits protein kinase A. *Molecules, 24*(8), 1567. https://doi.org/10.3390/molecules24081567. Epub 2019/04/24. PubMed PMID: 31009996.
84. Reed, J., Kinzel, V., Cheng, H. C., & Walsh, D. A. (1987). Circular dichroic investigations of secondary structure in synthetic peptide inhibitors of cAMP-dependent protein kinase: A model for inhibitory potential. *Biochemistry, 26*(24), 7641–7647. Epub 1987/12/01. PubMed PMID: 3427097.
85. Lei, J., Tang, X., Chambers, T. C., Pohl, J., & Benian, G. M. (1994). Protein kinase domain of twitchin has protein kinase activity and an autoinhibitory region. *The Journal of Biological Chemistry, 269*(33), 21078–21085. Epub 1994/08/19. PubMed PMID: 8063727.
86. Allen, B. G., & Walsh, M. P. (1994). The biochemical basis of the regulation of smooth-muscle contraction. *Trends in Biochemical Sciences, 19*(9), 362–368. Epub 1994/09/01. PubMed PMID: 7985229.
87. Kemp, B. E., Pearson, R. B., Guerriero, V., Jr., Bagchi, I. C., & Means, A. R. (1987). The calmodulin binding domain of chicken smooth muscle myosin light chain kinase contains a pseudosubstrate sequence. *The Journal of Biological Chemistry, 262*(6), 2542–2548. Epub 1987/02/25. PubMed PMID: 3818608.
88. Lukas, T. J., Mirzoeva, S., Slomczynska, U., & Watterson, D. M. (1999). Identification of novel classes of protein kinase inhibitors using combinatorial peptide chemistry based on functional genomics knowledge. *Journal of Medicinal Chemistry, 42*(5), 910–919. https://doi.org/10.1021/jm980573a. Epub 1999/03/12. PubMed PMID: 10072688.
89. Taylor, S. S., Buechler, J. A., & Yonemoto, W. (1990). cAMP-dependent protein kinase: Framework for a diverse family of regulatory enzymes. *Annual Review of Biochemistry, 59*, 971–1005. https://doi.org/10.1146/annurev.bi.59.070190.004543. Epub 1990/01/01. PubMed PMID: 2165385.
90. Ohno, S., Kawasaki, H., Imajoh, S., Suzuki, K., Inagaki, M., Yokokura, H., Sakoh, T., & Hidaka, H. (1987). Tissue-specific expression of three distinct types of rabbit protein kinase C. *Nature, 325*(7000), 161–166. https://doi.org/10.1038/325161a0. Epub 1987/01/08. PubMed PMID: 3808073.
91. Kubo, K., Ohno, S., & Suzuki, K. (1987). Primary structures of human protein-kinase-C beta-I and beta-Ii differ only in their C-terminal SEQUENCES. *FEBS Letters, 223*(1), 138–142. https://doi.org/10.1016/0014-5793(87)80524-0. PubMed PMID: WOS:A1987K563400027.
92. Coussens, L., Parker, P. J., Rhee, L., Yang-Feng, T. L., Chen, E., Waterfield, M. D., Francke, U., & Ullrich, A. (1986). Multiple, distinct forms of bovine and human protein kinase C suggest diversity in cellular signaling pathways. *Science, 233*(4766), 859–866. Epub 1986/08/22. PubMed PMID: 3755548.

93. Ohno, S., Akita, Y., Konno, Y., Imajoh, S., & Suzuki, K. (1988). A novel phorbol ester receptor/protein kinase, nPKC, distantly related to the protein kinase C family. *Cell, 53*(5), 731–741. Epub 1988/06/03. PubMed PMID: 3370672.
94. Ono, Y., Fujii, T., Ogita, K., Kikkawa, U., Igarashi, K., & Nishizuka, Y. (1988). The structure, expression, and properties of additional members of the protein kinase C family. *The Journal of Biological Chemistry, 263*(14), 6927–6932. Epub 1988/05/15. PubMed PMID: 2834397.
95. Takio, K., Wade, R. D., Smith, S. B., Krebs, E. G., Walsh, K. A., & Titani, K. (1984). Guanosine cyclic 3′,5′-phosphate dependent protein kinase, a chimeric protein homologous with two separate protein families. *Biochemistry, 23*(18), 4207–4218. Epub 1984/08/28. PubMed PMID: 6091741.
96. Wernet, W., Flockerzi, V., & Hofmann, F. (1989). The cDNA of the two isoforms of bovine cGMP-dependent protein kinase. *FEBS Letters, 251*(1-2), 191–196. Epub 1989/07/17. PubMed PMID: 2546820.
97. Hanley, R. M., Means, A. R., Ono, T., Kemp, B. E., Burgin, K. E., Waxham, N., & Kelly, P. T. (1987). Functional analysis of a complementary DNA for the 50-kilodalton subunit of calmodulin kinase II. *Science, 237*(4812), 293–297. Epub 1987/07/17. PubMed PMID: 3037704.
98. Bennett, M. K., & Kennedy, M. B. (1987). Deduced primary structure of the beta subunit of brain type II Ca2+/calmodulin-dependent protein kinase determined by molecular cloning. *Proceedings of the National Academy of Sciences of the United States of America, 84*(7), 1794–1798. https://doi.org/10.1073/pnas.84.7.1794. Epub 1987/04/01. PubMed PMID: 3470758; PMCID: PMC304527.
99. Tobimatsu, T., Kameshita, I., & Fujisawa, H. (1988). Molecular cloning of the cDNA encoding the third polypeptide (gamma) of brain calmodulin-dependent protein kinase II. *The Journal of Biological Chemistry, 263*(31), 16082–16086. Epub 1988/11/05. PubMed PMID: 2846534.
100. Tobimatsu, T., & Fujisawa, H. (1989). Tissue-specific expression of four types of rat calmodulin-dependent protein kinase II mRNAs. *The Journal of Biological Chemistry, 264*(30), 17907–17912. Epub 1989/10/25. PubMed PMID: 2553697.
101. Olson, N. J., Pearson, R. B., Needleman, D. S., Hurwitz, M. Y., Kemp, B. E., & Means, A. R. (1990). Regulatory and structural motifs of chicken gizzard myosin light chain kinase. *Proceedings of the National Academy of Sciences of the United States of America, 87*(6), 2284–2288. https://doi.org/10.1073/pnas.87.6.2284. Epub 1990/03/01. PubMed PMID: 2315320; PMCID: PMC53671.
102. Takio, K., Blumenthal, D. K., Edelman, A. M., Walsh, K. A., Krebs, E. G., & Titani, K. (1985). Amino acid sequence of an active fragment of rabbit skeletal muscle myosin light chain kinase. *Biochemistry, 24*(22), 6028–6037. Epub 1985/10/22. PubMed PMID: 3841288.
103. Rellos, P., Pike, A. C., Niesen, F. H., Salah, E., Lee, W. H., von Delft, F., & Knapp, S. (2010). Structure of the CaMKIIdelta/calmodulin complex reveals the molecular mechanism of CaMKII kinase activation. *PLoS Biology, 8*(7), e1000426. https://doi.org/10.1371/journal.pbio.1000426. Epub 2010/07/30. PubMed PMID: 20668654; PMCID: PMC2910593.
104. Payne, M. E., Fong, Y. L., Ono, T., Colbran, R. J., Kemp, B. E., Soderling, T. R., & Means, A. R. (1988). Calcium/calmodulin-dependent protein kinase II. Characterization of distinct calmodulin binding and inhibitory domains. *The Journal of Biological Chemistry, 263*(15), 7190–7195. Epub 1988/05/25. PubMed PMID: 2835367.
105. Hanson, P. I., Kapiloff, M. S., Lou, L. L., Rosenfeld, M. G., & Schulman, H. (1989). Expression of a multifunctional Ca^{2+}/calmodulin-dependent protein kinase and mutational analysis of its autoregulation. *Neuron, 3*(1), 59–70. Epub 1989/07/01. PubMed PMID: 2619995.
106. Ishida, A., Kameshita, I., Okuno, S., Kitani, T., & Fujisawa, H. (1995). A novel highly specific and potent inhibitor of calmodulin-dependent protein kinase II. *Biochemical and Biophysical Research Communications, 212*(3), 806–812. https://doi.org/10.1006/bbrc.1995.2040. Epub 1995/07/26. PubMed PMID: 7626114.

107. Braun, A. P., & Schulman, H. (1995). A non-selective cation current activated via the multifunctional Ca(2+)-calmodulin-dependent protein kinase in human epithelial cells. *The Journal of Physiology, 488*(Pt 1), 37–55. Epub 1995/10/01. PubMed PMID: 8568664; PMCID: PMC1156699.
108. House, C., & Kemp, B. E. (1990). Protein kinase C pseudosubstrate prototope: Structure-function relationships. *Cellular Signalling, 2*(2), 187–190. Epub 1990/01/01. PubMed PMID: 2400634.
109. Ricouart, A., Tartar, A., & Sergheraert, C. (1989). Inhibition of protein kinase C by retro-inverso pseudosubstrate analogues. *Biochemical and Biophysical Research Communications, 165*(3), 1382–1390. Epub 1989/12/29. PubMed PMID: 2514686.
110. Dominguez, I., Diaz-Meco, M. T., Municio, M. M., Berra, E., Garcia de Herreros, A., Cornet, M. E., Sanz, L., & Moscat, J. (1992). Evidence for a role of protein kinase C zeta subspecies in maturation of Xenopus laevis oocytes. *Molecular and Cellular Biology, 12*(9), 3776–3783. https://doi.org/10.1128/mcb.12.9.3776. Epub 1992/09/01. PubMed PMID: 1508183; PMCID: PMC360243.
111. Bogard, A. S., & Tavalin, S. J. (2015). Protein kinase C (PKC)zeta pseudosubstrate inhibitor peptide promiscuously binds PKC family isoforms and disrupts conventional PKC targeting and translocation. *Molecular Pharmacology, 88*(4), 728–735. https://doi.org/10.1124/mol.115.099457. Epub 2015/07/23. PubMed PMID: 26199377; PMCID: PMC4576679.
112. Moon, T. M., Sheehe, J. L., Nukareddy, P., Nausch, L. W., Wohlfahrt, J., Matthews, D. E., Blumenthal, D. K., & Dostmann, W. R. (2018). An N-terminally truncated form of cyclic GMP-dependent protein kinase Ialpha (PKG Ialpha) is monomeric and autoinhibited and provides a model for activation. *The Journal of Biological Chemistry, 293*(21), 7916–7929. https://doi.org/10.1074/jbc.RA117.000647. Epub 2018/04/01. PubMed PMID: 29602907; PMCID: PMC5971464.
113. Kemp, B. E. (1990). Peptides and protein phosphorylation (322p). Boca Raton: CRC Press.
114. Chu, Q., Moellering, R. E., Hilinski, G. J., Kim, Y.-W., Grossmann, T. N., Yeh, J. T.-H., & Verdine, G. L. (2015). Towards understanding cell penetration by stapled peptides. *Medicinal Chemistry Communication, 6*, 111–119. https://doi.org/10.1039/C4MD00131A.
115. Kutchukian, P. S., Yang, J. S., Verdine, G. L., & Shakhnovich, E. I. (2009). All-atom model for stabilization of alpha-helical structure in peptides by hydrocarbon staples. *Journal of the American Chemical Society, 131*(13), 4622–4627. https://doi.org/10.1021/ja805037p. Epub 2009/04/02. PubMed PMID: 19334772; PMCID: PMC2735086.

Novel Peptide-Based Inhibitors of Protein Kinases

Justin M. Holub

Abstract Protein kinases are a class of enzymes that modulate the function and activity of other proteins through phosphorylation. Protein kinases regulate many aspects of cellular metabolism including signal transduction, transcription, translation, cell-cycle progression, and biosynthesis. Owing to their profound influence over such critical cellular processes, mutations or aberrant expression of protein kinases can have major implications on cell health and viability. Indeed, dysfunctional protein kinase activity has been linked to such pathological conditions as neurodegeneration, inflammation, autoimmunity, and cancer. Despite their therapeutic importance, our ability to target discrete protein kinases using small-molecule-based inhibitors has been hindered due to high degrees of structural similarity among protein kinase active sites. Recently, peptides have emerged as powerful, yet selective, modulators of protein kinase activity by virtue of their ability to mimic highly specific substrate-interaction domains of protein kinases. This chapter provides an overview of the development and application of novel peptide-based protein kinase inhibitors. The goal here is to highlight how the various binding modes of peptide-based kinase inhibitors and efforts to enhance their binding affinities have contributed to the understanding of the complex nature of protein kinase–substrate interactions. Furthermore, the therapeutic relevance of peptide-based kinase inhibitors is explored, focusing on the advantages and limitations of such molecules as they are applied in the treatment of kinase-mediated disease.

Keywords Protein kinase · Peptide · Protein kinase inhibitor · Peptide-based therapeutic · Protein kinase substrate · Peptide-based kinase inhibitor · Protein kinase interaction domain · Protein-protein interactions

J. M. Holub (✉)
Department of Chemistry and Biochemistry, Ohio University, Athens, OH, USA

Molecular and Cellular Biology Program, Ohio University, Athens, OH, USA

Edison Biotechnology Institute, Ohio University, Athens, OH, USA
e-mail: holub@ohio.edu

P. Shapiro (ed.), *Next Generation Kinase Inhibitors*,
https://doi.org/10.1007/978-3-030-48283-1_8

Introduction

Protein kinases are a major class of regulatory enzymes that catalyze the transfer of phosphate groups from nucleotides to other proteins. This process, known as phosphorylation, results in significant physicochemical changes to the protein being phosphorylated and can be used as a means to regulate the functional activity of the modified protein. The human protein kinase superfamily is composed of over 500 genes, which constitutes roughly 2% of the entire human genome [1]. It has also been estimated that up to 30% of all human proteins are regulated through some kinase activity [2]. Protein kinases are involved in many aspects of cellular metabolism, controlling elements of transcription, translation, sensory responses, signal transduction, cell-cycle progression, differentiation, and cell death. Given their role as key regulators of cellular processes, it is perhaps not surprising that dysregulated kinase activity is associated with disease pathogenesis. In fact, aberrant kinase function can result in pathological conditions including diabetes, inflammation, neurodegeneration, and cancer [3–6]. As a consequence, protein kinases are now widely considered to be important targets for therapeutic intervention. Approximately 175 protein kinases are definitively linked to human disease; however, only a small subset of these kinases have been successfully targeted using inhibitor-based therapies [7]. This has prompted many drug discovery programs to aggressively pursue novel protein kinases, and it is now projected that members of the human protein kinase superfamily account for nearly 35% of all new targets screened by the global pharmaceutical industry.

Contemporary strategies for inhibiting protein kinase activity fall into three general categories: (1) using small molecules to compete for the nucleotide-binding site of the protein kinase [8], (2) clearing the kinase through antibody-mediated deactivation [9], and (3) inhibiting kinase-substrate interactions using molecules that mimic protein interaction domains [10]. For many years, it was widely accepted that targeting the nucleotide-binding site of a protein kinase with a small-molecule-based inhibitor was the most effective way to inhibit kinase activity. Indeed, the vast majority of protein kinase inhibitors currently available are small molecules that have been designed to compete with ATP for the nucleotide-binding pocket. However, high degrees of structural similarity among protein kinase catalytic domains have made targeting specific kinases with small-molecule-based ATP analogs a major challenge. On top of that, only a small subset of protein kinases associated with human disease are currently viewed as highly sought-after targets [11]. It has also been reported that patients treated with small-molecule-based kinase inhibitors can develop resistance to such drugs due to high mutation rates within the ATP-binding pocket of the target kinase [12]. Collectively, these issues have impeded our ability to treat kinase-related diseases using small-molecule-based therapies, and there is now considerable effort focused on developing highly selective and pharmacologically potent inhibitors of protein kinases that are capable of circumventing such resistance mechanisms.

One alternative strategy to small-molecule-based kinase inhibition has been to develop antibodies against protein kinases [9, 13, 14]. The primary objective here is to use antibodies to target and clear aberrant or dysfunctional protein kinases from the biological environment using a stimulated immune response. Antibodies are able to achieve an extremely high level of selectivity against specific biomolecular targets; however, there are significant technical and physiological drawbacks that hinder antibody-based approaches to drug development. For example, the large-scale production of therapeutic antibodies is often costly, and recombinant expression of antibodies can result in end-product heterogeneity [15]. In addition, full-length antibodies are relatively large biomolecules (~150,000 Da) that are not cell permeable, which effectively limits their application to targeting serum proteins or proteins that contain extracellular domains. Unfortunately, many protein kinases associated with human disease are intracellular proteins that lack extracellular domains and are unable to be targeted using antibody-based therapeutics.

Over the past 30 years, researchers have been developing synthetic peptides as a means to inhibit protein kinase activity. The rationale in this approach is that protein kinases can be inhibited by physically disrupting the protein-protein interactions that are required for successful kinase function. Due to their biomimetic nature and synthetic tractability, peptides are able to display large, solvent-exposed epitopes that can be engineered to target wide, shallow binding grooves on biomolecular surfaces. This notion is contrary to small molecules that generally target deep-binding pockets within enzymes or receptors. As a result, synthetic peptides have been used to inhibit biomolecular interactions that have proven difficult or impossible to target using small molecules [16]. In addition to their sequence specificity, peptide scaffolds can be engineered to fold into structures that mimic the architectures of protein-interaction domains [17, 18]. In this context, peptides that structurally mimic the interaction domain of protein kinase substrates can, in theory, be designed to inhibit virtually any protein kinase-substrate interaction. Furthermore, modular synthetic strategies used to generate peptides in situ allow for exquisite control over the final primary sequence. Using rational design, peptide-based mimetics of protein kinase substrates can be developed to include the phosphorylation site and the flanking amino acid residues that facilitate highly specific substrate recognition. Taken together, these features may allow for extraordinary specificity among peptide-based kinase inhibitors for targeting discrete kinases within complex biological environments. Furthermore, peptide oligomers range in size from around 2000 to 8000 Da, placing them between small-molecule- and protein-based therapeutics with respect to mass. By occupying this unique "middle space," peptides are ideally positioned among other drug candidates for enhanced target specificity and cell permeability. Moreover, it has been suggested that targeting protein interaction domains with peptide-based constructs may increase the likelihood of selective inhibition as such interaction surfaces have greater evolutionary divergence than ligand-binding pockets bound by small molecules [19].

This chapter will focus on the design, synthesis, and characterization of novel peptide-based kinase inhibitors that have shown success in inhibiting kinase activity. It will also cover applications of such peptide-based kinase inhibitors as potential therapeutics and as chemical genetics agents to study kinase function. Specific topics include (1) peptide-based inhibition of kinase-substrate interactions, (2) enhancing the specificity of small-molecule-based kinase inhibitors with bifunctional peptide ligands, and (3) utilizing peptides to disrupt interactions between kinases and cell-targeting (anchoring) proteins. Finally, current methods to enhance the efficacy of novel peptide-based kinase inhibitors for use in the clinic are explored.

General Organization of Protein Kinase Catalytic Domains

Protein kinases exert their effects by transferring phosphate groups from nucleotides, such as ATP, to side chains of other proteins. Such transphosphorylation events occur most commonly on serine (Ser), threonine (Thr), and tyrosine (Tyr) residues, and to a lesser extent on histidine (His) residues [20]. Protein kinases are broadly classified based on the side chain they phosphorylate. For example, protein serine/threonine kinases phosphorylate Ser/Thr residues, and protein tyrosine kinases phosphorylate Tyr residues. Certain kinases, such as the mitogen-activated protein kinase kinase (MAPKK), can phosphorylate Ser/Thr or Tyr residues and are, therefore, classified as dual-specificity kinases [21]. Despite having low sequence homology among different family members, the structures of protein kinase catalytic domains are strikingly similar. Comparative crystallographic, NMR, and computational modeling studies have indicated that the catalytic domains of many seemingly unrelated kinases have nearly identical three-dimensional architectures [22, 23]. This domain, colloquially referred to as the "kinase domain," is approximately 300 amino acids in length and is composed of an N-terminal lobe, a short oligomeric hinge region, and a C-terminal lobe [10, 24] (Fig. 1a). The N-terminal lobe is comprised of a five-stranded β-sheet (β1-5) and two α-helices (αB and αC) while the C-terminal lobe is largely α-helical and contains four short β-strands. The hinge region allows for flexibility between the two lobes and is required for catalytic function [25, 26]. A highly conserved cleft between the two lobes binds the donor ATP molecule from which the phosphate is transferred. In most Ser/Thr kinases, the substrate protein binds the C-terminal lobe of the kinase domain along a wide, shallow platform that serves as a complementary docking site for the substrate recognition domain (Fig. 1b) [24, 27]. Importantly, the substrate binds in a conformation that positions the hydroxyl group of the target phosphorylation site near the γ-phosphate of the bound ATP (Fig. 1c). In some protein kinases, the platform binding the substrate can be partially formed by a flexible polypeptide sequence known as the activation loop (A-loop). Many kinases become activated upon phosphorylation of one or more residues within their A-loop sequences, making the A-loop itself an important regulatory element of protein kinases [27]. In general, the structural organization of substrate-binding sites in Tyr kinases is similar to that of Ser/Thr kinases; however, there are slight differences in the positioning of the nucleotide and substrate. For instance, the target Tyr side chain is larger than Ser/Thr residues, and it extends approximately 4 Å further into the kinase catalytic domain [22].

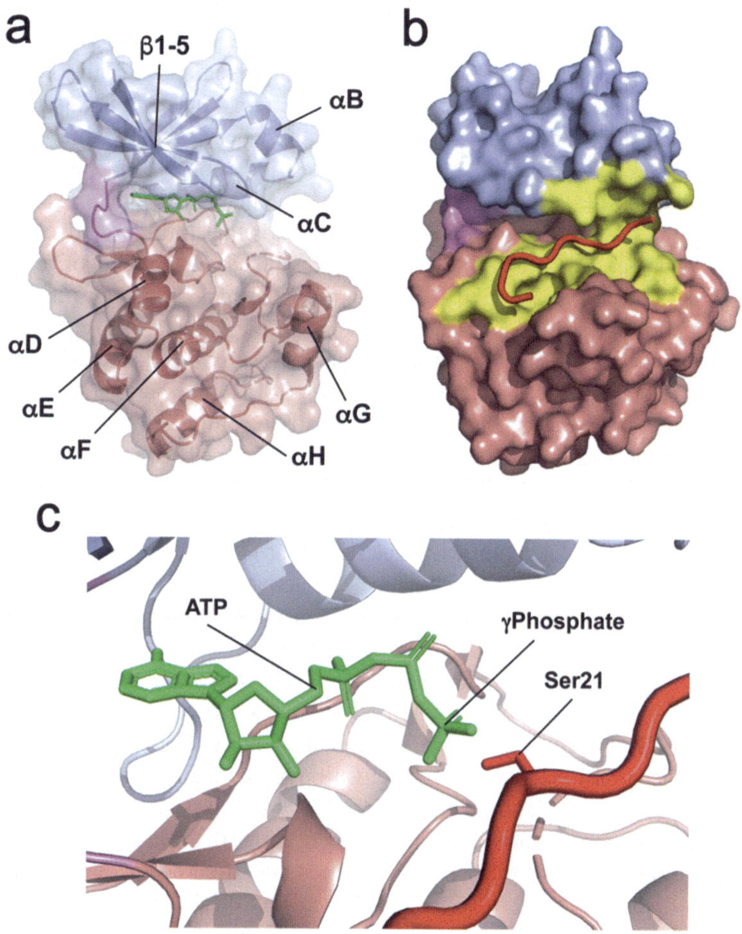

Fig. 1 Three-dimensional structure of a protein kinase catalytic domain. (**a**) Crystal structure of cAMP-dependent protein kinase bound to ATP (PDB ID: 1ATP). The N-terminal lobe is shown in light blue, the hinge region is depicted in magenta, and the C-terminal lobe is colored salmon. A bound ATP molecule is shown in green. Major secondary structure components for the N- and C-terminal lobes are indicated. (**b**) Surface rendering of cAMP-dependent protein kinase bound to inhibitor peptide PKI (residues 15–24) (PDB ID: 2GFC). The N-terminal lobe is shown in light blue, the hinge region is depicted in magenta, and the C-terminal lobe is salmon. The bound PKI substrate molecule is shown in red. The substrate-binding surface for the N- and C-terminal lobes is shown in yellow. (**c**) ATP-binding pocket of cAMP-dependent protein kinase showing ATP (green) and proximal phosphorylatable Ser residue of target substrate (red)

The catalytic activity of protein kinases is primarily controlled by amino acids that are distributed throughout the N- and C-terminal lobes. Within the N-terminal lobe, catalytic and stabilizing residues are primarily localized within the P-loop (also known as the glycine-rich loop or nucleotide-binding loop), strand β3, and helix αC. Within the C-terminal lobe, catalytic and stabilizing residues are located along the catalytic loop (strands β6 and β7) and the A-loop, which consists of about 20 amino acids located between strand β8, helix αE, and helix αF. Interestingly, these structural elements have been observed to contain regions of highly conserved sequence homology across a large number of protein kinases. For instance, the P-loop includes a consensus sequence of GxGxΦG where x is any amino acid and Φ is Tyr or Phe while the catalytic loop contains strictly conserved D or N residues [28]. Surprisingly, the N-terminal lobe of the protein kinase catalytic domain is highly dynamic despite being comprised of β-strands that form a relatively ridged antiparallel β-sheet. This flexibility is thought to enhance the effects of regulatory proteins that control kinase activity [29]. On the other hand, the C-terminal lobe is thought to be much less dynamic and serves as the docking platform for protein or polypeptide substrates. Typically, protein kinase substrates will interact with their cognate kinase catalytic domains through a short 10–15 amino acid sequence known as the "consensus sequence." During kinase-substrate complexation, the N-terminal region of the consensus sequence binds in a shallow groove between helices αD, αF, and αG of the C-terminal lobe. Conversely, the C-terminus of the consensus sequence binds in a configuration such that the residue adjacent to the phosphorylation site is buried in a pocket (known as the P + 1 loop) located within the C-terminal domain of the kinase "activation segment." The activation segment is an important regulatory element in protein kinases as its conformation influences both substrate binding and catalytic efficiency [28, 29]. Structurally, the activation segment is flanked on either side by short amino acid sequences that act as anchoring regions. In many kinases, these anchoring regions contain a conserved magnesium-binding Asp-Phe-Gly (DFG) sequence at the N-terminal anchor and an APE, ALE, or SPE sequence at the C-terminal anchor. The activation segment also contains the A-loop, which has the most variability among protein kinases in terms of length and sequence. The A-loop contains Ser, Thr, or Tyr residues that can be autophosphorylated or phosphorylated by other protein kinases and effectively controls the catalytic activity of the enzyme [27, 30]. The specific residue that becomes phosphorylated is known as the "primary phosphorylation site" and can form strong structure-inducing hydrogen bonds or electrostatic interactions with other side chains once covalently linked to a phosphate. Depending on its phosphorylation state, the primary phosphorylation site controls the catalytic activity of the kinase by structurally organizing the active site, activation loop, and binding surface for substrate recognition [22, 31].

Rationale for Using Peptide-Based Molecules to Inhibit Protein Kinases

In spite of a high degree of structural homology among their catalytic domains, protein kinases demonstrate remarkable selectivity with regard to their target substrates [10, 32]. Certainly, such specificity becomes apparent when one observes the enormous number of individual proteins that are targeted and phosphorylated by specific protein kinases. The specificity of a protein kinase is primarily controlled by the substrate-binding region located along the N- and C-terminal lobes (Fig. 1b). In contrast to the highly conserved ATP-binding site, the substrate-binding regions of protein kinases exhibit remarkable diversity. As described above, this region forms a shallow platform that serves as a complementary binding site for the target substrate that will ultimately become phosphorylated [23, 33]. Owing to the remarkable specificity between protein kinases and their target substrates, researchers are currently exploring ways to directly interfere with such interactions as a way to affect kinase inhibition [34, 35]. It should be noted, however, that while much is known regarding the structure and function of protein kinase nucleotide-binding sites, comparatively little is known about the vastly diverse substrate-binding regions. Consequently, novel peptide-based kinase inhibitors may not only hold significant therapeutic potential but may also be used as chemical genetics agents to better understand the molecular nature of kinase-substrate interactions.

Depending on their specific function, protein kinases may interact with various substrates including small molecules, peptides, proteins, nucleic acids, or other biomolecules. In fact, many protein kinases contain additional sites outside the nucleotide-binding site that may be targeted for allosteric or competitive inhibition [36, 37]. Kinase-substrate binding interactions are often established through large, shallow surface areas that have proven difficult or impossible to target using small molecules. One promising approach to inhibit kinase function has been to inhibit such interactions using peptide-based mimetics of kinase-substrate interaction domains. In theory, oligopeptides can be designed to mimic any region of a protein interaction domain due to their sequence specificity and ability to adopt three dimensional structures in solution [17, 18, 38]. Furthermore, because kinase specificity is often relegated through substrate-binding interactions, such peptide-based mimetics may be able to target discrete protein kinases with greater specificity compared to small-molecule inhibitors that target the nucleotide-binding site of the kinase catalytic domain.

Inhibiting Kinase-Substrate Interactions Using Synthetic Peptides

The remarkable selectivity that protein kinases exhibit for their substrates is primarily determined by the "substrate recognition motif" that contains specialized physicochemical features that influence substrate selection. To enhance specificity, substrate recognition motifs of protein kinases are composed of amino acids which form topological surfaces that are complementary to the kinase-binding domains of cognate substrates. It has, therefore, been reasoned that synthetic peptides derived from such substrate (or kinase) recognition motifs may act as inhibitors of kinase-substrate interactions. There are currently three generalizable approaches for inhibiting protein kinase activity with peptides that mimic protein interaction domains (Fig. 2). The first strategy involves using peptides that are derived directly from interaction domains of protein kinases or their substrates. Such peptides are often designed to compete for kinase-substrate interaction sites near the kinase catalytic domain (Fig. 1a). A second approach employs the use of so-called pseudosubstrate peptides that are derived from autoinhibitory domains that lie outside the kinase catalytic domain (Fig. 2b). Notably, pseudosubstrate-based kinase inhibitors have been designed to disrupt interactions between protein kinases and their own A-loop. The third strategy involves using synthetic peptides to disrupt the interactions between protein kinases and protein complexes that are required for kinase activation (Fig. 2c). It should be mentioned that such peptides inhibit the activation of protein kinases without directly targeting the active site or autoinhibitory domain of the kinase itself.

Peptide-Based Kinase Inhibitors That Compete with Protein Substrates

As mentioned above, the biomimetic nature and sequence specificity of synthetic peptides facilitates their development as mimetics of protein interaction domains. Over the past 30 years, many such "substrate-based" kinase inhibitors have been reported that directly interfere with the interactions between protein kinases and their cognate substrates [39–42]. In order to compete directly for the protein kinase active site, substrate-based kinase inhibitors are often designed as direct sequence mimetics of the substrate consensus sequence. Such peptides are usually designed to include the phosphorylation site and flanking residues that are critical for specific kinase recognition. The roots of this approach can be traced back to a seminal paper from the early 1970s in which Ashby and Walsh reported on the discovery of a 76-amino acid protein (designated PKI, for *p*rotein *k*inase *i*nhibitor) that co-precipitated with protein kinase A (PKA) [43, 44]. This heat-stable inhibitor was found to act by binding to the catalytic subunit of PKA, and it was demonstrated that this protein could inhibit the activity of PKA in several tissues, including heart, brain, kidney, liver, thymus, and muscle. Despite high inhibitory efficacy, the mechanism of PKI-based kinase inhibition was not established until several years later. In 1986, Cheng et al. used an in vitro kinase activity assay to demonstrate that certain oligopeptides derived from the kinase-binding domain of PKI were effective at inhibiting PKA [40]. These oligopeptides were derived from the canonical RRN*S*L consensus sequence of PKI and contained an Ala residue in place of the phosphor-acceptor Ser. Such peptides were effective at inhibiting PKA activity at a K_i as low as 0.2 nM. More recent crystallography studies have verified that a 20-residue synthetic peptide derived from the PKI consensus sequence interacts with PKA within its active site cleft even in the presence of small-molecule-based inhibitors that target the nucleotide-binding site [33, 45]. Moreover, the co-crystal structure showed

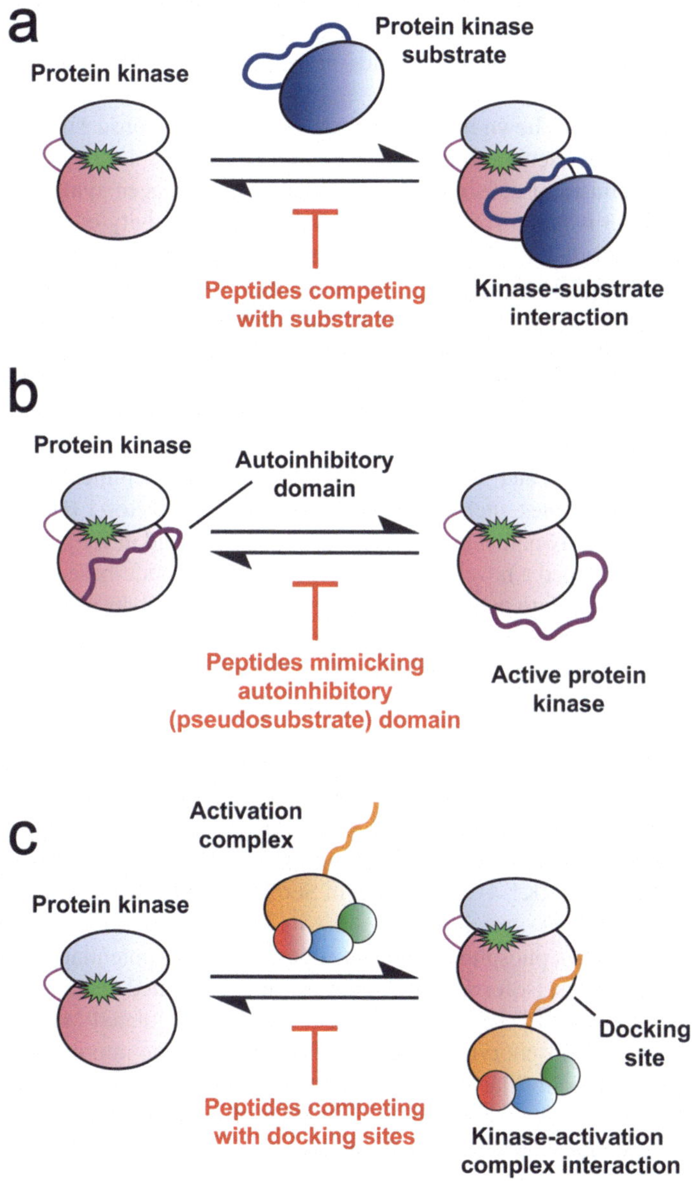

Fig. 2 Various strategies for peptide-based inhibition of protein kinases. (**a**) Peptides that compete with protein kinase substrates for the substrate-binding surface can inhibit kinase-substrate interactions. (**b**) Peptides that mimic autoinhibitory domains of protein kinases can inhibit kinase activity by rescuing the inactive state following removal of the autoinhibitory domain. (**c**) Peptides that compete with docking sites (D-sites) can effectively inhibit interactions between protein kinases and their activation complexes. Bound ATP molecule is shown as a green multipoint star

that specific residues within the consensus sequence are important for kinase recognition and specificity. The PKI peptide (residues 5–24) is now commercially available and is marketed as a selective peptide-based inhibitor of PKA that exhibits a K_i of 2.3 nM [46].

Other studies have shown that peptides derived from the consensus sequence of the cAMP-response-element-binding (CREB) protein can be developed as tools to study the mechanism of substrate phosphorylation by glycogen synthase kinase-3 (GSK-3). GSK-3 is a Ser/Thr kinase that modulates the activity of many proteins through phosphorylation [47]. An early report from Fiol et al. showed that a 13-amino-acid peptide derived from the *SXXXS*[p] consensus sequence of CREB could be used to map the specific site within CREB that is phosphorylated by GSK-3 [48]. In this study, it was demonstrated that the first Ser in the CREB consensus sequence was the site phosphorylated by GSK-3 and that the second (prephosphorylated) Ser acts as a priming site. It was also shown here that phosphorylation of the priming site was required for GSK-3 to phosphorylate the second Ser within the consensus sequence. Later studies showed that synthetic peptides derived from primed GSK-3 substrates, including CREB and heat shock factor-1 (HSF-1), could be developed as highly potent inhibitors of GSK-3 in vitro and in vivo. For example, Plotkin et al. developed a novel class of phosphorylated peptide-based inhibitors of GSK-3 that compete with natural substrate [42]. Here, the authors showed that peptides derived from the GSK-3-binding regions of HSF-1 activated glycogen synthase 2.5-fold over background in HEK293 cells and increased glucose uptake in primary mouse adipocytes. The mechanism of action was presumed to be through inhibition of GSK-3.

Peptides have also been used as substrate-based inhibitors of protein kinases that have been implicated in neurodegenerative disease. Alqaeisoom et al. recently reported on the development of a peptide-based kinase inhibitor that suppresses the activity of the microtubule affinity regulating kinase (MARK) proteins [39]. The MARK proteins (MARK1-4) are a family of Ser/Thr kinases that phosphorylate the microtubule-associated protein tau within its microtubule-binding repeat (R) domains [49]. Tau is a phosphoprotein that contains up to 79 potential phosphorylation sites on its longest isoform, 30 of which are phosphorylated under normal physiological conditions [50]. Unfortunately, aberrant or dysregulated MARK activity can result in hyperphosphorylated tau isoforms that aggregate into insoluble oligomers known as neurofibrillary tangles. Such tau aggregates have been suspected as the pathological agents responsible for the onset of neurodegenerative disorders, including Alzheimer's disease [51, 52], and kinases involved in tau phosphorylation are now considered important targets for therapeutic intervention. In this study, the authors designed a 13-amino-acid peptide (designated tR1) that was a direct sequence mimetic of the tau R1 domain (residues 244–274), a region known to be phosphorylated by MARK2. The tR1 peptide was found to selectively inhibit the MARK2-mediated phosphorylation of tau at Ser262 both in vitro and in cultured primary neurons at concentrations as low as 1 μM. Because tR1 was designed as a direct sequence mimetic of the tau R1 domain, these results strongly suggested that tR1 acts to inhibit kinase activity by directly competing with the R1-binding site of

MARK2. Furthermore, tR1 was found to be selective for MARK family proteins as it did not inhibit kinases such as GSK-3β from phosphorylating tau at other sites.

Pseudosubstrate-Based Kinase Inhibitors

In addition to competing directly for the substrate-binding site of protein kinases, peptide-based kinase inhibitors have also been developed from autoinhibitory sequences that are located outside the kinase catalytic domain. Many protein kinases are retained in catalytically inactive states by autoinhibitory regions known as "pseudosubstrate domains" [53] and become active only following interaction with a ligand or phosphorylation. Such activation typically occurs through the displacement of the autoinhibitory domain by a peptide substrate or phosphorylation of priming sites within the autoinhibitory region. Structurally, the pseudosubstrate domain is a short sequence of amino acids that mimics the substrate of the protein kinase and extends into the binding cavity of the catalytic domain. In many cases, the corresponding phosphor-acceptor residue of the kinase substrate is replaced by a nonphosphorylatable amino acid within the pseudosubstrate sequence. Mutations or deletions within the pseudosubstrate domain can result in kinase isoforms that are constitutively active, leading to dysfunctional or aberrant kinase signaling [54, 55]. It has, therefore, been reasoned that synthetic peptides designed to mimic pseudosubstrate domains can be used to maintain hyperactive kinases in their inactive states and may serve as potential therapeutics in the treatment of kinase-related disease.

Over the past several decades, considerable effort has been invested in developing peptide-based kinase inhibitors that are derived from pseudosubstrate domains. Indeed, oligopeptide sequences derived from pseudosubstrate domains represent arguably one of the largest classes of peptide-based kinase inhibitor reported in the literature. The concept of developing pseudosubstrate-based peptides as kinase inhibitors has been explored since the late 1980s. Historically, such constructs were used to determine the roles these domains played in regulating kinase activity [56, 57]. However, more recent studies have utilized pseudosubstrate-based peptides to directly inhibit the activity of protein kinases. One of the earliest examples of this approach was reported in 1993 by Eichholtz et al [41]. In this study, the authors developed a short peptide derived from the pseudosubstrate region of PKC (residues 20–28) as an inhibitor of PKC-mediated phosphorylation of protein substrates. Earlier studies that used synthetic peptides derived from the pseudosubstrate domain of PKC to inhibit of PKC activity in vitro had been reported [57]; however, their use in vivo was found to be somewhat limited due to membrane impermeability. In the Eichholtz study, the authors demonstrated that myristoylated peptides derived from the pseudosubstrate domain of PKC were effective at inhibiting the PKC-mediated phosphorylation of myristoylated alanine-rich C kinase substrate (MARCKS) proteins and suppressing activation of phospholipase D in human fibroblasts. These inhibitory effects were not observed in nonmyristoylated peptides, indicating that myristoylation could be used to enhance the cell permeability and inhibitory activity of novel peptide-based kinase inhibitors.

A similar peptide-based kinase inhibitor derived from the pseudosubstrate domain of PKC was used by Walaas et al. in 1997 to study whether PKC is linked to the insulin-mediated translocation of glucose transporters in living cells [58]. It had been shown previously that broad-spectrum kinase inhibitors, such as staurosporine and sphingosine, inhibited insulin-stimulated glucose transport [59]. However, such inhibitors lack specificity and were, therefore, unable to link PKC definitively to this phenomenon. The authors of the Walaas study noted that synthetic peptides derived from the PKC pseudosubstrate domain act as highly specific inhibitors of PKC and hypothesized that such peptides could be utilized to study how PKC affects the insulin-mediated translocation of GLUT4. In this report, Walaas et al. showed that the PKC pseudosubstrate peptide was able to inhibit the insulin-mediated increase of GLUT4 in the plasma membranes of SLO-permeabilized rat adipocytes in a concentration-dependent manner. This translocation effect was specifically linked to PKC as PKI-derived inhibitor peptides of PKA had no effect on PKC activity or GLUT4 translocation. More subtly, this study underscored the importance of utilizing highly specific inhibitors to elucidate the effects of select protein kinases on cellular functions.

In addition to inhibiting Ser/Thr kinases, pseudosubstrate-based kinase inhibitors have also been developed against tyrosine kinases. Using a rational design approach, Kamath et al. developed a potent and specific peptide-based inhibitor of the protein tyrosine kinase $p60^{c\text{-}Src}$ [60]. The $p60^{c\text{-}Src}$ protein is a cytoplasmic nonreceptor tyrosine kinase that is a product of the proto-oncogene c-Src [61]. Using a known peptide substrate for c-Src as a template, the authors developed a series of pseudosubstrate-based peptides that were able to inhibit the activity of $p60^{c\text{-}Src}$ at concentrations as low as 0.6 μM when tested in in vitro phosphorylation assays. The inhibitory hexapeptide sequence (CIYKYY) was modeled from the $p60^{c\text{-}Src}$ substrate MIYKYYF following an alanine scan that identified I^2, Y^3, Y^6, and F^7 as residues critical for activity. In contrast, no inhibition was detected in either Lyn or Lck tyrosine kinases, indicating that this peptide is selective for $p60^{c\text{-}Src}$. This study was notable because it was one of the first reports to expand the utility of peptide-based kinase inhibitors beyond Ser/Thr kinases by demonstrating that such constructs could be used to inhibit protein tyrosine kinases.

Inhibitory peptides based on pseudosubstrate domains have also been used as molecular tools to study conformational changes within protein kinases. Crystallographic data have shown that the catalytic subunit of PKA undergoes dramatic structural changes upon binding to nucleotides or inhibitors [62]. To investigate the underlying molecular mechanisms of these conformational changes, Zimmerman et al. published a study where they used surface plasmon resonance (SPR) to monitor binding of two separate pseudosubstrate inhibitors to PKA in the presence of nucleotides and divalent metal ions [63]. Here, the authors used the heat-stable PKA inhibitor peptide PKI [40] and a truncated form of the bovine type I regulatory (R) subunit (RIα-92–260) in a detailed binding study that evaluated how nucleotides and metal ions influence the binding of PKA to pseudosubstrate-based peptide inhibitors. Interestingly, the authors reported that binding of each peptide to PKA was dependent on the concentration of divalent metal ions and independent on the concentration of nucleotides. High-resolution crystal structures of PKA had previously shown that the catalytic domain contains two metal ion–binding sites; however, the importance of these metal ions on substrate binding had not yet been elucidated. In this work, the authors demonstrated that a stable complex between the PKA catalytic subunit, the pseudosubstrate inhibitor, and type I regulatory subunit (RI) only occurred in the presence of both ATP and Mg^{2+}. Furthermore, the authors showed that the concentration of Mg^{2+} had almost no influence on the association rate constant. However, the authors did observe that the dissociation rate of PKI from PKA was strongly influenced by Mg^{2+} ions. Specifically, higher concentrations of ions (up to 10 mM) caused the fast dissociation phase (ranging from 8×10^{-2} to 2×10^{-2} s^{-1}) to transiently modulate to a slow dissociation phase (ranging from 1.5×10^{-4} to 5×10^{-4} s^{-1}). The authors speculated that the influence of higher concentrations of Mg^{2+} on the dissociation rate constant may be attributed to the occupation of the second metal-binding site in the catalytic subunit. Importantly, this study demonstrated the utility of using pseudosubstrate peptide-based kinase inhibitors as tools to study the conformational changes and structural dynamics of protein kinase catalytic domains.

In 2015, Harrington et al. published a report on the development of single molecule, nanopore-based assays for the evaluation of Pim kinase inhibitors [64]. Pim kinases are a family of constitutively active Ser/Thr kinases that promote growth factor–independent cell proliferation through the phosphorylation of cellular proteins. There is considerable interest in developing selective inhibitors of Pim kinases as their overexpression has been linked to a number of solid-tissue cancers and leukemias [65]. In this elegant study, the authors applied a novel engineering technique known as "stochastic sensing" to produce heptameric alpha-hemolysin (αHL) pores that contained a single subunit that included a peptide sensor element (Fig. 3). By monitoring the current flow through a single pore in an artificial membrane under applied potential, the authors were able to monitor the binding of analytes to the pore or membrane. This unique assay was then used to develop a pseudosubstrate-based analog of the Pim protein consensus sequence (designated "Pimtide") as the sensor element. The authors were able to measure the binding of Pim-1 to the pseudosubstrate-based peptide in the presence of ATP without subsequent phosphorylation of the substrate. This approach was used to observe synergistic binding of the kinase to the pseudosubstrate-based sensor in the presence of ATP and to further evaluate competitive ATP-based inhibitors of Pim kinases. Notably, the authors were able to identify a potent small-molecule-based inhibitor that previous kinase activity assays had been unable to identify.

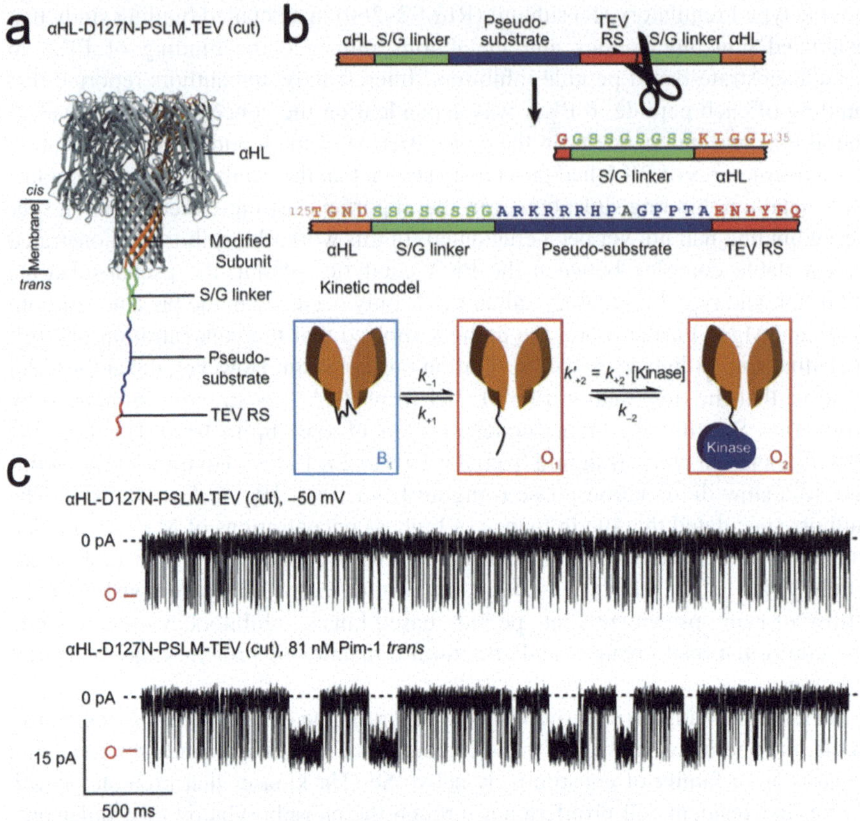

Fig. 3 Design and characterization of a single-molecule engineered nanopore sensor. (**a**) Schematic illustration of the protease-cleaved sensor indicating the location of the pseudosubstrate element (purple) flanked by Ser/Gly linkers (green) and a TEV protease recognition site (red). (**b**) Design of the TEV protease-cleavable *trans* loop fusion within the nanopore sensor. Kinetic model for the analysis of the observed current signal through the nanopore sensor in the presence of the Pim-1 peptide is shown below the bar diagram of the *trans* loop fusion. State B_1 corresponds to the blocked current level of the pore due to occlusion by the attached peptide. State O_1 corresponds to the open pore that is not bound to a kinase, and O_2 corresponds to the open pore with a kinase molecule bound to the sensor peptide. (**c**) Representative current traces of the nanopore sensor under an applied potential of −50 mM before (above) and after (below) the addition of 81 nM Pim-1 in the chamber. Figure adapted with permission [64]

Peptide-Based Kinase Inhibitors Targeting Docking Sites

Aside from ligand-induced structural changes within their catalytic subunits, the activities of protein kinases are also regulated through interactions with large, multiprotein complexes that work in concert to control kinase function [66]. In general, the regions of protein kinases that participate in interactions with other regulatory proteins are distinct from the nucleotide- or substrate-binding sites. These areas, colloquially known as "docking sites," promote association between kinases and other biomolecules including protein substrates, peptide regulators, small-molecule metabolites, or activation complexes [10]. Docking sites are believed to tether otherwise low-specificity catalytic domains of protein kinases to cognate substrates and enhance the specificity of signal transmission between cells [67]. Due to their significant level of influence over the activation of protein kinases, docking sites are now being exploited as a means to modulate protein kinase activity. In this context, peptide-based molecules that mimic the structures and sequences of docking sites have been shown to act as selective inhibitors of kinase function.

Docking interactions between protein kinases and other proteins can occur at multiple nodes along kinase signaling pathways [68]. For example, docking interactions are prominent at several steps of the mitogen-activated protein kinase (MAPK) signaling cascade (Fig. 4). This well-studied pathway is critical to the transmission of signals received at the cell surface by growth factors, hormones, or developmental regulators. Stimulation of the MAPK signal transduction cascade ultimately leads to the regulation of important biological processes including gene expression [69]. While other proteins are involved in the MAPK signaling cascade, the MAPK protein (originally called *e*xtracellular signal-*r*egulating *k*inase [ERK]) plays a crucial role by phosphorylating multiple downstream substrates such as RSK, MSK, MNK, and MK5 [70]. Importantly, docking interactions between proteins involved in these networks, including the MEK-mediated activation of MAPK, are critical for proper resolution of this signaling cascade. It has been shown previously that MEK proteins and their MAPK substrates contain short docking motifs, often referred to as "D-sites," that bind to complementary regions on MAPK [71]. Over the past 10 years, researchers have used such docking sites to design peptide-based kinase inhibitors that disrupt interactions between protein kinases and proteins that target the D-site. For example, in 2009 Bardwell and coworkers used synthetic peptides based on D-sites derived from MEK proteins to characterize the selectivity of the interaction between MEK proteins and MAPKs [72]. Because D-sites are found in both MEK proteins and MAPK substrates, the authors reasoned that peptides derived from either protein may inhibit MAPK binding. In this study, the authors developed a small library of peptides modeled from the D-sites of several MEK proteins including MEK1, MEK2, MKK3, MKK4, and MKK6. The MEK D-site sequence consists of a cluster of basic residues, a short amino acid spacer and motif comprised of a hydrophobic-*X*-hydrophobic amino acid sequence: $K/R_{2-3}–X_{1-6}–\phi–X–\phi$ (where X constitutes any amino acid and ϕ constitutes any hydrophobic amino acid). Using this model sequence as a starting point, the authors developed a small library of MEK D-site peptides that were able to inhibit the phosphorylation of various downstream MAPK targets including MEF2A, ATF2, and Elk-1. The authors utilized competitive inhibition assays to quantify the binding of specific D-site peptides to target MAPK proteins. Peptides derived from MEK protein–docking sites were able to inhibit MAPK proteins from phosphorylating substrates at concentrations in the low-to-mid μM range. These results indicated that similar MAPK D-sites are shared among different MEK proteins and MAPK substrates. The authors also hypothesized that because D-sites of human MEK proteins are derived

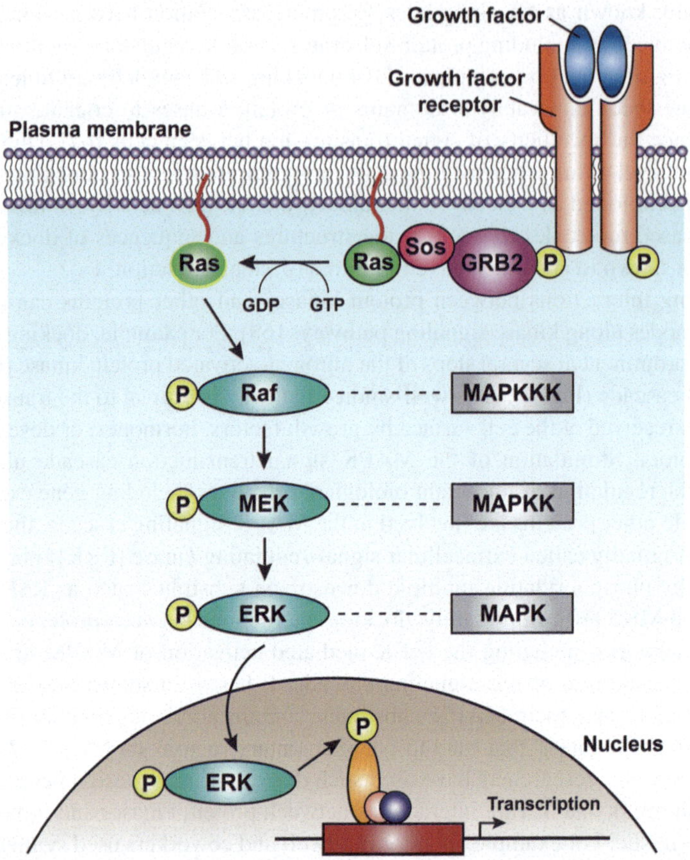

Fig. 4 The MAPK/ERK signal transduction cascade. Growth factors stimulate the MAPK/ERK pathway though interaction with growth factor receptors on the cell surface. Ligand binding initiates phosphorylation of the growth factor receptor, which leads to the activation of the small G-protein Ras via interaction with GRB2 and adaptor proteins. Subsequent downstream phosphorylation of key proteins Raf (MAPKKK), MEK (MAPKK), and ERK (MAPK) results in activated ERK translocating to the nucleus where it initiates transcription of growth factor–responsive genes by phosphorylating specific transcription factors. Figure adapted from Kim et al. [127]

from a similar sequence class (K/R_{2-3}–X_{1-6}–ϕ–X–ϕ), D-sites may only contribute to binding energy and not to specificity. However, results from this study suggested that peptides derived from MEK protein D-sites are moderately selective for their cognate MAPK substrates and contribute to overall kinase specificity. Taken together, these findings support a "double selection" model of kinase-substrate interaction in which docking sites and catalytic domains jointly contribute to kinase recognition.

Peptides that inhibit protein kinase activity by targeting docking sites have also been developed against c-Jun N-terminal kinase (JNK) proteins. JNK1 is abnormally elevated in certain tissues under diabetic conditions, which can cause constitutive activation of the JNK pathway. Because activation of the JNK pathway interferes with the function of β-cells and mitigates insulin action [73], it has been speculated that JNK1 plays an important role in establishing insulin resistance. In 2004, Kaneto et al. reported on the development of a novel, 20-amino-acid JNK-inhibitory peptide derived from the JNK-binding domain of the JNK-interacting protein-1 (JIP1) [74]. To enhance cell permeability, the authors covalently linked the peptide inhibitor to a 10-amino-acid carrier peptide based on the HIV-TAT sequence [75, 76]. To assess cell uptake and delivery, the peptide was further conjugated to a fluorescein isothiocyanate (FITC) tracer. Following development of the JIP1-HIV-TAT-FITC construct, the authors treated diabetic mice with the peptide at 10 mg/kg and monitored its accumulation in insulin target organs including the liver, fat, and muscle. The authors also found that the nonfasting blood glucose levels in mice treated with the JIP1-HIV-TAT-FITC peptide were significantly lower than untreated controls. The authors further demonstrated that glucose tolerance in JIP1-HIV-TAT-FITC-treated mice could be ameliorated. These results support the notions that the JNK pathway is involved in the exacerbation of diabetes and that suppression of the JNK pathway could be a viable therapeutic route to treat blood glucose disorders.

In 2016, a highly selective inhibitor of PKC delta (δPKC) based on glyceraldehyde-3-phosphate dehydrogenase (GAPDH) was identified by Qvit et al [77]. GAPDH is a known substrate of δPKC and plays a (noncatalytic) role in inducing mitochondrial elimination under oxidative stress [78]. In this study, the authors were interested in elucidating the mechanism by which oxidative stress inhibits the protective GAPDH-mediated elimination of damaged mitochondria. Using rational design, Qvit and coworkers developed a peptide (designated ψGAPDH) that was a direct sequence mimetic of the GAPDH-docking site on δPKC. The authors reasoned that the ψGAPDH-docking site on δPKC may have an analogous sequence to GAPDH similar to how the pseudosubstrate domain of δPKC mimics the phosphor acceptor sequence within the substrate. Here, it was determined that the ψGAPDH peptide inhibited δPKC-GAPDH interactions and subsequent phosphorylation of GAPDH in vitro at concentrations as low as 1 μM. In addition, the authors showed that the ψGAPDH peptide could be used to inhibit GAPDH oligomerization and GAPDH-mediated glycolytic activity. It was also demonstrated in this study that the ψGAPDH peptide did not affect the phosphorylation of five other δPKC substrates in whole-cell lysates. Finally, the authors showed that a ψGAPDH peptide conjugated to the cell-permeable peptide TAT (47–57) acted as an inhibitor of the elimination of damaged mitochondria in cardiac H9C2 cells following oxidative stress. This result suggested a possible therapeutic use for this peptide to treat complications associated with cell injury.

Similar strategies have been used to develop peptide-based kinase inhibitors that are directly derived from docking sites on the kinase itself. In this approach, the inhibitory peptide does not target the kinase but rather the docking site of the protein complex to which the kinase binds. One of the earliest examples of this strategy was reported in 2002 by Kelemen et al. [79] Here, the authors were interested in disrupting the interaction between the MAPK protein ERK and its cognate upstream kinase

MEK. The authors reasoned that a peptide derived from docking domains of either protein could theoretically block activation of the downstream protein kinase. To evaluate this hypothesis, the authors developed a 13-amino-acid peptide corresponding to the N-terminus of MEK1 (MPKKKPTPIQLNP), a region known to be involved in facilitating MEK-ERK interactions [80]. This peptide was designed specifically to bind and inhibit ERK activation in vitro and in cultured mammalian cells. In vitro fluorescence anisotropy studies showed that the peptide bound ERK with a K_d of approximately 77 nM and that the peptide co-precipitated with ERK proteins from whole-cell lysates. Furthermore, the authors showed that the MEK1-derived peptide inhibited growth factor–stimulated ERK activation in PC12 cells at concentrations between 5 and 50 μM but did not affect the activity of other kinases in similar assays. In order to facilitate translocation of the peptide across the cell membrane, the authors developed a series of modified ERK inhibitor peptides that contained translocation sequences derived from HIV-TAT or antennapedia [75, 81]. Studies evaluating cell uptake showed that fluorescently labeled MEK1 peptides containing the transduction domains were internalized by NIH 3T3 cells and were distributed throughout the cytosol in patterns that were similar to inactive (cytoplasmic) ERK but different from active (nuclear) ERK. The authors also found that the cell-permeable peptides were able to inhibit ERK activation in growth factor–stimulated NIH 3T3 and PC12 cells at concentrations ranging from 29 to 45 μM. Finally, the authors confirmed the inhibitory effects of the MEK1 peptide by observing a significant decrease in the transcriptional activity ELK1, a downstream effector of ERK. Notably, these results were among the first examples of using a peptide-based kinase inhibitor that was derived directly from a kinase to inhibit the phosphorylation (activation) of a downstream substrate.

Another example of using kinase-derived peptides to inhibit signal transduction includes a report by Niv et al. In this study, the authors analyzed specific subdomains of various protein kinases and studied their involvement in protein-protein interactions. This technology, dubbed “KinAce,” was used as a platform to develop inhibitory peptides that could modulate kinase-dependent signaling pathways [82]. More specifically, the KinAce strategy combines bioinformatics and crystallographic data to identify sequence variability within structurally conserved regions of protein kinase catalytic domains. Regions of interest included subdomain V (the αD region), the loop between subdomains IX and X (the HJ loop), and subdomain X (the αG helix). The variable sequences were then used as leads in the development of highly specific peptide-based kinase inhibitors. Importantly, the structured regions identified by KinAce are common to all protein kinases and share similar architectures. Despite sharing a common three-dimensional framework across multiple protein kinases, the authors showed that the KinAce regions contained patches of hypervariable sequences that were interspaced with highly conserved residues. Interestingly, it was shown that the conserved regions are often buried within the kinase active site, while the variable regions are solvent-exposed. The authors reasoned that this variability may be important for recognition of specific kinase substrates and that peptides derived from these regions could be effective at blocking upstream kinase activity. In this study, short myristoylated peptides derived from the target regions of the Tyr kinases c-Kit and Lyn, and the Ser/Thr kinases PDK1 and PKB were developed. For their inhibition studies, the authors synthesized a library of peptide oligomers derived from subdomains V and IX-X. Importantly, the peptides were designed to span the entire KinAce region and partially overlap. Furthermore, each peptide included several residues from the variable binding sites. The authors derived and synthesized an average of 15–30 peptides each from the protein kinases c-Kit, Lyn, PDK1, and PKB and found that 33% of the peptides derived from HJ-αG, αD, or both regions had some inhibitory activity. More specifically, the authors showed that a peptide derived from the αD region of c-Kit selectively inhibited SCF-induced transphosphorylation with an IC_{50} value of 7 μM. Peptides derived from the HJ-αG region of PDK1 significantly reduced the phosphorylation of PKB in DU-145 prostate cancer cells and inhibited cell proliferation at concentrations in the low- to mid-μM range. Furthermore, the authors demonstrated that peptides derived from the HJ-αG region of PKB successfully inhibited the phosphorylation of the PKB substrate GSK3. Finally, the authors showed that a peptide derived from the subdomain III of HJ-αG region of Lyn was effective at inhibiting phosphorylation of Syk and Lyn in a dose-dependent manner, yielding 80–90% inhibition at concentrations of 5 μM. Notably, none of the screened peptides had any inhibitory effect on other kinases from which they were not derived. The authors were keen to note that in addition to being used to develop highly effective peptide-based kinase inhibitors, the KinAce approach could be extended to be used as a way to screen discrete regions of kinases for their contribution to specific diseases (KinScreen). For example, the peptides developed using KinAce could potentially be used to rapidly test the influence of certain kinases on the growth, differentiation, and metabolism of cancer cells. In this context, inhibition of some metabolic process by a KinAce peptide may indicate a connection between that pathway and the specific region of the kinase from which the peptide was derived.

More recently, Oguiza and coworkers showed that a peptide derived from the NEMO-binding domain (NBD) of nuclear factor-κB kinase (IKK) could protect against diabetes-associated neuropathy and atherosclerosis in mouse models of type 1 diabetes [83]. The IKK complex is formed by two catalytic subunits (IKKα and IKKβ) and a regulatory subunit (NF-κB essential modulator [NEMO]). Both IKKα and IKKβ share a high degree of structural homology; each is composed of an N-terminal kinase domain, a central leucine zipper/helix-loop-helix dimerization domain, and a carboxy-terminal NEMO-binding domain [84]. The N-terminus of NEMO binds to the NBD sequences on IKK, leaving the rest of NEMO accessible for interacting with regulatory proteins. Structurally, the NBD peptide developed by Oguiza et al. is a single peptide oligomer comprised of three distinct regions: an N-terminal octalysine (K_8) cell-penetrating peptide, a short diglycine linker (GG), and a C-terminal sequence mimetic of the NEMO inhibitory peptide. Notably, this peptide construct inhibited the canonical NF-κB pathway and ameliorated renal dysfunction in diabetic mice. Interestingly, the authors observed that the NBD peptide did not affect the metabolic severity of diabetes, which was evidenced by no significant change in hyperglycemia, lipid profile, or body weight in treated versus untreated mice. However, the authors found that the NBD peptide did demonstrate renal histological improvement without any observable toxicity, liver damage, or other obvious side effects. Kidneys from NBD-peptide-treated mice displayed decreased intranuclear NF-κB activity and reduced atherosclerotic plaque size compared to untreated controls. More specifically, the authors observed that the in vitro treatment of cultured vascular smooth muscle cells with NBD peptides showed reduced nuclear translocation of the p65 subunit after high glucose stimulation. Real-time PCR showed that the NBD peptide inhibits the expression of NF-κB-dependent genes including Ccl2, Ccl5, and Tnfα. Furthermore, the authors detected indirect action of the NBD peptide on systemic inflammation, which was evidenced by reduced splenic expression of proinflammatory TH1 cytokines but not antiinflammatory Th32 genes. Taken together, these results suggested that the NBD peptide is capable of ameliorating NF-κB-dependent inflammation and can inhibit detrimental physiological effects of diabetes, including renal damage and atherosclerosis. These results also indicated that peptide-based kinase inhibitors do not necessarily need to compete with docking sites on protein kinases to affect inhibition of their function. Instead, they may be able to inhibit the formation of protein kinase complexes by mimicking a docking region of one of the individual complex components. This strategy may be exploited to affect (indirect) inhibition that only affects the kinase function when it is in the presence of a larger complex, thus enhancing selective activity of the kinase inhibitor.

It is perhaps worth noting that disrupting the docking interactions between protein kinases and their activation complexes can be used as a means to prevent the phosphorylation of downstream substrates without significantly affecting the overall activity of the kinase itself. This is because protein kinases bound to larger complexes often function differently than their free-form state [85]. In this context, signaling pathways that require kinases to be bound to larger protein complexes may be functionally separated from other cascades that are regulated by the free-form kinase. Selectively inhibiting interactions between kinases and their activation complexes may, therefore, be used as a means to block phosphorylation of one substrate but not another. Furthermore, as the studies outlined in this section have indicated, peptides that block interactions between protein kinases and their activators may be more effective at inhibiting overall kinase activity than those that block interactions between the kinase and its cognate substrates. This is likely because protein kinase substrates (and by extension their peptide-based mimetics) have comparatively low affinity for protein kinases. Targeting regions of higher binding affinity, such as those between protein kinases and their activator proteins, may facilitate the development of higher-affinity binders that inhibit kinase activity with greater specificity. Moreover, such constructs may be useful as tools to help dissect the complexities of redundant or parallel kinase signaling cascades in living systems.

Inhibiting Kinase Activity Using Hetero-Bivalent Peptides

Despite an increasing number of reports documenting the efficacy of peptide-based kinase inhibitors, targeting the nucleotide-binding pocket of protein kinases with small molecules remains the most widely used approach to suppress kinase activity. Nevertheless, the specificity of such small-molecule-based kinase inhibitors is often poor due to the high degree of structural similarity between protein kinase catalytic domains [10, 24]. This issue has prompted researchers to explore alternative approaches to enhance the specificity and efficacy of small-molecule-based kinase inhibitors. One promising strategy has been to design bivalent constructs that covalently link peptide mimetics of kinase substrates to small molecules that target the nucleotide-binding site. In principle, such "hetero-bivalent" inhibitors can simultaneously target the nucleotide-binding pocket and the substrate-binding domain located on the surface of the kinase [86] (Fig. 5). This strategy, therefore, allows for targeting of the protein kinase with a high-affinity (but low specificity) small molecule and a highly specific (but low affinity) peptide-based substrate mimetic.

One of the earliest applications that used hetero-bivalent constructs to affect kinase inhibition was reported in 1991 when Ricouart et al. developed a bifunctional ligand designed to inhibit protein kinase C (PKC) [87]. In this work, an inhibitor comprised of a short pseudosubstrate peptide (Ser-Arg_6) designed to target the substrate-binding site of PKC was covalently linked to an isoquinoline-5-sulfanamide ATP mimetic through a β-Ala linker. In vitro phosphorylation assays showed that the bisubstrate inhibitor was 67-fold more potent than the isoquinoline-5-sulfanamide alone. Notably, the enhanced potency was only observed when the two substrate components were linked, demonstrating the utility of the bivalent approach for inhibiting kinase activity.

More recent studies have used similar bivalent ligands to enhance the specificity of broad-spectrum kinase inhibitors such as staurosporine and PP2. Staurosporine is an alkaloid natural product that acts as an inhibitor of numerous kinases including PKA, PKC, CK1, CK2, and MAPK [88]. Staurosporine competes for the nucleotide-binding pocket of protein kinases and has been shown to have higher affinity for certain kinases compared to ATP [89]. In an effort to enhance specificity of this broad-spectrum kinase inhibitor, Meyer et al. conjugated staurosporine to a cyclic peptide ligand that was highly specific for PKA [90]. In this study, the authors used an innovative strategy to design a hetero-bivalent peptide-based kinase inhibitor that required no previous structural or sequence data. The inhibitor was initially developed by covalently linking a highly promiscuous analog of staurosporine to the protein Jun and generating a cyclic peptide library that was covalently linked to the protein Fos. Association of the two ligands was then afforded through the natural self-assembly of the Fos and Jun proteins (Fig. 6a). Phage display was then used to select for cyclic peptides that displayed micromolar affinity for PKA. The selected peptide was identified and subsequently conjugated to staurosporine though a PEG linker to generate the final bisubstrate conjugate (Fig. 6b). The authors observed that the respective inhibitory potency of the hetero-bivalent ligand increased 93-fold

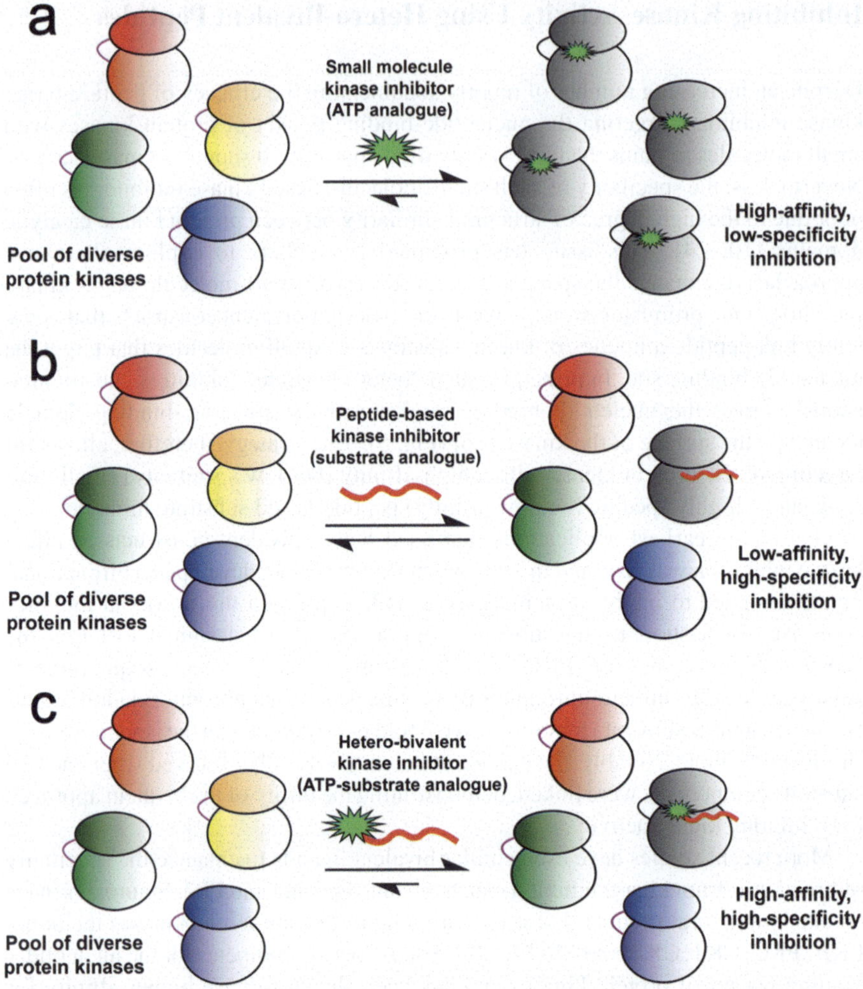

Fig. 5 Rationale for the design of hetero-bivalent peptide-based kinase inhibitors. (**a**) Small-molecule-based kinase inhibitors designed to target the ATP-binding pocket often exhibit high-affinity, nonspecific inhibition. (**b**) Peptide-based kinase inhibitors targeting the substrate-binding region of protein kinases will generally achieve highly specific targeting but suffer from low-affinity interactions. (**c**) Hetero-bivalent kinase inhibitors simultaneously target the ATP-binding pocket and substrate-binding region of protein kinases, ultimately leading to high-affinity, highly specific inhibition

over staurosporine and 21,000-fold compared to nonconjugated peptide. Moreover, the bivalent inhibitor showed remarkable in vitro selectivity toward PKA over a panel of six different kinases including ASK1, c-Src, and Mnk2 (Fig. 6c). Importantly, this strategy demonstrated the efficacy of enhancing the specificity of broad-spectrum kinase inhibitors by conjugating them to peptides that target specific sites within kinase catalytic domains.

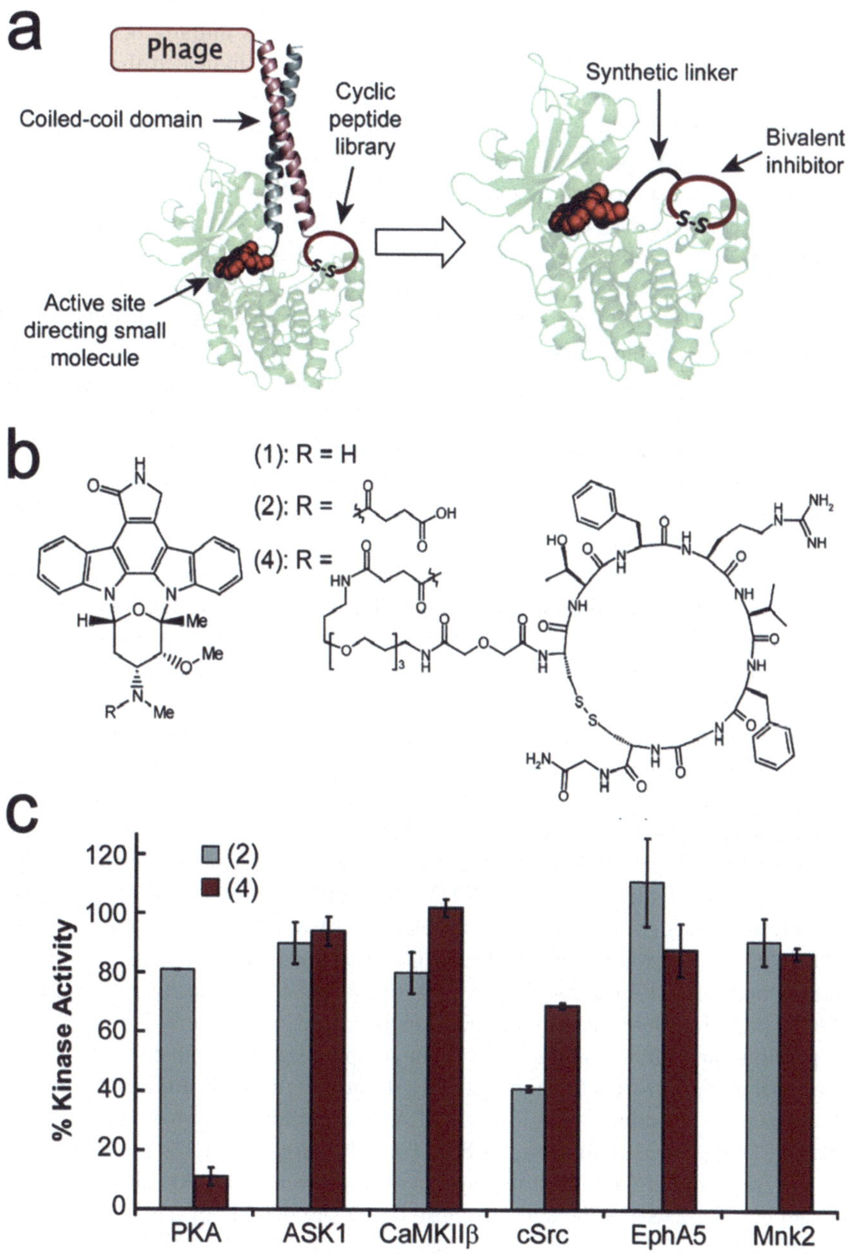

Fig. 6 Design and activity of a hetero-bivalent peptide-based kinase inhibitor for targeting protein kinase A (PKA). (**a**) Noncovalent tethering of staurosporine with a phage display peptide library through a coiled-coiled Fos-Jun heterodimer. (**b**) Chemical structures of hetero-bivalent peptide conjugates used to target PKA. (**c**) Activity screen targeting six different kinases shows significant inhibition of PKA by inhibitor **4**, but not with compound **2**. Inhibition of kinase activity was found to be selective for PKA. Figure adapted with permission [90]

PP2 is a pyrazole-based small molecule that has seen use in cancer research as an inhibitor of Src family kinases. While this compound was initially believed to be specific for Src family kinases, more recent studies have indicated that this compound is nonselective and can inhibit other kinase families with similar efficacy [91]. In 2015, Brandvold et al. used a derivative of PP2 and a Src peptide substrate to develop a highly specific, cell-permeable bisubstrate inhibitor of c-Src [92]. In this study, click chemistry was used to covalently link an alkyne-containing PP2 derivative to a consensus c-Src substrate sequence through a 1,2,3 triazole linkage. To facilitate conjugation, the authors replaced the phosphorylatable Tyr within the peptide sequence with a 4-aminophenylalanine residue that was subsequently acylated with an azide-functionalized linker. The authors obtained a K_d value of 0.28 nM for this inhibitor, which was 1300-fold more potent than the PP2 derivative and 1100-fold more potent than the peptide fragment alone. To evaluate specificity, the bisubstrate compound was screened in an in vitro competitive binding assay against 213 kinases. Here, the authors found that only two kinases (c-Src and a close homolog c-Yes) were bound by the bisubstrate inhibitor. To enhance the biological efficacy of the inhibitor, the authors appended the substrate with a polyarginine (Arg_9) tag that is commonly used to enhance the cell permeability of peptides and proteins [76]. The authors noted that the addition of the Arg_9 tag did impart cell permeability to the construct but had little impact on its affinity for c-Src. Furthermore, the cell-permeable bisubstrate construct inhibited the growth of the c-Src-dependent cancer cell lines HT-29 and SKBR3 but did not impact on the growth of c-Src-independent cell lines MCF-7 and T47D.

Researchers have also used peptide-based bisubstrate ligands as inhibitors of effector kinases along the Ras-RAF-MEK-ERK signaling cascade (Fig. 4). A recent study by Lechtenberg et al. used a structure-guided approach to develop a potent and selective inhibitor of ERK1/2 [93]. In this work, the authors linked a small molecule known to target the ATP-binding site of ERK1/2 to a peptide that would target the D-recruitment site (DRS) of ERK1/2. The small molecule chosen for the study was FR180204, a pyrazole-based semiselective ERK inhibitor that targets ERK2 with an IC_{50} of approximately 1 μM [94]. Despite relatively low binding affinity, the authors noted that FR180204 displays 10- to 30-fold selectivity over related p38α MAPK proteins. Here, the authors developed two hetero-bivalent inhibitors based on previous structural analysis of ERK2 in complex with its cognate substrates. To develop the first construct (designated SP1), the authors used the minimal C-terminal D-site peptide (residues 119–130) of PEA15, a protein known to interact with ERK1/2 [95]. It was demonstrated here that SP1 targeted ERK2 with an IC_{50} of 0.7 μM, representing a modest increase in affinity over FR180204 alone. For their second construct (SP2), the authors chose the D-site peptide of the ERK substrate RSK1 (residues 713–729) that was appended with the HIV-TAT transactivation domain [75, 76]. Both peptides utilized a "reverse" binding mode [96] to target ERK; however only the RSK1 peptide construct employed an additional helical element when binding to the kinase. Interestingly, the RSK1-containing inhibitor showed a 50-fold increase in potency inhibiting ERK2 with an IC_{50} of 14 nM despite being appended with the HIV-TAT sequence. Following this observation, the authors used a structure-based approach to establish that the inhibitor binds both the ATP-binding site and the DRS of ERK. For their third construct (SP3), the authors used click chemistry to conjugate an alkyne-functionalized FR180204 molecule to the N-terminus of the RSK1 peptide through an azidolysine moiety. This final construct was not appended with the HIV-TAT sequence and was found to target active (phosphorylated) ERK2 with an IC_{50} of 25 nM. Finally, the authors performed an in vitro assay where they tested the selectivity of SP3 against 55 kinases of the CMGC branch. It was shown here that SP3 not only bound ERK1/2 with high affinity, but also several other related MAPKs that contain a DRS, such as JNK1, JNK2, JNK3, and p38α. Interestingly, SP3 was not able to target other CMGC kinases that do not contain a DRS, suggesting that SP3 may be developed as a potent, yet selective, inhibitor of kinases that contain these specific binding sites.

Inhibiting Interactions Between Protein Kinases and Anchoring Proteins

Protein kinases are often distributed among separate subcellular compartments as a means to regulate their activity. Sequestering protein kinases within distinct organelles, including nuclei or mitochondria, allows their association with localized substrates to be tightly controlled [97]. In general, the specific subcellular localization of protein kinases is mediated through the interaction with anchor (or adaptor) proteins that regulate the trafficking of kinases throughout the cell. One approach to inhibiting kinase activity has been to disrupt such interactions with peptides that mimic anchor protein interaction domains. Over the past 25 years, synthetic peptides that disrupt interactions between protein kinases and their associated anchor proteins have shown efficacy in inhibiting kinase function.

One of the first studies on inhibiting the activity of protein kinases using peptides derived from anchor proteins was reported by Ron et al. in 1995 [98]. In this work, the authors developed a peptide derived from RACK1, a PKC-binding protein that anchors activated PKC to the plasma membrane near its localized substrates. It had been shown previously that *r*eceptor for *a*ctivated *C*-*k*inase (RACK) proteins increased PKC activity by stabilizing the active state of the kinase [99]. Furthermore, it was demonstrated that RACK1 was not a substrate or an inhibitor of PKC. The regulatory domains of PKC proteins contain two common regions: C1 and C2 [26, 100]. The C1 region of PKC is known to mediate binding between PKC and diacylglycerol while the C2 region regulates calcium binding to the kinase. PKC interacts with lipids at the plasma membrane through its C1 domain; however, RACK1 was shown to interact with PKC within its C2 domain [98]. The RACK-binding domain of PKC is a short sequence of amino acids that is part of the larger N-terminal domain, which was previously thought to contain at least part of the RACK-binding site. To identify the RACK1-binding site of PKC, the authors used short synthetic peptides derived from the C2 region of PKC to disrupt interactions between recombinant RACK1 and fragments of PKC containing either C1 or C2 regions. Notably, they observed that some C2-derived peptides acted as inhibitors of hormone-induced translocation of PKC, indicating that the C2 region contains at least part of the RACK1-binding site. Using this approach, the authors mapped portions of the RACK1-binding site on PKC to amino acids 186–198 and 209–226 within the C2 region of PKC. Furthermore, peptides corresponding to these regions were shown to inhibit the translocation of C2-containing PKC isozymes in neonatal cardiac myocytes. These results indicated that the C2-derived peptides inhibited PKC function by binding to RACK1 and disrupting the RACK1/PKC interaction.

Similar approaches have been used to inhibit the activity of PKA in synaptic transmission. In an early report, Rosenmund et al. showed that peptide oligomers derived from the conserved kinase-binding region of A-kinase anchoring proteins (AKAPs) could be used to inhibit PKA-mediated phosphorylation of AMPA/kainite channels in cultured neurons [101]. In this study, the authors utilized a 24-amino-acid peptide derived from a conserved amphipathic helix common to the AKAP protein Ht31 to block binding of PKA to AKAP. Interestingly, a shorter (16-amino-acid) peptide derived from Ht31 did not block this interaction. The authors also demonstrated that treatment of cells with Ht31 peptides could inhibit the PKA-mediated regulation of AMPA/kainate currents, providing the first-ever evidence that PKA-anchoring proteins are crucial in the regulation of synaptic function. It had been shown previously that PKA-dependent phosphorylation is required to maintain the function of AMPA/kainite channels in hippocampal neurons [102]. In the Rosenmund study, the absence of ATP, or the presence of peptide-based inhibitors of PKA, caused the gradual decline of whole-cell currents evoked by kainite. These results indicated that PKA plays a crucial role in channel activity. To test the influence of AKAP proteins on localizing PKAs near the channel, inhibitor peptides derived from Ht31 were added to the cells and reduced AMPA/kainite-meditated currents to the same extent as other PKA-specific inhibitors, including PKI. The authors also noted that the effects of PKI and the Ht31 peptide were not additive, indicating that PKA localization to the channel is required for the modulation of AMPA/kainite-mediated currents.

The discovery of short peptides that disrupt interactions between PKA and AKAP has led to the development of novel molecular tools for evaluating PKA activity. For example, synthetic peptides that disrupt interactions between PKA and its regulatory subunit (RI) have been used to evaluate Type I PKA signaling. In 2006, Carlson et al. combined bioinformatics analyses and peptide-screening arrays to develop a high-affinity *RI a*nchoring *d*isruptor (RIAD) peptide that demonstrated >1000-fold selectivity for Type I PKA over Type II PKA [103]. In this study, the authors used a bioinformatic analysis approach on a set of dual-affinity AKAP-binding sequences to develop a synthetic peptide that binds PKA with higher affinity and greater specificity than any previously reported AKAP-derived peptide. More specifically, the authors utilized a *m*ultiple *e*M of *m*otif *e*licitation (MEME) algorithm [104] to screen the RI-binding sites of PKA for anchoring proteins that bind RIα. Based on comparisons to corresponding sites within sample proteins of a nonredundant database, the authors identified regions of amino acid similarity and used bioinformatics software to predict side chains that were most likely to occupy a particular site. To facilitate this process, the linear PKA R domain-binding sequences of D-AKAP1, AKAP149, ezrin, and two sites from AKAP82 were aligned and analyzed. A position-dependent scoring matrix (PDSM) consensus sequence of 20 amino acids was then identified. Further optimization of the peptide was performed using two-dimensional peptide arrays, and it was determined that strategic placement of acidic residues afforded peptides that retained RIα binding but bound poorly to RIIα. The resultant 18-amino-acid RIAD peptide was shown to bind Type I PKA with high selectivity. Following further optimization, cell-permeable RIAD peptides were shown to selectively uncouple cAMP-mediated inhibition of T-cell function and inhibited progesterone synthesis at the mitochondria in steroid-producing cells.

RIAD peptides have also been employed to suppress PKA-mediated immune responses. Antitumor treatments based on the infusion of T-cells expressing chimeric antigen receptors (CAR T-cells) are still largely ineffective on solid tumors. However, recent work has focused on developing RIAD peptides to inhibit PKA-mediated inhibition of T-cell receptor (TCR) activation. This inhibition process requires PKA to localize to the immune synapse via binding to the AKAP protein ezrin. In 2016, Newick et al. generated a line of T-cells that expressed RIAD peptides to determine whether RIAD peptides derived from AKAP proteins could blunt the negative effects of PKA on T-cell activation [105]. These cells (dubbed CAR-RIAD T-cells) showed increased TCR signaling following treatment with adenosine in vitro and showed enhanced killing of tumor cells compared to those treated with CAR T-cells alone. Furthermore, when injected into mice, the antitumor efficacy of murine CAR-RAID T-cells was substantially enhanced compared to control mice treated with only CAR T-cells. It was also shown that CAR-RIAD T-cells migrated more efficiently to chemokines and had better adherence to cell matrices. The authors concluded that RIAD peptides augment CAR T-cell efficiency by inhibiting the PKA-mediated inhibition of TCR activation. This landmark study underscored the physiological relevance of PKA-anchoring proteins in disease pathogenesis and demonstrated that peptide-based inhibition of PKA activity may be a viable route for developing therapeutics that inhibit the growth and propagation of cancer cells.

Another example of an inhibitor designed to disrupt the interactions between protein kinases and their anchoring proteins includes a peptide that corresponds to residues 188–226 of the FRAT1 protein. FRAT1 is a mammalian protein that acts as a co-regulator of the WNT signaling pathway [106]. FRAT belongs to a family of GSK3-binding proteins that positively regulates the WNT signaling pathway by inhibiting GSK3-mediated phosphorylation of β-catenin. In 1999, Thomas et al. developed a peptide derived from the GSK3-binding domain of FRAT1 (designated "FRATtide") that binds GSK3 and prevents its interaction with Axin [107]. In this study, the authors demonstrated that FRATtide significantly reduced the activity of GSK3α and GSK3β isolated from human serum. It was also shown that FRATtide blocked the interaction between GSK3 and the C-terminal domain of Axin (residues 281–500), suggesting that the binding sites on GSK3 for FRAT1 and Axin may overlap. Notably, FRATtide was found not to suppress GSK3 activity toward other substrates, including glycogen synthase and eIF2B. This is likely because phosphorylation of each of these substrates is independent of Axin and dependent on "priming" phosphorylations. This specific result may explain why essential cellular functions of GSK3 can continue to be observed despite suppression of β-catenin phosphorylation.

Subsequent studies with FRATtide-based molecules have helped to elucidate disparate mechanisms of GSK3 inhibition. The structure of FRATtide in complex with GSK-3β has been elucidated, and these studies revealed that the activation loop of uncomplexed (phosphorylated) GSK-3β adopts a similar conformation to that of the FRATtide-bound from [108]. Interestingly, the activation loop of GSK3β in complex with FRATtide was found to adopt similar conformations to those activation loops of related kinases CDK2 and ERK2. A sulfate ion was also found to be present near the activation loop of the FRATtide-GSK3β complex and is thought to occupy the site of the phosphoserine residues within "primed" substrates. The co-crystal structure showed that the FRATtide forms a helix-turn-helix motif when bound to the C-terminal lobe of the kinase domain (Fig. 7). Importantly, these data showed that the FRATtide binds near, but does not obstruct, the substrate-binding channel of GSK-3β. Combined with previous reports that showed that FRATtide blocks the association between GSK3β and Axin [107], the authors of this study concluded that the Axin-binding site on GSK-3β overlaps with the binding site of FRATtide. Furthermore, the proximity of the Axin-binding site to the active site of GSK3β provides structural evidence how Axin acts as a scaffolding protein that promotes β-catenin phosphorylation.

More recently, the FRATtide peptide was included in a study that used diverse peptide-based kinase inhibitors to elucidate the function of a novel C-terminal

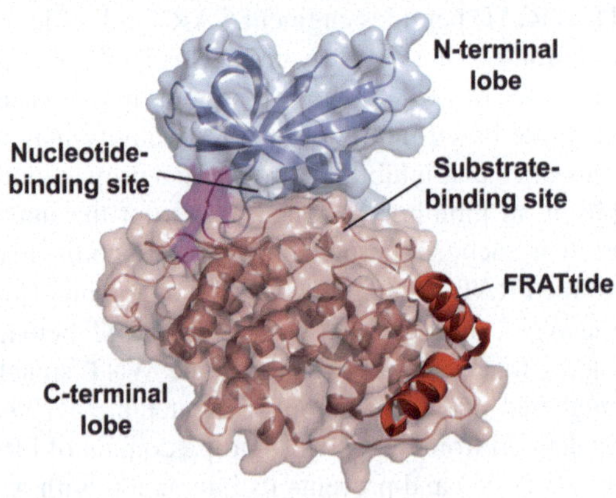

Fig. 7 Co-crystal structure of glycogen synthase kinase-3 beta (GSK-3β) catalytic domain bound to the inhibitory FRATtide peptide (PDB ID: 1GNG). The N-terminal lobe of GSK-3β is shown in light blue, the hinge region is depicted in magenta, and the C-terminal lobe is colored salmon. The FRATtide peptide (residues 1–39) is shown in red. The positions of the nucleotide-binding site and the substrate-binding region of GSK-3β are indicated

scaffold-binding region of GSK-3β [109]. In this study, the authors utilized mutated versions of GSK3β to determine the binding mechanisms of peptides derived from three GSK-3β-binding proteins. Specifically, these peptides were derived from Axin (AxinGID), FRAT1 (FRATtide), and GSKIP (GSKIPtide). To determine which amino acids are critical for imparting selectivity to other binding partners, the authors focused on installing point mutations within the extreme C-terminal helix domain of GSK-3β (residues 339–383). Interestingly, it was determined that specific GSK-3β interacting proteins bound to this region with at least five distinct binding modes, which further highlighted the versatile role GSK-3β plays in cellular signaling. To classify each binding mode, the authors used specific characteristics of each GSK-3β mutant (V267G and Y288F) bound to their respective interacting partners. For example, the binding mode of GSK-3β to AxinGID, hNinein, and Dyn-like protein was categorized into one group, and GSKIP, FRATtide, CABYR, and Astrin were classified as four individual groups. Briefly, these modes were characterized by the ability for each respective GSK-3β-binding protein to interact with the various GSK-3β mutants. Here, AxinGID, hNinein, and Dyn-like protein all interacted positively with wild-type GSK-3β and GSK-3β(Y288F) but did not bind GSK-3β(V267G). On the other hand, GSKIP interacted positively with wild-type GSK-3β and GSK-3β(Y288F), and only weakly to GSK-3β(V267G). FRATtide interacted strongly with wild-type GSK-3β and GSK-3β(V267G) but did not bind GSK-3β(Y288F). CABYR was found to interact strongly with all three GSK-3β variants. Astrin only interacted with the wild-type GSK-3β and was unable to bind either of the mutants. In addition, the authors showed that AxinGID, Dyn-like protein, and hNinein possessed independent binding modes through C-terminal truncation assays and serial site-directed mutagenesis of the GSK-3β C-terminal domain.

Enhancing the Clinical Efficacy of Peptide-Based Kinase Inhibitors

From a drug design standpoint, peptides are generally considered less desirable than small molecules as potential lead compounds. This is largely because peptide-based molecules have intrinsic physicochemical properties that limit their application in vivo. For instance, most peptides do not readily cross cell membranes or the blood-brain barrier, which can limit their application to extracellular targets. Moreover, peptides shorter than 15 amino acids are often intrinsically disordered in solution and are, therefore, highly susceptible to degradation by serum or cytoplasmic proteases [110, 111]. Finally, longer peptides can trigger immune responses when administered in vivo [112, 113], leading to rapid clearance or inflammation. Despite these challenges, recent advancements in peptide synthesis techniques and high-throughput screening procedures have allowed researchers to develop peptides that circumvent many of these issues [114, 115]. Consequently, peptides are becoming widely accepted as viable lead compounds for drug development, and many pharmaceutical companies are beginning to invest more heavily in the development of peptide-based therapeutics [116].

It could also be argued that it is precisely the synthetic tractability and biomimetic nature of peptides that make them ideal candidates for drug development. As several of the studies outlined in this chapter have demonstrated, synthetic peptide-based kinase inhibitors can be modified in various ways to enhance their therapeutic efficacy. For instance, the membrane permeability of peptide-based kinase inhibitors can be enhanced by installing hydrophobic moieties, which can be achieved by either including a higher percentage of hydrophobic amino acids within the primary sequence [117] or by appending lipophilic functionalities to the peptides during synthesis [118]. In the context of peptide-based kinase inhibitors, several groups have successfully employed myristoylation strategies to enhance the membrane permeability of inhibitory peptides that target cytosolic kinases [41, 119]. In addition to installing hydrophobic moieties, peptides can also be engineered for efficient cell internalization by installing cationic amino acids into their primary sequence or by appending the peptide with protein transduction sequences such as Tat, poly-Arg, or antennapedia [76]. This strategy has been applied to several novel peptide-based kinase inhibitors that have successfully targeted cytosolic kinases including JNK1 and ERK [74, 93]. Recent evidence has also shown that certain peptides can be used to shuttle small molecules, peptides, and even full-length proteins across the blood-brain barrier [120]. While it has yet to be applied in practice, conjugating such "shuttling" peptides to peptide-based kinase inhibitors may be an effective approach to deliver highly selective antagonists that target kinases involved in neurodegenerative disease.

The proteolytic stability of peptides can also be enhanced by linking medium-length polymer chains, including PEG, PG, PVP, and PHPMA, to the peptide in order to increase its half-life in vivo [121]. This strategy has been used extensively to enhance the bioavailability of numerous peptide- and protein-based therapeutics [122–124]. In addition, the immunogenicity of peptide-based therapeutics may be reduced by removing potentially cross-reactive B- or T-cell epitopes from peptide sequences. Recent advancements in protein sequence database management and computational prediction software have allowed researchers to identify such epitopes and have facilitated the sequence-based rational design of peptide-based therapies that display reduced immunogenicity [125]. Importantly, testing of other peptide-specific triggers of immune responses, such as aggregation potential, post-translational modifications, or excipient effects, must be conducted when developing final formulations of peptide-based therapies. While these approaches have been used to enhance the efficacy of many peptide-based therapeutics for use in the clinic, their specific application to peptide-based kinase inhibitors remains limited. This is likely because the overall market share occupied by peptide-based kinase inhibitors compared to other classes of therapeutic peptides approved for clinical use is still relatively small. Nevertheless, this situation presents a unique development opportunity as chemically modified peptide-based kinase inhibitors that display enhanced biological efficacy represent a virtually untapped market in the context of next-generation therapeutics.

Conclusions and Perspectives

The ability to inhibit discrete protein kinases with high selectivity represents one of the greatest challenges facing modern molecular biology. Despite the enormous wealth of knowledge that has been amassed on protein kinases since they were first discovered in 1954 [126], the scientific community is still actively searching for molecules that are able to inhibit protein kinases without significant cross-reactivity. While many small-molecule-based kinase inhibitors that target the nucleotide-binding site with high affinity have been developed, these compounds often suffer from limited selectivity due to a high degree of structural similarity among protein kinase active sites. Furthermore, antibodies that target protein kinases are able to target distinct kinases with high efficiency, but their relatively large size limits their application to kinases that contain extracellular domains.

Since the late 1980s, peptides have emerged as promising candidates as inhibitors of protein kinases due to their synthetic tractability, midrange size, and ability to mimic protein interaction domains. In this chapter, three generalized classes of peptide-based kinase inhibitors were introduced, and different mechanisms through which peptides can affect kinase inhibition were discussed. It is also worth mentioning that the successful development of many of the kinase inhibitors outlined herein has required the collective work of researchers across many scientific disciplines. Considering the multitude of approaches and tremendous collaborative efforts that are being made to develop peptide-based kinase inhibitors, chances are high that researchers will soon make breakthroughs that greatly enhance the efficacy of such molecules for use in vitro and in the clinic. Finally, peptide-based kinase inhibitors are noteworthy because they not only represent formidable constructs that have high therapeutic potential but also may be used as tools to help researchers better understand the complex nature of kinase-substrate interactions. Ultimately, this knowledge will lead to a more profound understanding of kinase function on a molecular level and will facilitate the development of innovative medicines that will effectively treat kinase-mediated disease.

References

1. Manning, G., Whyte, D. B., Martinez, R., Hunter, T., & Sudarsanam, S. (2002). The protein kinase complement of the human genome. *Science (New York, N.Y.), 298*, 1912–1934. https://doi.org/10.1126/science.1075762.
2. Ubersax, J. A., & Ferrell, J. E., Jr. (2007). Mechanisms of specificity in protein phosphorylation. *Nature Reviews Molecular Cell Biology, 8*, 530–541. https://doi.org/10.1038/nrm2203.

3. Hanahan, D., & Weinberg, R. A. (2011). Hallmarks of cancer: The next generation. *Cell, 144*, 646–674. https://doi.org/10.1016/j.cell.2011.02.013.
4. Karin, M. (2005). Inflammation-activated protein kinases as targets for drug development. *Proceedings of the American Thoracic Society, 2*, 386–390. https://doi.org/10.1513/pats.200504-034SR. discussion 394-385.
5. Mass, E., et al. (2017). A somatic mutation in erythro-myeloid progenitors causes neurodegenerative disease. *Nature, 549*, 389–393. https://doi.org/10.1038/nature23672.
6. Musi, N. (2006). AMP-activated protein kinase and type 2 diabetes. *Current Medicinal Chemistry, 13*, 583–589.
7. Klaeger, S., et al. (2017). The target landscape of clinical kinase drugs. *Science (New York, N.Y.), 358*(6367), eaan4368. https://doi.org/10.1126/science.aan4368.
8. Roskoski, R., Jr. (2016). Classification of small molecule protein kinase inhibitors based upon the structures of their drug-enzyme complexes. *Pharmacological Research, 103*, 26–48. https://doi.org/10.1016/j.phrs.2015.10.021.
9. Fauvel, B., & Yasri, A. (2014). Antibodies directed against receptor tyrosine kinases: current and future strategies to fight cancer. *MAbs, 6*, 838–851. https://doi.org/10.4161/mabs.29089.
10. de Oliveira, P. S., et al. (2016). Revisiting protein kinase-substrate interactions: Toward therapeutic development. *Science Signaling, 9*, re3. https://doi.org/10.1126/scisignal.aad4016.
11. Elkins, J. M., et al. (2016). Comprehensive characterization of the published kinase inhibitor set. *Nature Biotechnology, 34*, 95–103. https://doi.org/10.1038/nbt.3374.
12. Lovly, C. M., & Shaw, A. T. (2014). Molecular pathways: Resistance to kinase inhibitors and implications for therapeutic strategies. *Clinical Cancer Research: An Official Journal of the American Association for Cancer Research, 20*, 2249–2256. https://doi.org/10.1158/1078-0432.Ccr-13-1610.
13. Reshetnyak, A. V., et al. (2013). Structural basis for KIT receptor tyrosine kinase inhibition by antibodies targeting the D4 membrane-proximal region. *Proceedings of the National Academy of Sciences of the United States of America, 110*, 17832–17837. https://doi.org/10.1073/pnas.1317118110.
14. Swain, S. M., et al. (2013). Pertuzumab, trastuzumab, and docetaxel for HER2-positive metastatic breast cancer (CLEOPATRA study): Overall survival results from a randomised, double-blind, placebo-controlled, phase 3 study. *The Lancet Oncology, 14*, 461–471. https://doi.org/10.1016/s1470-2045(13)70130-x.
15. Kunert, R., & Reinhart, D. (2016). Advances in recombinant antibody manufacturing. *Applied Microbiology and Biotechnology, 100*, 3451–3461. https://doi.org/10.1007/s00253-016-7388-9.
16. Tsomaia, N. (2015). Peptide therapeutics: Targeting the undruggable space. *European Journal of Medicinal Chemistry, 94*, 459–470. https://doi.org/10.1016/j.ejmech.2015.01.014.
17. Holub, J. M. (2017). Small scaffolds, big potential: Developing miniature proteins as therapeutic agents. *Drug Development Research, 78*, 268–282. https://doi.org/10.1002/ddr.21408.
18. Jochim, A. L., & Arora, P. S. (2009). Assessment of helical interfaces in protein-protein interactions. *Molecular BioSystems, 5*, 924–926. https://doi.org/10.1039/b903202a.
19. Hanold, L. E., Fulton, M. D., & Kennedy, E. J. (2017). Targeting kinase signaling pathways with constrained peptide scaffolds. *Pharmacology & Therapeutics, 173*, 159–170. https://doi.org/10.1016/j.pharmthera.2017.02.014.
20. Besant, P. G., Tan, E., & Attwood, P. V. (2003). Mammalian protein histidine kinases. *The International Journal of Biochemistry & Cell Biology, 35*, 297–309.
21. Dhanasekaran, N., & Premkumar Reddy, E. (1998). Signaling by dual specificity kinases. *Oncogene, 17*, 1447–1455. https://doi.org/10.1038/sj.onc.1202251.
22. Kornev, A. P., & Taylor, S. S. (2010). Defining the conserved internal architecture of a protein kinase. *Biochimica et Biophysica Acta, 1804*, 440–444. https://doi.org/10.1016/j.bbapap.2009.10.017.
23. Stout, T. J., Foster, P. G., & Matthews, D. J. (2004). High-throughput structural biology in drug discovery: Protein kinases. *Current Pharmaceutical Design, 10*, 1069–1082.

24. Scapin, G. (2002). Structural biology in drug design: Selective protein kinase inhibitors. *Drug Discovery Today, 7*, 601–611.
25. Bartova, I., Koca, J., & Otyepka, M. (2008). Functional flexibility of human cyclin-dependent kinase-2 and its evolutionary conservation. *Protein Science: A Publication of the Protein Society, 17*, 22–33. https://doi.org/10.1110/ps.072951208.
26. Steinberg, S. F. (2008). Structural basis of protein kinase C isoform function. *Physiological Reviews, 88*, 1341–1378. https://doi.org/10.1152/physrev.00034.2007.
27. Adams, J. A. (2003). Activation loop phosphorylation and catalysis in protein kinases: Is there functional evidence for the autoinhibitor model? *Biochemistry, 42*, 601–607. https://doi.org/10.1021/bi020617o.
28. Cowan-Jacob, S. W. (2006). Structural biology of protein tyrosine kinases. *Cellular and Molecular Life Sciences: CMLS, 63*, 2608–2625. https://doi.org/10.1007/s00018-006-6202-8.
29. Taylor, S. S., & Kornev, A. P. (2011). Protein kinases: Evolution of dynamic regulatory proteins. *Trends in Biochemical Sciences, 36*, 65–77. https://doi.org/10.1016/j.tibs.2010.09.006.
30. Czerwinski, R., et al. (2005). Characterization of protein kinase C theta activation loop autophosphorylation and the kinase domain catalytic mechanism. *Biochemistry, 44*, 9563–9573. https://doi.org/10.1021/bi050608q.
31. Kornev, A. P., Haste, N. M., Taylor, S. S., & Eyck, L. F. (2006). Surface comparison of active and inactive protein kinases identifies a conserved activation mechanism. *Proceedings of the National Academy of Sciences of the United States of America, 103*, 17783–17788. https://doi.org/10.1073/pnas.0607656103.
32. Miller, C. J., & Turk, B. E. (2018). Homing in: Mechanisms of substrate targeting by protein kinases. *Trends in Biochemical Sciences, 43*, 380–394. https://doi.org/10.1016/j.tibs.2018.02.009.
33. Zheng, J., et al. (1993). 2.2 A refined crystal structure of the catalytic subunit of cAMP-dependent protein kinase complexed with MnATP and a peptide inhibitor. *Acta Crystallographica Section D Biological Crystallography, 49*, 362–365. https://doi.org/10.1107/s0907444993000423.
34. Eldar-Finkelman, H., & Eisenstein, M. (2009). Peptide inhibitors targeting protein kinases. *Current Pharmaceutical Design, 15*, 2463–2470.
35. Kaidanovich-Beilin, O., & Eldar-Finkelman, H. (2006). Peptides targeting protein kinases: strategies and implications. *Physiology (Bethesda, Md.), 21*, 411–418. https://doi.org/10.1152/physiol.00022.2006.
36. Arencibia, J. M., et al. (2017). An allosteric inhibitor scaffold targeting the PIF-pocket of atypical protein kinase C isoforms. *ACS Chemical Biology, 12*, 564–573. https://doi.org/10.1021/acschembio.6b00827.
37. De Smet, F., Christopoulos, A., & Carmeliet, P. (2014). Allosteric targeting of receptor tyrosine kinases. *Nature Biotechnology, 32*, 1113–1120. https://doi.org/10.1038/nbt.3028.
38. Watkins, A. M., & Arora, P. S. (2014). Anatomy of beta-strands at protein-protein interfaces. *ACS Chemical Biology, 9*, 1747–1754. https://doi.org/10.1021/cb500241y.
39. Alqaeisoom, N., Qing, C., Arachchige, D., Colvin, R. A., & Holub, J. M. (2019). Inhibiting phosphorylation of tau (τ) proteins at Ser262 using peptide-based R1 domain mimetics. *International Journal of Peptide Research and Therapeutics*, 447–463, https://doi.org/10.1007/s10989-018-9689-6.
40. Cheng, H. C., et al. (1986). A potent synthetic peptide inhibitor of the cAMP-dependent protein kinase. *The Journal of Biological Chemistry, 261*, 989–992.
41. Eichholtz, T., de Bont, D. B., de Widt, J., Liskamp, R. M., & Ploegh, H. L. (1993). A myristoylated pseudosubstrate peptide, a novel protein kinase C inhibitor. *The Journal of Biological Chemistry, 268*, 1982–1986.
42. Plotkin, B., Kaidanovich, O., Talior, I., & Eldar-Finkelman, H. (2003). Insulin mimetic action of synthetic phosphorylated peptide inhibitors of glycogen synthase kinase-3. *The Journal of Pharmacology and Experimental Therapeutics, 305*, 974–980. https://doi.org/10.1124/jpet.102.047381.

43. Ashby, C. D., & Walsh, D. A. (1972). Characterization of the interaction of a protein inhibitor with adenosine 3′,5′-monophosphate-dependent protein kinases. I. Interaction with the catalytic subunit of the protein kinase. *The Journal of Biological Chemistry, 247*, 6637–6642.
44. Ashby, C. D., & Walsh, D. A. (1973). Characterization of the interaction of a protein inhibitor with adenosine 3′,5′-monophosphate-dependent protein kinases. II. Mechanism of action with the holoenzyme. *The Journal of Biological Chemistry, 248*, 1255–1261.
45. Bonn, S., et al. (2006). Structural analysis of protein kinase A mutants with Rho-kinase inhibitor specificity. *The Journal of Biological Chemistry, 281*, 24818–24830. https://doi.org/10.1074/jbc.M512374200.
46. Glass, D. B., Cheng, H. C., Mende-Mueller, L., Reed, J., & Walsh, D. A. (1989). Primary structural determinants essential for potent inhibition of cAMP-dependent protein kinase by inhibitory peptides corresponding to the active portion of the heat-stable inhibitor protein. *The Journal of Biological Chemistry, 264*, 8802–8810.
47. Doble, B. W., & Woodgett, J. R. (2003). GSK-3: Tricks of the trade for a multi-tasking kinase. *Journal of Cell Science, 116*, 1175–1186. https://doi.org/10.1242/jcs.00384.
48. Fiol, C. J., Mahrenholz, A. M., Wang, Y., Roeske, R. W., & Roach, P. J. (1987). Formation of protein kinase recognition sites by covalent modification of the substrate. Molecular mechanism for the synergistic action of casein kinase II and glycogen synthase kinase 3. *The Journal of Biological Chemistry, 262*, 14042–14048.
49. Drewes, G., Ebneth, A., Preuss, U., Mandelkow, E. M., & Mandelkow, E. (1997). MARK, a novel family of protein kinases that phosphorylate microtubule-associated proteins and trigger microtubule disruption. *Cell, 89*, 297–308.
50. Lee, V. M., Goedert, M., & Trojanowski, J. Q. (2001). Neurodegenerative tauopathies. *Annual Review of Neuroscience, 24*, 1121–1159. https://doi.org/10.1146/annurev.neuro.24.1.1121.
51. Alonso Adel, C., Mederlyova, A., Novak, M., Grundke-Iqbal, I., & Iqbal, K. (2004). Promotion of hyperphosphorylation by frontotemporal dementia tau mutations. *The Journal of Biological Chemistry, 279*, 34873–34881. https://doi.org/10.1074/jbc.M405131200.
52. Iqbal, K., Liu, F., Gong, C. X., Alonso Adel, C., & Grundke-Iqbal, I. (2009). Mechanisms of tau-induced neurodegeneration. *Acta Neuropathologica, 118*, 53–69. https://doi.org/10.1007/s00401-009-0486-3.
53. Kemp, B. E., Parker, M. W., Hu, S., Tiganis, T., & House, C. (1994). Substrate and pseudosubstrate interactions with protein kinases: Determinants of specificity. *Trends in Biochemical Sciences, 19*, 440–444.
54. Pears, C. J., Kour, G., House, C., Kemp, B. E., & Parker, P. J. (1990). Mutagenesis of the pseudosubstrate site of protein kinase C leads to activation. *European Journal of Biochemistry, 194*, 89–94.
55. Zhao, J., et al. (1998). The expression of constitutively active isotypes of protein kinase C to investigate preconditioning. *The Journal of Biological Chemistry, 273*, 23072–23079. https://doi.org/10.1074/jbc.273.36.23072.
56. House, C., & Kemp, B. E. (1987). Protein kinase C contains a pseudosubstrate prototope in its regulatory domain. *Science (New York, N.Y.), 238*, 1726–1728.
57. House, C., & Kemp, B. E. (1990). Protein kinase C pseudosubstrate prototope: Structure-function relationships. *Cellular Signalling, 2*, 187–190.
58. Walaas, O., Horn, R. S., & Walaas, S. I. (1997). The protein kinase C pseudosubstrate peptide (PKC19-36) inhibits insulin-stimulated protein kinase activity and insulin-mediated translocation of the glucose transporter glut 4 in streptolysin-O permeabilized adipocytes. *FEBS Letters, 413*, 152–156.
59. Nishimura, H., & Simpson, I. A. (1994). Staurosporine inhibits phorbol 12-myristate 13-acetate- and insulin-stimulated translocation of GLUT1 and GLUT4 glucose transporters in rat adipose cells. *The Biochemical Journal, 302*(Pt 1), 271–277. https://doi.org/10.1042/bj3020271.
60. Kamath, J. R., Liu, R., Enstrom, A. M., Lou, Q., & Lam, K. S. (2003). Development and characterization of potent and specific peptide inhibitors of p60c-src protein tyrosine kinase

using pseudosubstrate-based inhibitor design approach. *The Journal of Peptide Research: Official Journal of the American Peptide Society, 62*, 260–268.
61. Brickell, P., & The, M. (1992). p60c-src family of protein-tyrosine kinases: Structure, regulation, and function. *Critical Reviews in Oncogenesis, 3*, 401–446.
62. Huse, M., & Kuriyan, J. (2002). The conformational plasticity of protein kinases. *Cell, 109*, 275–282.
63. Zimmermann, B., Schweinsberg, S., Drewianka, S., & Herberg, F. W. (2008). Effect of metal ions on high-affinity binding of pseudosubstrate inhibitors to PKA. *The Biochemical Journal, 413*, 93–101. https://doi.org/10.1042/bj20071665.
64. Harrington, L., Alexander, L. T., Knapp, S., & Bayley, H. (2015). Pim kinase inhibitors evaluated with a single-molecule engineered nanopore sensor. *Angewandte Chemie (International ed. in English), 54*, 8154–8159. https://doi.org/10.1002/anie.201503141.
65. Swords, R., et al. (2011). The Pim kinases: New targets for drug development. *Current Drug Targets, 12*, 2059–2066.
66. Endicott, J. A., Noble, M. E., & Johnson, L. N. (2012). The structural basis for control of eukaryotic protein kinases. *Annual Review of Biochemistry, 81*, 587–613. https://doi.org/10.1146/annurev-biochem-052410-090317.
67. Grewal, S., Molina, D. M., & Bardwell, L. (2006). Mitogen-activated protein kinase (MAPK)-docking sites in MAPK kinases function as tethers that are crucial for MAPK regulation in vivo. *Cellular Signalling, 18*, 123–134. https://doi.org/10.1016/j.cellsig.2005.04.001.
68. Vinayagam, A., et al. (2011). A directed protein interaction network for investigating intracellular signal transduction. *Science Signaling, 4*, rs8. https://doi.org/10.1126/scisignal.2001699.
69. Seger, R., & Krebs, E. G. (1995). The MAPK signaling cascade. *FASEB Journal: Official Publication of the Federation of American Societies for Experimental Biology, 9*, 726–735.
70. Moens, U., Kostenko, S., & Sveinbjornsson, B. (2013). The role of mitogen-activated protein kinase-activated protein kinases (MAPKAPKs) in inflammation. *Genes, 4*, 101–133. https://doi.org/10.3390/genes4020101.
71. Remenyi, A., Good, M. C., & Lim, W. A. (2006). Docking interactions in protein kinase and phosphatase networks. *Current Opinion in Structural Biology, 16*, 676–685. https://doi.org/10.1016/j.sbi.2006.10.008.
72. Bardwell, A. J., Frankson, E., & Bardwell, L. (2009). Selectivity of docking sites in MAPK kinases. *The Journal of Biological Chemistry, 284*, 13165–13173. https://doi.org/10.1074/jbc.M900080200.
73. Nakatani, Y., et al. (2004). Modulation of the JNK pathway in liver affects insulin resistance status. *The Journal of Biological Chemistry, 279*, 45803–45809. https://doi.org/10.1074/jbc.M406963200.
74. Kaneto, H., et al. (2004). Possible novel therapy for diabetes with cell-permeable JNK-inhibitory peptide. *Nature Medicine, 10*, 1128–1132. https://doi.org/10.1038/nm1111.
75. Frankel, A. D., & Pabo, C. O. (1988). Cellular uptake of the tat protein from human immunodeficiency virus. *Cell, 55*, 1189–1193.
76. Wagstaff, K. M., & Jans, D. A. (2006). Protein transduction: Cell penetrating peptides and their therapeutic applications. *Current Medicinal Chemistry, 13*, 1371–1387.
77. Qvit, N., Joshi, A. U., Cunningham, A. D., Ferreira, J. C., & Mochly-Rosen, D. (2016). Glyceraldehyde-3-phosphate dehydrogenase (GAPDH) protein-protein interaction inhibitor reveals a non-catalytic role for GAPDH oligomerization in cell death. *The Journal of Biological Chemistry, 291*, 13608–13621. https://doi.org/10.1074/jbc.M115.711630.
78. Yogalingam, G., Hwang, S., Ferreira, J. C., & Mochly-Rosen, D. (2013). Glyceraldehyde-3-phosphate dehydrogenase (GAPDH) phosphorylation by protein kinase Cdelta (PKCdelta) inhibits mitochondria elimination by lysosomal-like structures following ischemia and reoxygenation-induced injury. *The Journal of Biological Chemistry, 288*, 18947–18960. https://doi.org/10.1074/jbc.M113.466870.

79. Kelemen, B. R., Hsiao, K., & Goueli, S. A. (2002). Selective in vivo inhibition of mitogen-activated protein kinase activation using cell-permeable peptides. *The Journal of Biological Chemistry, 277*, 8741–8748. https://doi.org/10.1074/jbc.M108459200.
80. Xu, B., Wilsbacher, J. L., Collisson, T., & Cobb, M. H. (1999). The N-terminal ERK-binding site of MEK1 is required for efficient feedback phosphorylation by ERK2 in vitro and ERK activation in vivo. *The Journal of Biological Chemistry, 274*, 34029–34035. https://doi.org/10.1074/jbc.274.48.34029.
81. Joliot, A., Pernelle, C., Deagostini-Bazin, H., & Prochiantz, A. (1991). Antennapedia homeobox peptide regulates neural morphogenesis. *Proceedings of the National Academy of Sciences of the United States of America, 88*, 1864–1868. https://doi.org/10.1073/pnas.88.5.1864.
82. Niv, M. Y., et al. (2004). Sequence-based design of kinase inhibitors applicable for therapeutics and target identification. *The Journal of Biological Chemistry, 279*, 1242–1255. https://doi.org/10.1074/jbc.M306723200.
83. Oguiza, A., et al. (2015). Peptide-based inhibition of IkappaB kinase/nuclear factor-kappaB pathway protects against diabetes-associated nephropathy and atherosclerosis in a mouse model of type 1 diabetes. *Diabetologia, 58*, 1656–1667. https://doi.org/10.1007/s00125-015-3596-6.
84. Zandi, E., Rothwarf, D. M., Delhase, M., Hayakawa, M., & Karin, M. (1997). The IkappaB kinase complex (IKK) contains two kinase subunits, IKKalpha and IKKbeta, necessary for IkappaB phosphorylation and NF-kappaB activation. *Cell, 91*, 243–252.
85. Tuganova, A., Klyuyeva, A., & Popov, K. M. (2007). Recognition of the inner lipoyl-bearing domain of dihydrolipoyl transacetylase and of the blood glucose-lowering compound AZD7545 by pyruvate dehydrogenase kinase 2. *Biochemistry, 46*, 8592–8602. https://doi.org/10.1021/bi700650k.
86. Gower, C. M., Chang, M. E., & Maly, D. J. (2014). Bivalent inhibitors of protein kinases. *Critical Reviews in Biochemistry and Molecular Biology, 49*, 102–115. https://doi.org/10.3109/10409238.2013.875513.
87. Ricouart, A., Gesquiere, J. C., Tartar, A., & Sergheraert, C. (1991). Design of potent protein kinase inhibitors using the bisubstrate approach. *Journal of Medicinal Chemistry, 34*, 73–78.
88. Karaman, M. W., et al. (2008). A quantitative analysis of kinase inhibitor selectivity. *Nature Biotechnology, 26*, 127–132. https://doi.org/10.1038/nbt1358.
89. Iyer, G. H., Taslimi, P., & Pazhanisamy, S. (2008). Staurosporine-based binding assay for testing the affinity of compounds to protein kinases. *Analytical Biochemistry, 373*, 197–206. https://doi.org/10.1016/j.ab.2007.11.004.
90. Meyer, S. C., Shomin, C. D., Gaj, T., & Ghosh, I. (2007). Tethering small molecules to a phage display library: Discovery of a selective bivalent inhibitor of protein kinase A. *Journal of the American Chemical Society, 129*, 13812–13813. https://doi.org/10.1021/ja076197d.
91. Brandvold, K. R., Steffey, M. E., Fox, C. C., & Soellner, M. B. (2012). Development of a highly selective c-Src kinase inhibitor. *ACS Chemical Biology, 7*, 1393–1398. https://doi.org/10.1021/cb300172e.
92. Brandvold, K. R., et al. (2015). Exquisitely specific bisubstrate inhibitors of c-Src kinase. *ACS Chemical Biology, 10*, 1387–1391. https://doi.org/10.1021/cb501048b.
93. Lechtenberg, B. C., et al. (2017). Structure-guided strategy for the development of potent bivalent ERK inhibitors. *ACS Medicinal Chemistry Letters, 8*, 726–731. https://doi.org/10.1021/acsmedchemlett.7b00127.
94. Ohori, M., et al. (2005). Identification of a selective ERK inhibitor and structural determination of the inhibitor-ERK2 complex. *Biochemical and Biophysical Research Communications, 336*, 357–363. https://doi.org/10.1016/j.bbrc.2005.08.082.
95. Mace, P. D., et al. (2013). Structure of ERK2 bound to PEA-15 reveals a mechanism for rapid release of activated MAPK. *Nature Communications, 4*, 1681. https://doi.org/10.1038/ncomms2687.

96. Luechapanichkul, R., et al. (2013). Specificity profiling of dual specificity phosphatase vaccinia VH1-related (VHR) reveals two distinct substrate binding modes. *The Journal of Biological Chemistry, 288*, 6498–6510. https://doi.org/10.1074/jbc.M112.449611.
97. Alto, N., Carlisle Michel, J. J., Dodge, K. L., Langeberg, L. K., & Scott, J. D. (2002). Intracellular targeting of protein kinases and phosphatases. *Diabetes, 51*(Suppl 3), S385–S388. https://doi.org/10.2337/diabetes.51.2007.s385.
98. Ron, D., & Mochly-Rosen, D. (1995). An autoregulatory region in protein kinase C: The pseudoanchoring site. *Proceedings of the National Academy of Sciences of the United States of America, 92*, 492–496. https://doi.org/10.1073/pnas.92.2.492.
99. Mochly-Rosen, D., Khaner, H., & Lopez, J. (1991). Identification of intracellular receptor proteins for activated protein kinase C. *Proceedings of the National Academy of Sciences of the United States of America, 88*, 3997–4000. https://doi.org/10.1073/pnas.88.9.3997.
100. Newton, A. C. (1995). Protein kinase C: Structure, function, and regulation. *The Journal of Biological Chemistry, 270*, 28495–28498. https://doi.org/10.1074/jbc.270.48.28495.
101. Rosenmund, C., et al. (1994). Anchoring of protein kinase A is required for modulation of AMPA/kainate receptors on hippocampal neurons. *Nature, 368*, 853–856. https://doi.org/10.1038/368853a0.
102. Wang, L. Y., Salter, M. W., & MacDonald, J. F. (1991). Regulation of kainate receptors by cAMP-dependent protein kinase and phosphatases. *Science (New York, N.Y.), 253*, 1132–1135.
103. Carlson, C. R., et al. (2006). Delineation of type I protein kinase A-selective signaling events using an RI anchoring disruptor. *The Journal of Biological Chemistry, 281*, 21535–21545. https://doi.org/10.1074/jbc.M603223200.
104. Bailey, T. L., Williams, N., Misleh, C., & Li, W. W. (2006). MEME: Discovering and analyzing DNA and protein sequence motifs. *Nucleic Acids Research, 34*, W369–W373. https://doi.org/10.1093/nar/gkl198.
105. Newick, K., et al. (2016). Augmentation of CAR T-cell trafficking and antitumor efficacy by blocking protein kinase A localization. *Cancer Immunology Research, 4*, 541–551. https://doi.org/10.1158/2326-6066.Cir-15-0263.
106. Li, L., et al. (1999). Axin and Frat1 interact with dvl and GSK, bridging Dvl to GSK in Wnt-mediated regulation of LEF-1. *The EMBO Journal, 18*, 4233–4240. https://doi.org/10.1093/emboj/18.15.4233.
107. Thomas, G. M., et al. (1999). A GSK3-binding peptide from FRAT1 selectively inhibits the GSK3-catalysed phosphorylation of axin and beta-catenin. *FEBS Letters, 458*, 247–251.
108. Bax, B., et al. (2001). The structure of phosphorylated GSK-3beta complexed with a peptide, FRATtide, that inhibits beta-catenin phosphorylation. *Structure, 9*, 1143–1152.
109. Howng, S. L., et al. (2010). Involvement of the residues of GSKIP, AxinGID, and FRATtide in their binding with GSK3beta to unravel a novel C-terminal scaffold-binding region. *Molecular and Cellular Biochemistry, 339*, 23–33. https://doi.org/10.1007/s11010-009-0366-0.
110. Bottger, R., Hoffmann, R., & Knappe, D. (2017). Differential stability of therapeutic peptides with different proteolytic cleavage sites in blood, plasma and serum. *PLoS One, 12*, e0178943. https://doi.org/10.1371/journal.pone.0178943.
111. Werle, M., & Bernkop-Schnurch, A. (2006). Strategies to improve plasma half life time of peptide and protein drugs. *Amino Acids, 30*, 351–367. https://doi.org/10.1007/s00726-005-0289-3.
112. Camacho, C. J., Katsumata, Y., & Ascherman, D. P. (2008). Structural and thermodynamic approach to peptide immunogenicity. *PLoS Computational Biology, 4*, e1000231. https://doi.org/10.1371/journal.pcbi.1000231.
113. Morrison, C. (2018). Constrained peptides' time to shine? *Nature Reviews Drug Discovery, 17*, 531–533. https://doi.org/10.1038/nrd.2018.125.
114. Hondowicz, B. D., et al. (2012). Discovery of T cell antigens by high-throughput screening of synthetic minigene libraries. *PLoS One, 7*, e29949. https://doi.org/10.1371/journal.pone.0029949.

115. Made, V., Els-Heindl, S., & Beck-Sickinger, A. G. (2014). Automated solid-phase peptide synthesis to obtain therapeutic peptides. *Beilstein Journal of Organic Chemistry, 10*, 1197–1212. https://doi.org/10.3762/bjoc.10.118.
116. *Global peptide therapeutics market, dosage, price & clinical trials insight 2024* (pp. 1–1250). PNS Pharma (2018).
117. Stone, T. A., & Deber, C. M. (2017). Therapeutic design of peptide modulators of protein-protein interactions in membranes. *Biochimica et Biophysica Acta—Biomembranes, 1859*, 577–585. https://doi.org/10.1016/j.bbamem.2016.08.013.
118. Avadisian, M., & Gunning, P. T. (2013). Extolling the benefits of molecular therapeutic lipidation. *Molecular BioSystems, 9*, 2179–2188. https://doi.org/10.1039/c3mb70147f.
119. Krotova, K., et al. (2006). Peptides modified by myristoylation activate eNOS in endothelial cells through Akt phosphorylation. *British Journal of Pharmacology, 148*, 732–740. https://doi.org/10.1038/sj.bjp.0706777.
120. Oller-Salvia, B., Sanchez-Navarro, M., Giralt, E., & Teixido, M. (2016). Blood-brain barrier shuttle peptides: An emerging paradigm for brain delivery. *Chemical Society Reviews, 45*, 4690–4707. https://doi.org/10.1039/c6cs00076b.
121. Qi, Y., & Chilkoti, A. (2015). Protein-polymer conjugation-moving beyond PEGylation. *Current Opinion in Chemical Biology, 28*, 181–193. https://doi.org/10.1016/j.cbpa.2015.08.009.
122. Abuchowski, A., McCoy, J. R., Palczuk, N. C., van Es, T., & Davis, F. F. (1977). Effect of covalent attachment of polyethylene glycol on immunogenicity and circulating life of bovine liver catalase. *The Journal of Biological Chemistry, 252*, 3582–3586.
123. Alters, S. E., et al. (2012). GLP2-2G-XTEN: A pharmaceutical protein with improved serum half-life and efficacy in a rat Crohn's disease model. *PLoS One, 7*, e50630. https://doi.org/10.1371/journal.pone.0050630.
124. Cleland, J. L., et al. (2012). A novel long-acting human growth hormone fusion protein (VRS-317): Enhanced in vivo potency and half-life. *Journal of Pharmaceutical Sciences, 101*, 2744–2754. https://doi.org/10.1002/jps.23229.
125. Paul, S., et al. (2013). Evaluating the immunogenicity of protein drugs by applying in vitro MHC binding data and the immune epitope database and analysis resource. *Clinical & Developmental Immunology, 2013*, 467852. https://doi.org/10.1155/2013/467852.
126. Burnett, G., & Kennedy, E. P. (1954). The enzymatic phosphorylation of proteins. *The Journal of Biological Chemistry, 211*, 969–980.
127. Kim, H. J., & Bar-Sagi, D. (2004). Modulation of signalling by Sprouty: A developing story. *Nature Reviews Molecular Cell Biology, 5*, 441–450. https://doi.org/10.1038/nrm1400.

Index

P. Shapiro (ed.), *Next Generation Kinase Inhibitors*,
https://doi.org/10.1007/978-3-030-48283-1

The manufacturer's authorised representative in the EU is Springer Nature Customer Service Centre GmbH, Europaplatz 3, 69115 Heidelberg, Germany. If you have any concerns regarding our products, please contact ProductSafety@springernature.com

Printed and bound by CPI Group (UK) Ltd, Croydon, CR0 4YY
05/10/2026
02228126-0003